NURSING A LOVED ONE AT HOME

A Care Giver's Guide

A *supportive, practical*
medical handbook for
all levels of care

By Susan Golden, R.N.
Foreword by Kenneth R. Barmach, M.D.

RUNNING PRESS
Philadelphia, Pennsylvania

Instructions for cardiopulmonary resuscitation and removing airway
obstructions (pages 203–206 and 208–211) are excerpted from the
Heartsaver Manual, ©1987 by the American Heart Association.
Reprinted by permission of the American Heart Association.

Canadian representatives: General Publishing Co., Ltd.,
30 Lesmill Road, Don Mills, Ontario M3B 2T6.

International representatives: Worldwide Media Services, Inc.,
115 East Twenty-third Street, New York, NY 10010.

10/91

9 8 7 6 5 4 3 2 1
Digit on the right indicates the number of this printing.

Library of Congress Cataloging-in-Publication Data
Golden, Susan
Nursing a Loved One at Home
Includes index.
1. Home nursing. I Title
RT61.G65   1988   649.8   87-43259
ISBN 0-89471-591-7 (lib. bdg.)
ISBN 0-89471-590-9 (pbk.)

Printed in the United States of America
Cover design by Toby Schmidt
Interior illustration by Richard Burke, except pages 204–206 and
208–209 from the *Heartsaver Manual* ©1987,
reproduced with permission
from the American Heart Association
Typography by Today's Graphics, Philadelphia

This book may be ordered by mail from the publisher.
Please include $2.00 for postage.
But try your bookstore first!
Running Press Book Publishers
125 South Twenty-second Street
Philadelphia, Pennsylvania 19103

C. I

This book is dedicated
to my patients.
They have touched my life
in so many ways, most of all
teaching me
courage and dignity.

Contents

Illustrations

Foreword

Many forces in America today make it likely that more and more of us will need to know how to provide nursing care at home. Government and private insurers now require that many types of surgery and diagnostic tests be performed on an outpatient basis and that expensive hospital stays be shortened. As the proportion of senior citizens increases, more individuals will need medical and custodial care. At the same time, advances in technology have produced sophisticated medical machines small enough and simple enough to be used at home.

Attitudes are changing, too. Many families are turning away from the impersonal, technical environment of the hospital and choosing to provide the more loving, individual care that can be given in the home. I believe that this trend toward home care actually may be safer for many patients because there is less risk of administrative errors or infections acquired in the hospital.

This safer, individualized, and loving nursing requires that the care giver be confident and well-informed. In this book, author Susan Golden provides a very clear and complete guide that will help in the preparation for and the day-to-day responsibilities of home-care nursing. I believe that this book also will improve communication between the care giver, the physician, and other members of the health care team as they work together to provide safe, complete, compassionate health care in the home.

KENNETH R. BARMACH, M.D.

Acknowledgments

I wish to thank all those who have offered their guidance and expertise: Dr. Kenneth R. Barmach, a board-certified internist on the staff of Pennsylvania Hospital, Philadelphia, for his insightful foreword; the American Heart Association, for supplying instructions in emergency lifesaving techniques; my publishers, Lawrence and Stuart Teacher, who recognized the need for this book; and my editor, Cynthia F. Roberts, whose invaluable assistance helped to see this project through. Thanks also to Sylvain, whose enthusiasm, support, and love made this book possible.

Preface

This book was written to help you plan, prepare, and carry out a home nursing program when your loved one is discharged from the hospital. In my experience as a home care nurse and consultant, I often see family members or friends who are happy to bring a loved one home, but also anxious and concerned about being capable of managing home care. It is my hope that the practical information, valuable resources, and nursing tips in this book will allay some of those fears.

After working in hospitals for ten years as a registered nurse, and often handling patient discharges, I entered the field of home health care. When I was no longer the nurse who was sending patients out of the hospital and never seeing them again, I began to see the problems some families face in making the transition from hospital to home. Instructions that patients receive in the hospital aren't always practical when applied at home. I found home care givers often were told what to do without being told *why* it's important. I believe an informed care giver will be a better care giver, and able to feel more confident about nursing a loved one at home.

The information in this book, no matter how useful, is not intended as a substitute for competent medical care by professionals. Make sure a home care plan is written for your patient before he or she leaves the hospital. Although I have tried to provide up-to-date instructions, always check with your health care team before attempting any procedure since techniques are constantly changing through rapid advances in medical technology.

High-tech home care is now a reality. We are seeing patients discharged into the home sooner than ever before. Thanks to modern medicine and home care support systems, families are able to realize their natural desire to have a loved one at home during recuperation from illness or injury. It's important to know that you are not alone in choosing home care for a loved one. The health care team, along with hospital social workers, home health-care agencies, community service organizations, and psychological support groups, are there for you as you undertake this loving commitment.

1 Before Your Loved One Comes Home

Public health policy, modern medical technology, and a growing respect for the value of tender loving care have combined in the past decade to make home care a valuable, viable option for families who want to bring a loved one home from the hospital. Your home is certainly a more natural environment than the hospital halls, and one more conducive to recovery. Home health care is hard work, but if you are determined to care for your loved one at home, you will find the rewards can far outweigh the obstacles.

Home care is a successful solution for many families, but it is *not* for everyone. Never commit yourself to a home care program without careful, rational planning. Make a thorough review of your finances, your time constraints, and your patient's care requirements. Of course, you want what's best for your loved one; this often means putting emotions aside while you consider the pros and cons of home care. This chapter will help you decide whether home care is right for you and your loved one by discussing the physical, financial, emotional, and medical aspects you must weigh before making such a commitment.

When considering a home care program, find out what your patient can expect: Is it full recovery, requiring only a period of convalescence; long-term care and rehabilitation, with limited return to prior activities; or long-term care with little hope of recovery? What type and level of care will be needed?

Will you be able to care for your loved one alone, or will you need help? What kind of financial assistance do you have or will you need? Is your insurance adequate? Meet with your patient's physician and members of the health care team to discuss discharge plans and needs. Take an active role to make a specific plan for discharge and home care.

The Health Care Team

Who are the members of the health care team? Although this varies from hospital to hospital, it generally includes the physician, nurses (floor nurses and specialized nurses), dietitians, therapists (speech, physical, occupational, or respiratory), social workers, discharge planners, you, and the patient's family. Find out who handles the discharge process in your hospital. Many hospitals have home care services that work in cooperation with community resources; some hospitals contract out home health care services.

Try to confine your patient's care to one physician who will supervise the health care team. Whenever possible, medical questions and reports should be directed toward the supervising physician only. In selecting your primary physician, consider the following: Can the doctor easily be reached in emergencies? Will he or she be able to make house calls if it is difficult to move the patient? Will the physician accept insurance payments for services rendered, or will you be responsible for paying the difference between the physician's fees and the insurance reimbursements?

Nursing Alternatives

Depending upon your patient's condition, you and the health care team will decide what kind of additional services will be needed. Check with your insurance company to see what nursing services are covered. Most insurance carriers will not pay for nursing services provided by a relative. Private duty nursing charges, either at the hospital or home, may not be reimbursed, or a limit is applied. These expenses can climb quickly, to as much as $6,000 a week for 24-hour nursing care!

If extra nursing care is necessary, consider hiring one of the following at-home nursing professionals:

Registered Nurse (R.N.):   Has completed two or more years of professional training and is licensed by the state to perform professional nursing duties under a doctor's orders.

Licensed Practical/Vocational Nurse (L.P.N., L.V.N.):   Has completed a minimum of one year of professional training and usually works under the supervision of a registered nurse. He or she may not be licensed to perform as many duties as a registered nurse.

Nurse's Aide or Homemaker: Probably has completed some form of medical training and can provide basic patient care, but is not a medical professional. Duties include bedmaking, baths, assisting with feedings, and may include light housekeeping and meal preparation for the patient.

Sitter: Usually has little or no medical training and generally is not allowed to do any direct patient care. The job of a sitter is to watch over the patient.

Nurses are not expected to perform household chores; their obligation is to the patient. Some nurses may offer to help with non-patient functions and do so at their own discretion. You are not necessarily obliged to provide meals for home nurses; check the nursing agency's policy on this.

In most cases, home nurses have been carefully screened by the agencies and you should feel comfortable leaving them alone in your home. I recommend, however, that you always put away any money or valuables whenever you have new people in your home. The director of the agency, usually a registered nurse, will meet you and your patient at the hospital or in your home. He or she will evaluate your home situation and the patient's equipment and staff requirements. During the interview, find out how the agency operates; ask about billing procedures and about whom to contact if you have concerns about insurance coverage or staffing. The agency will need doctor's orders before it can begin the patient's medical care.

Other types of nursing services include the Visiting Nurse Association (also listed as the Visiting Nurse Service or Visiting Nurse Society), which provides nurses who visit the patient to oversee care or perform procedures ordered by a physician. They visit many patients a day, so each visit is limited in time. These nurses do not offer around-the-clock or extended nursing services. Some nursing associations now have divisions specializing in high-tech nursing; ask about this if your loved one needs such care.

Certified home health agencies are licensed to care and bill for Medicare patients. Many private full-service home health care companies now provide nursing services, medical equipment, nutritional services, pharmaceutical services, and oxygen and respiratory equipment. Recently, these companies have started to provide specialists in some of the more sophisticated therapies, including IV therapy, nutritional therapy, and physical therapy. Some hospitals, as well as national companies such as Upjohn, Abbott, Staff Builders, and Continental Health Affiliates, now offer these services at home. You'll find home care companies in the telephone directory under "nursing" or "home health care."

Here is a list of things to ask when choosing a home care company:

1. What services does the company offer?
2. Where is the company located? Does it have local offices? Does it belong to a national network that can service a patient who frequently travels?
3. Is the staff accessible? Is there 24-hour emergency coverage?
4. Does the company offer frequent delivery schedules and prompt, reliable service?
5. Are the workers bonded and protected by malpractice insurance?
6. What are the workers' qualifications?
7. What type of screening process is used, and can the company offer references?
8. How does the company expect payment?

Many doctors and hospitals have been forming partnerships with home care companies and they stand to make a profit by recommending a service in which they have a financial interest. Your insurance company also may require you to use a particular home care company. Before signing a contract, make some cost comparisons, ask for references, and get referrals from friends or other health professionals. Home care companies are competing for your business; you may be able to negotiate changes in the standard contract that will work best for you. Do your research so you can take an active role in discharge planning and home care provisions.

Medical Procedures and Equipment

If a specific medical procedure is begun or continued in the home, be sure it has been demonstrated to you and that you have performed it correctly several times while in the presence of a medical professional. You should feel confident that you'll be able to perform this procedure when you're at home. Take notes, ask questions, and keep a file of brochures or literature on the procedures. In most cases, hospital patients are taught during the day shift, so you should try to make yourself available then. Even if the patient will be performing his own care, take time to learn the procedures, too. Get the names of products being used and where they can be purchased.

If your patient needs a special diet, can you provide it at home? Speak with the hospital dietitian. What medicines will the patient need? Discuss this with your physician and write down a complete list of the medications. Order in advance, so you'll have them on hand when your loved one comes home. Ask when and how each medication should be taken. Are there any special instructions? Which ones can be renewed without a prescription? Which must be given absolutely on time, and which can be skipped if there is a problem? Are there any side effects? The more information you have, the more reassuring the move from the hospital to home will be.

When working with a medical equipment supplier or nursing agency, be sure to determine what supplies and equipment will be provided and what you will need to have on hand. Order ahead, so supplies are at home when your patient arrives. Some equipment from the hospital, such as restraints or pressure mattresses, may have been purchased and are yours to take home when your loved one is discharged. Usually a hospital social worker or home care coordinator will be available to help you with these details.

Most electrical medical equipment has three-pronged (grounded) plugs. If your electrical outlets aren't equipped for these plugs, you'll need to buy adapters at a hardware store. You may need to have an electrician determine whether the wiring in your home is suitable for such equipment. If your patient will be using home kidney dialysis, you may have to make changes in your household plumbing.

Most items can be ordered from a medical equipment supplier, which can be found in the telephone directory. Look for basic supplies at your pharmacy. When choosing an equipment supplier, ask these questions:

1. Will the firm bill your insurance company directly, so you will not have to pay out of pocket? (Some insurance companies cover only 80% of these costs and you must pay the other 20%.)
2. How quickly can the company fill an order, and will they deliver?
3. Will the delivery staff set up equipment?
4. What other services are offered?
5. Can someone be reached after hours in an emergency?

If your patient is on Medicare and you are ordering equipment, you probably will be asked the following:

1. What is needed and why?
2. How long will your patient need the equipment?
3. Did the doctor recommend this equipment? (It probably won't be covered unless ordered by a doctor.)

All equipment covered for reimbursement under Medicare must meet these criteria: the equipment can withstand repeated use; it is used primarily for medical purposes; it is not generally useful to a person in the absence of an illness or injury.

Your local Social Security office should have a list of reimbursable items, along with a price list noting an allowable charge on each item. Include the costs of shipping and taxes on the total bill. You and the physician must complete the appropriate forms before you'll receive reimbursement; you may have to remind your physician to follow through. When ordering supplies or filling out Medicare forms, be sure to let all parties know if your patient is being treated for a work-related injury involving Worker's Compensation.

Insurance Coverage

I cannot overemphasize the importance of reviewing costs *before* your patient is discharged. Health care is expensive and someone will have to pay—hopefully, not you! Often, when patients are discharged, little thought has been given to finances. You may have an emotional commitment to getting your loved one home—and rightfully so—but the actual cost to you cannot be ignored. Sometimes, because of these costs, home care is not feasible.

Before discharge, look at your health insurance policy to see what benefits it provides. Unfortunately, many people learn about benefits only after a family member gets sick or has an accident. Read your policy carefully, including the fine print. Here are some important areas to consider in your review:

1. What is the deductible, and must it be met annually?
2. Does the policy pay 100% of costs, or only 80%? Sometimes policies pay 100% of costs only after expenses reach a certain point; if so, find out what that threshold is.

3. Are there limits on the policy? Some contain a cap on expenses that can be confining if your loved one has a long-term illness or needs multiple surgeries.
4. Is coverage limited for "catastrophic diseases," such as cancer or AIDS?
5. Will doctors' fees and costs for diagnostic tests be paid outside of the hospital?
6. Will your insurance cover new or experimental therapies? Many policies will not reimburse you for drugs or treatments that haven't been widely adopted in the medical field.

Are home health care benefits part of your insurance package? Some plans stipulate that a patient must be hospitalized for a certain length of time before home care will be reimbursed. If you have home care benefits, look for the following:

1. Does it cover nursing care, both skilled and unskilled? What about visits from therapists (nutritional, physical, respiratory)?
2. Must you use a home health care agency designated by the insurer? You may be penalized if you choose one that doesn't have an agreement with your insurer.
3. Will medical equipment in the home be covered? Must you buy or rent the equipment?
4. Are costs of medications given at home reimbursed?
5. Does the insurance company require approval *before* you incur any medical costs? If so, you may not be reimbursed for expenses if you fail to get approval.

If any part of your policy is unclear, call your agent or representative. If some needed services are not covered or reimbursed, speak with a social worker or discharge planner at the hospital. Often, he or she can suggest ways of getting additional assistance.

Even if your insurance coverage is sound, you need to be thoroughly familiar with reimbursement policies so you are not saddled with mounting out-of-pocket expenses while waiting for a check to arrive. Whenever possible, consult your insurer before incurring major medical expenses. Explain the doctor's recommendations and find out what will be covered.

If your loved one is over 65 (or younger and meets certain criteria) Medicare will cover some costs. There are two parts to Medicare: Part A covers hospitalization charges; Part B covers physicians' bills, medical equipment, and other costs. Although Medicare is federally funded, you must pay extra to subscribe to Part B. If your patient is insured only by Medicare, you probably must use a certified home health care agency to be reimbursed for home care.

Medicaid assistance is for the indigent and applicants must meet strict standards on monthly income and total assets. As health care costs rise, consult your social worker or Medicaid representative if your patient is nearing eligibility. Medicaid is administered by the states, so check with local offices about eligibility. You may find out about other state programs that will benefit your loved one.

Many major medical policies have very poor coverage for home health care, but that is slowly changing as the need for home care grows. Home care companies usually check with your insurance company to be sure coverage is in place. You may be asked to make a deposit toward any therapy that isn't covered by insurance, or to sign a binding contract that makes you responsible for all uninsured charges. *Don't sign such a contract without a careful review; you may want your family lawyer to read it first.* Sometimes therapy costs are reimbursed while the patient is hospitalized, but not covered when the patient returns home. Ask for a bill of estimated charges; this can help you decide whether you and your family can afford out-of-hospital therapy for your loved one.

You may be able to assign benefits to the health care company, meaning the home care provider can bill the insurer directly. If your insurer allows it, I recommend this option because it keeps you from paying out of pocket, and it cuts down on your paper work and bookkeeping. Save all doctors' bills, pharmacy receipts, and other medical charges for your own records. If your insurance company requests them, send copies and keep the originals. If a claim is denied, find out why. Your social worker or health care company may be able to help you resubmit the claim when an error is made or documentation is missing.

Get all of your reimbursement questions answered before your loved one is discharged from the hospital. Don't let anyone rush you. Government cost-cutting changes now include incentives to get hospitals to discharge Medicare patients quickly. This is how it works: Diseases have been separated into categories known as diagnostic related groups (DRG). Gall bladder disease, for example, has an allotment of seven days' hospitalization for surgery. If the patient is discharged in five days, the hospital still receives reimbursement for a full seven days. If the patient stays longer than seven days, the government will not reimburse beyond the limit and the patient may be responsible for the difference. Be an advocate for your loved one if early discharge is recommended. Make sure care isn't compromised for the hospital's convenience and budget.

Assessing Your Home

In your haste to bring your loved one home, you may forget that it is not the comfortable, cozy place it was before illness or injury struck. Consider your patient's physical limitations: Will stairs be a problem? Is there access to bathrooms? Will you need to install air conditioning or air filtering equipment? If your loved one is in a wheelchair, is your house accessible—both inside and outside? Do you have enough room for recuperation and rehabilitation equipment? Will you need an extra refrigerator to store intravenous feeding solutions? Consult members of the health care team to determine whether your house is suitable for home recovery. Know as much as you can about your loved one's medical condition and requirements for recuperation; read appropriate chapters of this book *now* to determine whether your home could be hazardous to someone in frail health.

When you're planning the homecoming, don't forget about transportation. Will your patient be able to ride comfortably in your car, or is suitable mass transit available? Will your car hold a wheelchair, walker, or other equipment? Some community services provide transportation for the disabled.

A Care Giver's Concerns

You may feel overwhelmed by all of these details and perhaps you are concerned that you aren't capable of caring for your patient, or that you could cause him some harm. Express these fears to the health care team. Ask yourself: Do you really believe you can handle this commitment, or are you taking it on because you feel an obligation to a loved one? Can you and your family handle the financial burdens?

It won't be easy and there will be times when you feel you can't take another day. Don't take too much of that burden alone. Discuss your patient's care with the entire family; devise a plan that lets everyone take part. Map out a schedule, and set limits for all family members.

Remember also that your plan is not carved in stone—it can be changed if necessary. Accept offers of help from friends, relatives, or anyone else who would like to help.

Many community and volunteer services may be able to cover for you when you have to go out, or are there to offer emotional support. (See the Appendix for a list of community resources.) Keep in mind there may be interim hospitalizations. Use that time to catch up on your rest and do something for yourself—don't spend all your time running back and forth to the hospital. Keep your own well-being in mind.

Understanding Illness

The psychological aspects of an illness are many and you may find it easier to care for your patient if you understand some of them. Often, a patient who has been hospitalized a long time considers the hospital a safe and secure cocoon—she doesn't want to go home. The hospital gives her a sense of security; her needs are met, the doctors understand her illness, and she is unconditionally accepted. The hospital can be an escape for a patient who fears facing her friends, family, or co-workers. Maybe the patient has been disfigured by surgery and wants to hide. Perhaps she simply isn't ready to accept her illness and get on with life. Whatever the reason, it should be respected and the lines of communication should remain open.

When faced with serious illness or disability, many people go through a range of emotions that mirror the psychological stages Dr. Elisabeth Kubler-Ross recognized among the terminally ill in her landmark book, *On Death and Dying*. Your patient may pass through some, or all, of these stages before she accepts the diagnosis. The length of each phase will vary, and sometimes will exist side by side with another stage.

The most common reaction a patient has first is denial. Help your patient openly discuss her illness; don't support the denial. Understand the patient's need to cope in her own way and help her look realistically at the illness. Once your patient stops denying her illness, anger and frustration may surface. Look out; this anger may be directed at you! Although you may instinctively withdraw from the patient or become angry yourself, try to support her through this period. Help her express and understand her anger. Depression can follow; she may withdraw from you and the family. Be there for her with understanding and support. With time and patience, your loved one will reach a phase of acceptance and adaptation to her condition.

Be sensitive to your patient's needs. There may be times when she wishes to be alone, to do something for herself, or to be told how brave she is. Quite often when someone is sick, we tend to lose sight of her needs as a person, or what she was before she became ill. Pay attention to both verbal and non-verbal communication. Remember that you probably know the patient better than anyone on the health care team. Don't become so involved in being the care giver or nurse that you forget to be a wife or husband, sister or brother.

Dealing with the emotional aspect of illness is not easy. You may resent the new burden that has suddenly fallen upon you, and you may feel guilty about these feelings. They are normal; find some way to vent them. Just as your patient passes through stages, you must do the same. Take time to talk with your patient about how you both feel, good and bad. *Keep those lines of communication open.*

Find support systems or emotional outlets; they will become more important as time goes by. Get out of the house; make time for yourself. Investigate community resources; seek out local chapters of the American Cancer Society, the Multiple Sclerosis Society, or agencies with support groups where you'll meet others with similar problems. The American Red Cross offers courses in home care. Meals on Wheels or similar community groups may offer hot meals for the homebound. Seek professional counseling, if you need it. Don't become a silent martyr—if you don't ask for help, you are not apt to receive any!

Care Giver's Checklist

1. Discuss your patient's needs with the health care team and make necessary arrangements *before* your loved one comes home.

2. Evaluate nursing needs and home health care agencies.

3. Order equipment and medications before discharge; get training in special medical procedures from health professionals while your loved one is in the hospital.

4. Investigate community support systems for the patient, care giver, and family.

5. Be sensitive to the psychological effects of illness. Offer your patient love, support, encouragement, and keep open the lines of communication.

2 Setting Up Your Home Care Program

Deciding to care for a loved one at home takes thought, patience, and planning. If you believe that home care is best for you and your patient, start working with the health care team to adapt your home for medical care. Try to keep the household intact, so it feels more like a home than a hospital. Of course, this depends on how great your patient's home care needs will be.

If possible, your loved one should return to the room she occupied before her hospitalization. However, be sure to consider the following: Will stairs be a problem for you or the patient? Is easy access to a bathroom or telephone important? Is adequate ventilation or warmth a consideration?

Before you make any major structural changes, consider whether your patient's condition is temporary or permanent. Any structural changes you make for the patient may be tax deductible, and possibly will be reimbursed by your insurance company. Save all receipts and canceled checks. Get a letter from your doctor documenting the need for any changes or expenses you incur due to the patient's illness. If your patient is in a wheelchair, consider the access into and throughout the house. This should be considered not only for practical reasons, but for safety in case of an emergency such as a fire. (See the Appendix for companies that specialize in adapting your home for someone in a wheelchair.)

Try to keep the patient's room free of objects and obstacles on the floor. Look out for electrical wires, loose carpets, and area rugs that could trip your patient. It's useful to have a night-light, or to turn on a hall or bathroom light during the night.

Environment is so important to one's well-being. Little things such as noise, odors, or temperatures can aggravate a patient who is not feeling well. A clean, bright, and cheery environment is a big help to any patient.

If there are children at home, tell them what to expect and what their role will be. You might arrange for them to meet with the physician sometime before discharge to discuss the situation. Don't forget the family pet. Find out if there are limitations to the pet visiting or being around the patient.

Visitors usually are important in helping a patient to get well, but be sensitive to needs for quiet and rest. The same goes for telephone calls. Remember that visitors can leave the patient's side, but your patient may not be able to walk away. Perhaps you can make a "Do Not Disturb" sign for her to hang out when she wishes privacy or rest.

Supplies and Equipment

After you have adequately planned the physical setting and made changes, you can begin to assess what supplies will be needed. If your patient is recuperating and plans to be up and about, there is no reason why her own bed should not be used. If the patient is confined to bed or has special needs, consider getting a hospital bed. Some advantages are that the head, foot, and height of the bed can be adjusted, making it easier for the patient to change her position. A hospital bed also is easy on the care giver's back. Most of these beds come with safety rails; if not, you can request them. The adjustment mechanisms are operated manually or electrically.

You can rent or buy the bed from a medical supplier. If the bed is to be used for a long time, consider purchasing one. Many good bedding shops sell hospital-type beds that blend nicely in the home.

An overbed table is useful. The patient should have a nightstand next to the bed so she can have whatever she needs in easy reach. Get a bell so your patient can signal for help, or even a portable, inexpensive intercom system. This could allay any worry you may have about leaving the patient alone. Other useful items include a clock; fresh water and a cup; a television or radio; books; a wastebasket; and anything else the patient wants close by. Provide chairs for guests and a comfortable chair for your patient.

Review other needs with the health care team; there may be inexpensive ways to meet them. For example, a small chair can be turned into a backrest. A cardboard box can be cut away and used to lift sheets off the patient's feet and legs. Be creative! Improvise if you have to, even if it is just temporary until you get the proper equipment.

Be sure to have your patient's prescriptions filled before discharge. Store all medications as directed and keep them out of reach of children! If your patient is discharged in the morning, have her take her morning medications before leaving the hospital. Check with the nurse to find out what the next scheduled doses are. If you have a long car ride, perhaps the nurse can give you the medications you will need if you won't get home before they are due. (For additional medication information, see Chapter 8.)

Patient Safety

Most accidents can be prevented. Anticipate problems and know how to handle them. Keep a first aid kit on hand, stored in a safe place. Make a list of all important telephone numbers such as doctors, police, fire department, and rescue or ambulance squad. Ask your patient's doctor what potential emergencies could occur with your loved one and how to treat them. Do you and your family know cardiopulmonary resuscitation (CPR)? Courses in this lifesaving technique are offered in most communities. Be sure to read Chapter 16 in this book on medical emergencies.

Falls are one of the most common accidents in home care. If you are caring for a confused or unconscious patient, protect her from falling out of bed by using safety rails on the sides of the bed; keep them up whenever she is alone. If you do not have safety rails, use several high-backed chairs placed up against the bed. If you are using a hospital electric bed, always leave the height of the bed in the down position when you are not with the patient. Place objects within easy reach; patients often fall out of bed when trying to reach for something too far away. Patients who are sedated, taking sleeping medication, or pain-killers should be told not to get out of bed alone. Leave a urinal or bedpan close by so they will not get out of bed during the night.

If your patient has a fall, stay calm and do not move her immediately. Ask her to lie still while you try to find out what happened and if she is hurt. If you feel she is injured, keep her there, making her as comfortable as possible with a pillow or blanket, and call your physician for advice. Describe what you feel happened and what the injuries may be. If you feel you have a real emergency, call your ambulance/rescue squad.

If you are *absolutely* sure that your patient is not injured, you can slowly move her to a sitting position. After she sits up, help her stand and return to bed. If she is not able to get up, ask someone to help you move her. If you have any doubts about your patient's injuries, *do not move her*. Seek medical attention. It is a good idea to report any falls to your physician immediately. Frail bones can be broken even with the slightest fall, especially in the elderly. The doctor may want X-rays taken to be sure nothing has been broken.

A confused or disoriented patient may need to be restrained when she is left unattended. Most loved ones resist this. Restraints, or "posey restraints," are used only to protect the patient from harm to herself or others. If you feel your patient may need to be restrained, talk this over with your physician and get permission before you do so. A patient may need to be restrained if she pulls out tubes or catheters; scratches a wound, dressing, skin rashes, or sores; or if she is extremely confused and apt to fall or wander. Combative or extremely agitated patients must be restrained and, depending on the severity of the problem, may not be manageable at home.

Various types of restraints are available: soft wrist restraints can be used to keep a patient from pulling on a catheter or tube; vest and belt restraints prevent a patient from falling out of a wheelchair or bed; mitt restraints fit over the hands and prevent a patient from scratching irritated skin; and limb restraints limit movement, also preventing removal of tubes or catheters (figure 1). Most of these can be purchased from a medical supply store. If your patient used them in the hospital, they may have been purchased and belong to her. Have a professional show you how to use restraints. They should not be so tight that circulation is impaired, and they should never be used on a seizure-prone patient. During a seizure the patient's muscles become rigid and tense, and if the patient is restrained, it could cause fractures or other injuries. Use extreme caution on patients with respiratory difficulties or heart problems, and never apply restraints directly over wounds or intravenous catheters.

All restraints should be applied carefully. Tie a bow or knot that can be released easily in an emergency. Never restrict movement so much that a patient has trouble breathing or that circulation is blocked. The knot should not be the type that is apt to tighten up as the patient moves (figure 2). Soft, padded restraints are best; if you are using unpadded restraints, pad them with cotton wads or any other soft material.

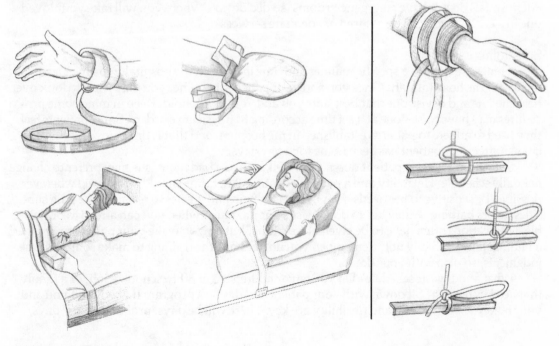

Fig. 1 Four types of restraints

Fig. 2 Tying restraints

Tell your patient why you are restraining her and be sure she understands that it is not a punishment. Change the restraints to different positions often to prevent skin irritation. Check for circulation problems. Is the skin cold to the touch; is the color unusual; or are there any changes in sensation? If the skin appears cold or blue, or the patient complains of a tingling sensation or numbness, loosen the restraint immediately. When the restraints are off, move the patient's hand, wrist, or leg to exercise it. Leave some slack in the restraints and tie your knot or bow under the bed mattress. It is not a good idea to tie the restraints onto the bedside safety rail. Take off the restraints whenever someone is with the patient. If your patient is apt to vomit, restrain her on her side only, and change her position often. If this is a new procedure, be sure to have a medical professional demonstrate the techniques before you proceed.

Fire safety should be a major concern. Smoking in bed is a fire hazard, so be extra-careful with patients who are confused or sedated and want to smoke. Do not leave such a patient alone with matches. Provide a large ashtray that will not spill. *No one* is allowed to smoke when oxygen is in use. Be sure you and your family have decided how your patient will escape in case of an emergency. If you have a fire and must move a bedridden patient, place her on a blanket or area rug and pull her to safety.

In regard to medical emergencies, a wise old doctor once told me that "unless a person won't stop bleeding, or has stopped breathing, most things can wait." You probably know this if you have ever spent time waiting to be seen in a hospital emergency room. I do not mean to say that if these two conditions do not exist, there is no emergency. However, you can remain calm and tend to the patient first, and then call the doctor.

If your patient's condition seems to be worsening or if you anticipate problems, act right away—do not wait to see what happens. If you need to call an ambulance, remember to give all necessary information, including your address. Often people forget the basics during a crisis. Try to describe the problem so rescue workers can prepare to care for your loved one. All hospitals do not have emergency rooms, so decide *now* where you will take your loved one in a crisis so you can be assured of adequate services.

Scheduling

Things are done in a specific manner and time interval in the hospital, mostly as a convenience for the hospital staff. Once you and your patient are home, you may want to look over her schedule and devise one that best suits you and your household. Keep in mind some procedures may have to be done at a set time according to physician's orders. Some patients feel they need to adhere to patterns established in the hospital, and that is fine, too. This may change after your patient has been home for a few days.

Sometimes, when a patient doesn't feel well, or had a bad night, she may prefer to change her daily schedule. Flexibility and a patient's control of her time should be allowed wherever possible. Be sensitive to her needs. Maybe she is in pain and wishes to rest until the pain subsides before bathing. Allow her to do so. Use your judgment when you can afford to be flexible. Medications often have to be given at a set time, but do you wake your patient to give her a vitamin pill? Probably not. Remember, you do not have the training to make some of these judgments, so plan with your doctor.

What about your schedule? Do you have children to get off to school, a job, or a family that needs attention? Sit down with your patient and devise a program that will suit you and your family. Organization and flexibility are key. There will be days, probably many days, when you won't follow this schedule. On those days, set priorities and work around those. If you find that you need help, reach out for it. Set limits for both the patient and the family, or you will find that you, too, need that hospital bed! If there are older children or others to help you, be sure to take advantage of their assistance. Don't get so caught up with physical chores that you forget behind that surgical dressing is someone you love. Often, your patient may need your love, or a good hug, much more than she needs her bed made or her teeth cleaned.

Sometimes, unrealistic plans are made in the quest to get your loved one home, or her health circumstances have changed. If you are overwhelmed, there are many home services available, and your physician or social worker should be able to help you find one.

Record Keeping

You will find it a big help to you, to the patient, and to the physician if you keep daily records of the following: patient vital signs; medications; special problems; fluid intake and output (if ordered by the doctor); diet; patient progress and activities; and anything else that relates to your patient's condition. It will help to have a written record, especially when your doctor is evaluating your patient's progress and response to treatment. Be sure to bring it along when you visit the doctor. Refer to sample charts throughout this book for examples of how to keep daily records.

When traveling, take a list of your patient's medications, a copy of her medical history, and other pertinent information. Have your patient carry an identification card with medical information, or ask her to wear a bracelet or medallion indicating medical problems.

Care Giver's Checklist

1. Look at your home through your patient's eyes. Is there easy access to the bathroom? Will rugs, furniture, or the children's toys create hazards? Is the environment bright, clean, and cheerful?

2. Consider major structural changes carefully before your patient comes home. Document the need for major changes for tax and insurance purposes.

3. Stock up on supplies, equipment, and medications.

4. Don't jeopardize your patient's recovery through disregard for safety. Keep a first aid kit on hand, post a list of phone numbers for emergency services, and map out a fire escape route for your patient.

5. Sit down with your patient and family to draw up a reasonable daily schedule. Charts may be helpful in keeping track of medications, feedings, dressing changes, and your patient's daily progress.

3 Day-to-Day Personal Care

Your loved one may be unable to do the simplest everyday activities during his recuperation. You may need to bathe your patient, brush his teeth, wash his hair, shave his whiskers, or trim his toenails. These time-consuming tasks, which he did so well before he became ill, are important to his sense of well-being. Try to perform them with a sense of love and concern; your patient probably is distressed about being unable to keep himself clean.

However, patients who need help with personal hygiene sometimes tend to regress or become dependent. Try not to nurture this; encourage as much independent activity as possible. It may be very hard for you to watch your patient struggle through a simple task, but you must remember how important it is that he continue to aim for independence.

Bed Making

If your patient can get out of bed alone or with your assistance, it's much easier to make the bed. There are many ways to make a bed, but in all cases, make sure the bottom sheet is tight around the mattress and the bed is wrinkle free (since wrinkles can cause skin irritation and eventually bed sores), that there are enough bedclothes to cover the patient's feet, and that top sheets are not too snug. Remember to turn the mattress from time to time, whenever it's convenient to do so.

If the patient is apt to soil the bed or is incontinent you'll want to protect the mattress with a shower curtain, plastic tablecloth, or large plastic garbage bag. Large absorbent pads are available from your medical supplier. You can provide additional protection by using a drawsheet. This is a flat sheet folded in half lengthwise and placed across the bottom sheet, between the patient's shoulders and knees. Tuck the drawsheet into both sides of the bed. The drawsheet can also serve as a lifting device to help position your patient in bed. If you wish to protect the bottom sheet surface, you can also add rubber or plastic sheeting between it and the drawsheet. Place a bedsheet over this so the plastic or rubber does not touch your patient. You can change only the drawsheet if it becomes soiled or covered with perspiration.

When your patient is confined to bed, linen changes become even more essential. You can make an occupied bed with or without help. If you are unassisted, use safety rails to prevent the patient from rolling out of bed.

If the bed can be elevated, raise it until you can work comfortably. Loosen all the linens from the mattress and have fresh sheets ready by the bedside. Place the bed in a flat position and ask your patient to roll all the way over to one side of the bed. Now push all the linens as far as you can underneath the patient, and place the fresh linens on the mattress in toward the patient. Have him roll over all of the linens; then remove the soiled ones and tuck the fresh ones tightly in place (figure 3). Completing one side at a time is faster for you and more comfortable for the patient. If he is unable to roll over without your help, grasp the drawsheet from the opposite side and pull your patient toward you.

If your patient cannot roll over, you can change the bed by working from top to bottom (figure 4). Raise the head of the bed and then pull all the linens down as far as you can and tuck them under the patient's buttocks. Ask your patient to lift up, either by holding his

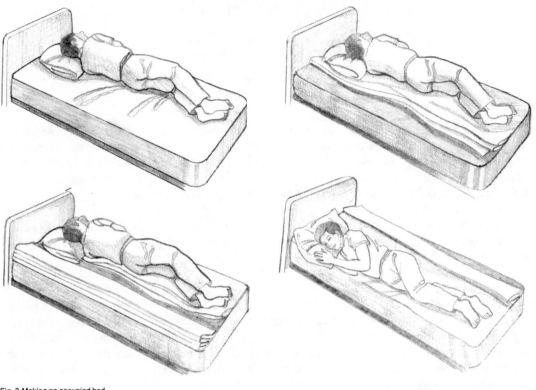

Fig. 3 Making an occupied bed

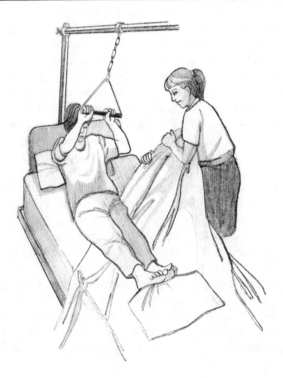

Fig. 4 Changing a bed from top to bottom

overhead trapeze, if he has one, or by doing a push-up with his upper body to lift his buttocks. Remove the dirty linens and replace them with clean sheets. Afterward, be sure to pull the linens taut.

To make a hospital or mitered corner (figure 5), tuck the bottom of the sheet under the mattress, then lift the side edge of the sheet about 12 inches from the mattress corner, and hold it at a right angle to the mattress. Now tuck in the bottom edge of the sheet left hanging below the mattress, drop the edge and tuck it under the mattress.

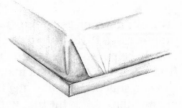
Fig. 5 Mitered corner

Remember to clean plastic mattress covers often with a mild soap-and-water solution if your patient is incontinent. Launder the sheets in the usual fashion, using a fabric softener to help prevent skin irritation. If the sheets are stained, try presoaking them (cold water for blood; hot water for stains such as urine or feces) and pre-spot with stain remover before machine washing. Adding bleach to the wash cycle will help remove the remains of the stain.

Bathing

The patient's bath is probably the most flexible aspect of his care. If you are pressed for time, it may be put off until later, unless of course the patient is soiled and needs immediate attention. If he is tired or in pain, don't worry about postponing the bath, or even skipping a day. For some patients, a bath or shower is not allowed, so consult with the doctor.

If your patient is able to get up, he should be encouraged to go into the bathroom to bathe by himself. You may need to help him get there. Allow him his privacy, but stay close in case he needs help. Never let your patient lock the door. If he is weak, set a chair next to the sink so he can sit down to wash. Bath seats and appliances for the tub or shower are available to assist patients (figure 6). You can also get special support bars for the bath. A removable shower spray is helpful, as the patient can sit in the shower and bring the spray down to his level. Use non-slip mats or strips to guard against falls.

Be very careful of the water temperature, especially if your patient can't reach the temperature controls. Bath thermometers are available at most pharmacies. A safe bath temperature is 100 to 110° F (37.8 to 43.3° C). If the water temperature in your house changes whenever someone turns on water elsewhere or flushes the toilet, notify others in the house when your patient is showering. Water temperature is a special consideration for patients who have circulatory problems, nerve disorders, or who are disoriented. They are not

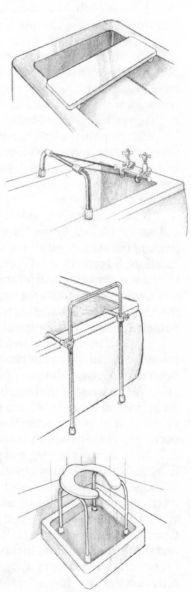
Fig. 6 Bath appliances

aware of differences in temperature and could easily be burned. Very hot water also causes blood vessels to dilate, which alters blood flow and can cause dizziness or fainting.

In helping a patient into the bathtub or shower, always adjust the water temperature first—never sit the patient in the shower and then turn on the water. When you turn off the shower, shut off the hot water first. To help your loved one into or out of the bath, stand behind him, beside the tub, with your arms around his waist. Have him grasp his own wrist while you hold his forearms with your hands. Help your patient step into the tub and lower him while keeping your back straight, bending at the knees. Reverse this process to get him out of the bathtub. You may also face the patient and offer support with your arms as he steps into and out of the tub.

If your patient cannot go into the bathroom, you can set up a bath area on a table beside the bed. You'll need a basin for water, soap, washcloth, towel, mirror, comb, and other supplies. Set these up within easy reach of the patient and allow him to bathe himself. You may have to assist with his back or other areas he cannot reach. Water cools quickly, so try to replace it with warm water midway through the bath. Insure the patient's privacy by choosing a time when you and he will have few interruptions.

Elderly patients tend to have dry, fragile skin. Perhaps these patients should bathe only every other day; you can alternate with a sponge bath. Avoid excessive use of soap. Bath oils in the water will help keep dry skin from becoming drier. Apply lotions after the bath. Avoid the use of rubbing alcohol, as it is very drying. Hypoallergenic products may be best for your patient's skin.

If your patient is unable to help bathe himself, you will most likely have to give him a full bath in his bed, unless there is a way to move him into the bathtub. You will need all of the supplies mentioned above. A bed bath not only cleanses the body but will stimulate circulation and provide mild exercise. Use this time to look for changes in skin condition, temperature, rashes, and joint mobility. Keep the patient covered with a light blanket or sheet, uncovering each area only when you wash it. This will keep the patient warm and maintain his privacy. During the bath, the room should be warm and free of drafts. If your patient is in an electric hospital bed, raise it to a level that makes the bathing easy for you.

Begin at the head and work downward. It's easier if you make a mitt from a facecloth by folding it in half over your hand and tucking the four corners into the center. Start with the eyes, working from the inner portion out, using a separate part of the washcloth for each eye. Wash the rest of the face, being firm but gentle. Rinse and dry each area well. Now wash and dry the chest and both arms, from the wrists to the upper arm. If your patient is large, lift up excess skin folds to wash them, being extra careful to dry them well. Skin breakdown can occur anywhere two body surfaces touch.

Now uncover one leg and place it, bent at the knee, with the foot flat on the bed. Use firm, smooth strokes to help stimulate blood flow. Do not massage the leg, as this can dislodge blood clots that may have formed as a result of inactivity. Don't forget to dry between each toe! Cover the leg and repeat with the other leg.

Lower the head of the bed after you have bathed and dried the patient's legs and feet. Change the bath water and ask the patient to turn onto his side or stomach. Wash his back and then put some lotion in the palm of your hand (to warm it up) and massage his back. (You don't have to worry about blood clots there.) Use long, firm strokes, giving special attention to any reddened areas.

Now bathe the rectal area, avoid contaminating the genitals, and be sure to remove all soap. Change the bath water again and get a fresh washcloth. Have the patient turn on his back and bathe the genitals, avoiding the rectal area. It is sometimes refreshing for a female patient to be placed on a bedpan and have warm water poured over the genitals.

After the bath, you may wish to soak the patient's hands and feet in a basin of warm, soapy water. Apply some light talcum powder, but not so much that it cakes. Now give your patient a fresh gown and help him put on anything else that was removed before the bath. You can change the bedridden patient's bed at this time, as well. The patient may be tired after his bath and need to rest.

Some patients connected to certain medical apparatus will be unable to take a full bath. The doctor may allow these patients to be temporarily disconnected; be sure to check on this first. Intravenous and some other tubes may or may not be allowed to get wet. Casts must never get wet. As a general rule, if a dressing or cast becomes wet, it must be changed. If you have permission to bathe the patient but are told to keep an area dry, place plastic wrap around it. In most cases you will not be able to immerse the wrapped part, but this offers some protection against moisture.

Personal Hygiene

Encourage your loved one to participate in a regular routine of good grooming—from head to toes.

Mouth Care.　　　Oral hygiene is important to all of us, especially to those who cannot look after this themselves. Be sure to inspect your patient's mouth while doing mouth care. Mouth sores can indicate loose-fitting dentures, or problems with medications or diet. Report any problems to the health care team.

Good oral hygiene not only makes the patient feel better, but will enhance his taste for food and will aid in good nutrition. Naturally, the patient should be allowed to manage this on his own, if he can. He may need your assistance if he must do this at the bedside. He should have a kidney-shaped basin (like those used in the hospital) or something similar to rinse into. Wrap a towel or piece of plastic under the patient's chin to keep him and his bed dry.

If your patient can sit up and cooperate, bring all of the equipment to the bedside. Brush his teeth, moving the brush away from the gumline, using a gentle, firm, up-and-down motion. After brushing, give him a gentle mouthwash solution so he can rinse thoroughly.

It is particularly important that good oral hygiene be provided to comatose patients, as they often breathe only through their mouths, which causes dryness and cracking. Cleanse the mouth using swabs dipped in a solution of warm water and baking soda, or warm water and mouthwash; some dentists recommend equal parts of baking soda and salt mixed with enough hydrogen peroxide to make a paste (this cleans the teeth and helps combat gum disease). It's especially important for comatose patients to sit upright so that they do not choke. Swab the mouth thoroughly after washing the teeth and gums.

Another tool for cleaning the teeth and the inside of the mouth is a tongue depressor or popsicle stick with the tip wrapped in a gauze pad four inches square. Tape the edges of the pad to hold it in place. Dip this into your mouthwash solution and swab around the inside of the mouth several times, being sure to remove any food residue or caked mucus. Try wrapping gauze around your first two fingers to gently clean away food. Be careful not to make your patient gag.

Another means of oral hygiene, especially for the patient who cannot open his mouth wide, is the Water Pik. The Water Pik provides a pulsating flow of solution that helps break up and remove food particles. The solution should be warm water and mouthwash, or warm water and salt. Check with your doctor to see which solution he or she feels is best for your patient; it may be that some solutions should not be used, especially on patients undergoing radiation and chemotherapy treatments. If there are any mouth sores, avoid salt solutions and mouthwash, which would irritate the condition. A sponge-tipped device is available for patients with irritated gums. If you see any bleeding from the gums, report it to your physician.

For the patient with an extremely dry mouth, commercially available lemon and glycerin swabs are refreshing and help generate saliva (a few sucks on a lemon or orange will accomplish the same thing). Keep the swabs refrigerated, as they are even more refreshing when cool. If the patient has been on oxygen or is breathing through his mouth, his lips will be especially dry; apply petroleum jelly or lip balm. Quite often, a comatose or stroke patient will need frequent suctioning of excess mucus; this is discussed in Chapter 11.

Dentures.   If your patient is unconscious, dentures should be removed, as they may slip back and cause choking or airway obstruction. Wash your hands before and after handling dentures. You can use a piece of tissue or gauze to grasp them. To remove dentures, place your thumb and forefinger in the patient's mouth, feeling for the outer ridge of the denture. Exert a slight downward pressure to break the suction and pull the denture plate out. The same process can be used for partial plates. Clean the dentures with whatever solution the patient is accustomed to using, or use warm water. Be sure the water is not too hot, as this may warp the dentures. Clean dentures at least once a day using a special denture brush, which is softer than a regular toothbrush. If the dentures have metal parts, do not soak them in cleansing solution, as this can break down the surface. For the same reason, never soak dentures in mouthwash. Be careful not to drop them.

While the dentures are out, you can perform mouth care by cleaning the gums with a sponge dipped in warm water and mouthwash or baking soda and water. Dentures can be reinserted by reversing the removal process. Patients who are able to eat solid or semi-solid foods should have their dentures in place. Loose-fitting dentures can cause poor appetite. If dentures are removed too long, gums can recede, resulting in a poor fit.

Eyes.   Cleansing the eye area is extremely important. Remember that if you clean both eyes with the same section of towel, you may be transferring organisms from one eye to the other; this is known as "cross-contamination." For this reason, family members should never share towels.

To prevent cross-contamination, use a different section of the washcloth for each eye. Clean each eye from the inner section out using one smooth stroke, not a rubbing back-and-forth action. If there is excess crust formation, you can loosen it by soaking a cotton ball in warm water, wringing it out, and resting it over the eye for a short period. Be sure to remove any caked-on crust from the lid and eye surface.

The comatose patient may rest without shutting his eyes, which causes the eye to become dry and irritated. Lubricants and artificial tears are available for this problem. These can be applied after you have cleansed the eye. (Again, check with your doctor first!)

Another way to soothe the comatose patient's eyes is to gently place cotton balls moistened with warm water on the eyelids and secure them with a non-allergenic tape. Change the cotton balls as often as necessary. To apply eye ointments and medications, refer to Chapter 8. Some medications cause side effects such as double or blurry vision. If your patient develops any eye-related side effects, tell the doctor.

If your patient wears glasses and is unable to put them on himself, don't forget to do this for him. Remember to check eyeglass prescriptions and get regular eye care. In caring for the immediate condition, other aspects of care are often overlooked.

Ears.   Ears can be cleaned using a dry cotton swab to clean the outer ear canal. Do not put the tip of the swab in the inner ear, as you can do harm or cause irritation. If there is an excessive amount of wax, moisten the swab with warm water to try to dislodge it. If the patient is complaining of ear pain or loss of hearing, excess wax may have become lodged in the ear canal, and this may require medical attention.

If your patient wears a hearing aid, don't forget to put it in place, and remember to change batteries as needed. If the patient is hard of hearing in one ear, speak into the good ear, and face the patient as you do so.

Hair.   If he is well enough to get up and if the doctor approves, the patient can wash his own hair. The patient confined to home may wish a haircut or styling. Some hairdressers have portable equipment and will come to your home. This is bound to be a special treat for your patient and something he will enjoy. For patients who cannot wash their hair, there are a number of dry shampoos available in the drugstore. These are powders you sprinkle onto the hair and comb through—they really work, too! If the patient is going to spend a long time confined to bed and has long hair, it might be a good idea to cut his hair to an easier-to-manage length.

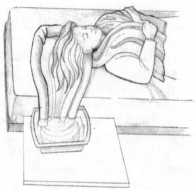

Fig. 7 Washing hair in bed

When you shampoo your patient's hair in bed, you will want to prevent him and the bed from getting soaked. There are a variety of devices you can buy in a medical supply store specifically for this purpose, or you can construct your own (figure 7). First place a large plastic garbage bag, shower curtain, or plastic tablecloth under the patient's head and torso. Arrange one section of the plastic to run down the side of the bed into a bucket. Roll a big towel or blanket into a U-shaped log. This goes under the patient's head and shoulders and the plastic cover. You can now shampoo the patient's head without fear of soaking the mattress.

Inspect the scalp for any skin breakdown or irritation. You may have to cut off matted hair—that's why brushing and combing are important. Brushing also helps improve scalp circulation.

Shaving.   Use either an electric or safety razor, whichever is most comfortable for you (but do not use a safety razor on a patient who has blood clotting problems or who is on anticoagulant therapy).

To use an electric razor, check first to see that it has been cleaned from its last use. If the patient uses a pre-shave, apply that first. Shave, moving the razor firmly in a circular motion until the surface feels smooth. Now apply an aftershave lotion or talcum.

If you are using a safety razor, your patient will need to sit. Be sure you have proper lighting, and that the blade is clean and fresh. You can soak the beard with a warm, wet cloth or apply a pre-shave solution to soften the beard. Note the direction the beard is growing; you'll stroke in that direction. Now apply either shaving cream or a soapy lather to the beard. Begin with your razor at the sideburn, using firm, smooth, downward strokes. Shave toward the center of the chin. If your patient is able, ask him to stretch his upper lip so you can shave that area. To shave the neck, work up toward the chin. Rinse the razor frequently.

Now, rinse the entire face and neck, using a fresh basin of water, and apply aftershave or whatever the patient prefers. Don't forget to rinse the razor well and apply fresh blades as needed. If you make a cut or nick, apply pressure. A styptic pencil or a piece of toilet paper applied to the area can help stop the bleeding. Apply a mild antiseptic after the bleeding has stopped.

Nails and Feet. Hands and feet can be soaked in a basin of warm water, about 115° F (46° C). Be sure the water is not too hot; always test it yourself before offering it to your patient. Patients with impaired circulation or sensation will not know if the water is too hot. Soaking the feet for about ten minutes will help to cleanse and loosen dry skin. After soaking, remove the feet from the basin and place on a clean towel. Dry around each nail surface and between each toe. Remove any debris. After you bathe the feet, apply a lotion. Clean under the nail beds by using a manicurist's blunt orange stick. Do not use nail scissors or clippers; you may cut the patient, causing additional problems or infection. If the nails are long, try shaping them with a nail file or emery board. File straight across the nail. Never try to cut the nails of a diabetic or a patient with impaired circulation.

If your patient's nails have been neglected or if he has other foot problems, call in a podiatrist. Many will make house calls, and their visits may be covered by insurance.

During foot care, observe skin temperature, color of nail beds (they should be pink), ingrown toenails, corns or bunions, any redness, or skin breakdown. Mention these conditions to your physician.

Clean and Sterile Techniques

Throughout this book, I will refer to clean or sterile techniques in describing medical procedures that you may be performing daily. *Clean technique* refers to the cleanest of circumstances: clean equipment, clean counter tops, clean hands, and a clean environment. Equipment from the dishwasher is considered clean, not sterile.

In *sterile (aseptic) technique,* anything touching the patient must be sterile (absolutely free of microorganisms). There are variations to sterile procedure; some doctors require only sterile equipment, others want the care taker to wear sterile gloves, cap, face mask, and protective gown. The extent of sterile technique will depend on the patient's condition.

When sterile technique is required, make a conscious effort to keep anything sterile from touching anything unsterile. Equipment or materials can be assumed sterile only if they arrive sealed and labeled as sterile; do not use anything that has been opened. If an item is contaminated, discard it and use a new one.

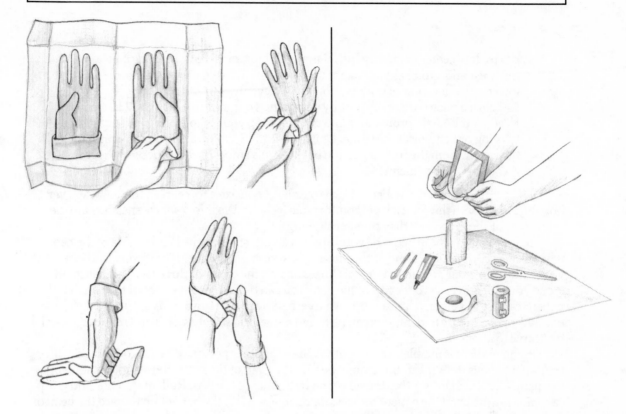

Fig. 8 Putting on sterile gloves

Fig. 9 Sterile field and equipment

Sterile gloves are required for some types of patient care. They come in different sizes in a sealed package. Applying sterile gloves is not an easy task (figure 8). Never touch the outside surface of the gloves. When you open the package, you will find the cuffs already are turned down. Take one glove by the cuff and put it on. Pick up the second glove by placing your gloved hand inside the rolled-down cuff of the second glove (between the cuff and outer surface; only the sterile surfaces will touch one another). While still holding the under cuff of the second glove, slide it onto your hand. Unfold the cuffs, being sure not to contaminate the outer surface of the gloves.

Put your gloves on only *after* you have prepared all of your equipment; once they are on, you cannot touch anything that is not sterile unless you discard the gloves and put on a new pair. It's helpful to have someone hand equipment to you during a sterile procedure.

A sterile field is a sterile towel or paper towel placed flat on a working surface. As long as the top of the towel remains sterile, you can empty all of your sterile equipment—gauzes, sponges, instruments—onto the field before you put on the gloves. When you break open the packages, let the equipment fall onto the sterile field without touching it (figure 9). If your health care team recommends sterile technique at home, have a medical professional demonstrate the procedure before you attempt it alone.

Moving Your Patient

There is a correct and an incorrect way to move or lift a patient. The wrong way can hurt your back, so it is important to learn proper body mechanics. Follow these three principles:

1. Keep a low center of gravity by flexing your hips and knees, instead of bending at the waist and letting all the weight fall in one area. By bending your knees and lowering your center of gravity, you help to evenly distribute the weight.
2. Establish a wide base of support by spreading your legs about 10 to 12 inches.
3. Keep your body in proper alignment by moving your whole body and not just twisting or bending at the waist. Lean into the object you are lifting by shifting the weight from the front leg to the back leg in a smooth, continuous motion. Avoid jerky movements.

When you lift something, bend down to its level and exert force from there. Whenever possible, work with things at a level comfortable for you. Wear low shoes; sneakers are the safest type of shoes because they prevent slipping.

To lift your patient in bed if he is able to assist you, stand at the head or side of the bed, wherever access is easiest. Bend at the knees, place your arms under his armpits, and interlock your arms. Ask your patient to bend his knees and on the count of three have him push off while you pull him toward the top of the bed. You can tie a rope to the foot of the bed that the patient can use to help pull himself up. An overbed trapeze (figure 10) is useful for the obese, paralyzed, or fracture patient; this can be found at medical supply stores and requires a special bedframe to attach it.

If your patient is unable to help, but you have another person to assist you, you can lift the patient on his drawsheet. If possible, be sure the head of the bed is flat so you're not working against gravity. Untuck the drawsheet on both sides of the bed. Roll up the ends and grasp each side firmly. Bend the patient's knees, if possible, and lift the patient up toward the head of the bed (figure 11).

To lift a dependent patient up in bed without the help of another person, stand or kneel at the head of the bed, grasp the patient under his armpits and around the chest, bend his knees and slide him toward you in a smooth motion (figure 12). (If the headboard is removable, it will make lifting easier. Headboards on most hospital beds are removable.)

You can use several methods to prevent the patient from slipping back down in the bed. Tuck pillows between the foot of the bed and the patient's feet; this will keep the feet in proper alignment as well. A footboard also can be used; order one from a medical supply store or make one (figure 13). If your patient is sitting, place pillows in the gap between his feet and the bed's footboard. Be sure to cover the footboard with a blanket or other soft covering.

To turn your patient to one side, you may need only to give him a gentle push or pull. A bedside safety rail or something steady for the patient to hold will help. If your patient has an abdominal incision and turning is uncomfortable, he can place a pillow over his abdomen and hold it there while turning. A fracture patient may require special turning techniques, which is discussed in Chapter 13.

If your patient cannot turn without assistance, untuck the drawsheet on the side opposite the direction he will be turning. Go to the side the patient is to turn to, reach over the patient and grab the edges of the drawsheet, pulling the patient toward you. You can keep your patient on that side by placing a pillow lengthwise between the shoulders and the buttocks, then gently easing the patient back into it. Be sure the patient is not lying on his arm, hand, or shoulder. If your patient is unconscious or confused, keep the safety railing up. (How to place your patient in various positions will be discussed later in this chapter.) If you do not have extra pillows, you can use a blanket rolled up like a log.

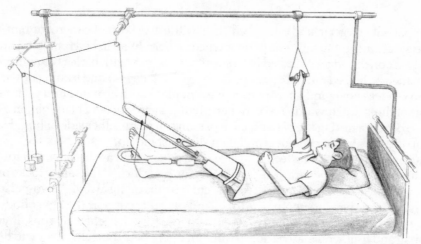

Fig. 10 Overbed trapeze

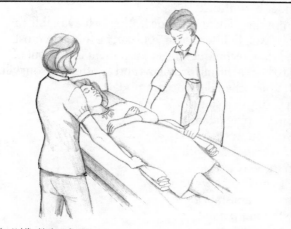

Fig. 11 Lift with drawsheet

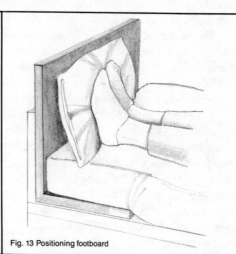

Fig. 13 Positioning footboard

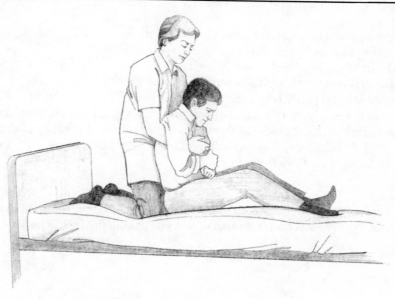

Fig. 12 One-person lift

If your patient can get in and out of bed with a little assistance, be there for him, especially if he is weak and apt to fall. The patient who has been lying in bed for a long time should get up slowly, sit on the edge of the bed for a short period first, with his legs dangling over the side. He can then be helped out of bed. Support him by facing him and leaning down to his height with your legs apart and knees bent; have him place both arms around your neck, and on the count of three, lift upward. You can then pivot him around and place him in a chair. If there are two of you assisting the patient, each person can sit on either side of him. Have him put one arm on each of your shoulders and then slowly stand up.

You can use the above lifting techniques to get a patient into a wheelchair. Before placing the patient in a wheelchair, be sure you have it nearby, have locked the safety locks on each side, and have turned the wheels inward to prevent it from rolling away. A two-person lift can be used by having one person support the torso and the other support the lower body and legs. If the patient's legs are paralyzed, gently lower them into the wheelchair stirrups. If your patient is small and frail, you may be able to lift him out of bed yourself. Be sure to bend your knees and waist, and have the patient place both of his arms around your neck. Put one of your arms around his back and the other under his buttocks.

Be careful of your back when you attempt this. There is a wide leather belt available to support your lower back. This is the same belt weight lifters wear, and can be found in most sports shops. You can use many of the same lifting techniques to get the patient in and out of the shower, tub, and cars. If there are going to be real lifting problems and another person will be home to assist you later on, why not shift your schedule to accommodate this?

Whenever your patient is going from a sitting to a standing position, you should prevent his feet from slipping out in front of him by blocking them with the side of your foot. If your patient is unsteady, be sure he has tight-fitting shoes with rubber soles. Often, bedroom slippers get in the way and cause the patient to slip or lose his balance. If you believe your patient may be too weak to walk, even with your assistance, do not try it. If you happen to be walking with your patient and he starts to fall or you can no longer carry his weight, try to grab him under each arm and gently ease him onto the floor or chair.

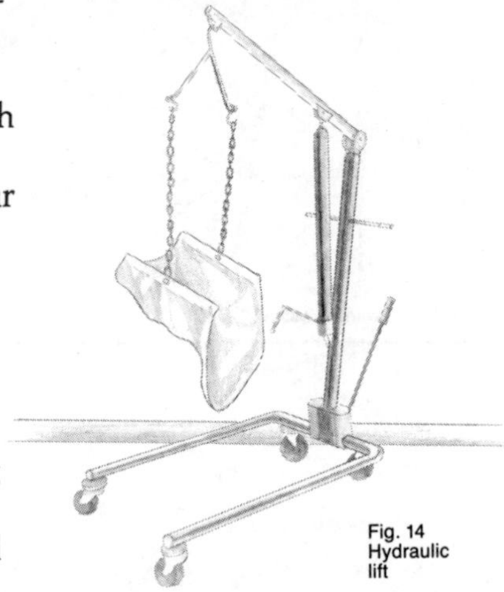

Fig. 14
Hydraulic
lift

Moving a patient who cannot assist you can be tricky, especially if the patient is larger than you. If you will be using any of the techniques described above, have them demonstrated to you in the hospital before discharge. Special lifts are available to lift patients in and out of bed or bathtub (figure 14). For the paralyzed or permanently disabled patient, there are motorized or hydraulic lifts and special wheelchairs made for shower use. In addition, there are a number of specialty companies and organizations that can help you adapt your home to meet your patient's needs. (See the appendix for a list of resources.)

Walking

Walking is essential to the patient's recovery. Work within set goals and limitations, helping your patient progress. This is one area where you should not be too flexible; it is important that the patient get up and move each day, even if some days it is only to go from the bed to the chair. Encourage him to keep moving.

Walkers and canes help the patient who is only partially weight-bearing or who needs assistance with balance. A walker is safer than a cane for the patient who is weak or unsteady. When using a walker, place it directly in front of the patient, place your foot in front of its base and one of your hands on the top of the frame to prevent it from moving. Ease the patient into an upright position in front of the walker. To use a walker, the patient must first place it in front of him, plant it firmly on the floor and then walk into it. (I cannot tell you how many patients I've seen prancing down hospital hallways, holding their walkers in the air in front of them.)

If your patient is a stroke victim or has a cast on one side, support the weakened side. Many times a stroke patient will have the affected arm in a sling to prevent it from swinging and upsetting his balance.

If your patient is using a cane, the cane should have a rubber tip on the bottom and should be the right size, as should the walker. The handle should be level with the hip joint. (Walker and cane heights can easily be adjusted.) The cane is held with the hand of the unaffected side if the patient has had a stroke; if the patient has a cast or something wrong with one leg, he should hold the cane on the other side. The cane should be placed about four to six inches in front of the patient.

Crutches should be adjusted to the appropriate height, leaving at least two finger-widths of space between the top of the crutch and the patient's armpit. A crutch should never rest directly under the armpit, where there is a bundle of nerves that could be damaged. Place both crutches about six to eight inches in front of your patient. Then, with his weight distributed by his hands, the patient should swing his legs up to the crutches and then repeat the process.

Any patient who is new to this or who appears unsteady should be "spotted" by standing behind or in front of your patient. Be prepared to break a fall by easing your patient gently into the bed, a chair, or onto the floor. Another way to spot your unsteady patient is to walk behind him with a good grip on his pants belt.

Positioning

Body positioning and proper alignment are essential to everyone, but most important for those with impaired movement (figure 15). Frequent changes of position, movement, exercise, and turning can help provide overall comfort and help promote normal body functions. They also can prevent bedsores, respiratory problems, and limited joint movement.

The basic body positions are:

Supine: lying flat on the back, face turned upwards.

Prone: lying flat on the stomach, face to one side.

Lateral: lying on the side, head turned to the side.

Fowler's: reclining on the back, in a semi-sitting position.

Semi-Fowler's: reclining on the back, with the bed only slightly elevated.

High Fowler's: sitting upright.

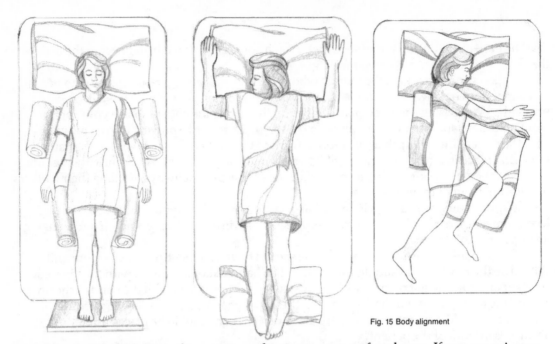

Fig. 15 Body alignment

A patient should change his position at least every two to four hours. If you are using an electric hospital-type bed, you can easily achieve any number of positions. With a standard bed you will have to improvise: pillows are useful to support and elevate a patient; the back of a chair, turned upside down and padded with pillow, can be a backrest. There are also many commercial backrests and supporters. A rolled-up blanket or towel can be used to support various parts of the body and to prevent an arm or leg from rolling or dropping.

If the patient has a favorite sleeping position, help him find it. If your patient is unconscious, you will have to alternate positions. Keep in mind that skin surfaces should never touch one another.

Care Giver's Checklist

1. Your patient may not be able to care for himself and will need help bathing and attending to personal hygiene. Don't forget mouth, eye, skin, and ear care.

2. Avoid back strain by learning the right way to lift your patient from a bed or wheelchair.

3. Proper positioning of your patient will increase comfort, discourage bedsores, and promote normal body functions.

4. Keep your patient's bed fresh and wrinkle-free. Use a drawsheet to protect bedding and as a lifting device for patient positioning.

5. Movement, walking, and exercise are essential to recovery. Work with the health care team to establish goals and limitations, and encourage your loved one to get moving!

4 Daily Activities for Home Care Patients

To maintain some degree of independence and to participate in society, your patient should carry out as many activities of daily living as possible. These include dressing, eating, personal hygiene, toileting, getting in and out of bed, walking, and performing manual tasks. The patient's goal is to care for himself in his daily routine without depending on others.

You and other members of the health care team can teach and guide your patient through daily activities, but ultimately he must learn to do them himself. Since everyone is different, self-care techniques need to be flexible and adapted to the patient's needs and life-style. Many patients cannot perform commonplace activities easily, so you'll need a great deal of common sense, patience, and a little creativity. Often, performing even a simple task requires concentration and considerable effort. You must be not only a care taker, but also a "coach" who emphasizes your patient's assets and progress, while listening to him, encouraging him, and sharing in his satisfactions and triumphs as he progresses.

Dressing

When illness or a disability makes it necessary to adapt clothing to your patient's needs, much help is available. If you can sew, you can alter his own clothes. There are also many items on the market adapted to special patient needs.

A patient who is able to dress independently should be allowed to do so. If he needs your help, let him try to do as much as possible for himself, providing help only when he needs it. If your patient would like to be dressed, don't deny him this; it is important to his sense of well-being. Choose clothes that are easy to get on and off. If the patient is apt to be incontinent or need the bedpan or commode, choose clothes with easy access. For a woman, a dress or skirt with a slit in the back makes sense. Pants with elastic waistbands are easy to get up and down. A sweat suit or jogging suit is comfortable and easy to launder.

A patient who can dress himself may have some special limitations; he may be arthritic, have limited movement in one arm, or be paralyzed from the waist down. Work within those limitations to allow as much independent activity as possible. The patient with weak or arthritic hands or arms will find it difficult to put on heavy shoes that require lacing. Perhaps he could wear loafers or slippers. Many sneakers come with Velcro™ fasteners and are good, safe walking shoes. Provide clothes that open in front and are easy to get on and off. Clothes with zippers or Velcro fasteners are easier than buttons for some patients. Stop and look at your patient's problems and limitations and then choose clothing that will work for him. Often, a slight adjustment here or there will make an item wearable.

If your patient is confined to bed or dependent on you, consider the ease of getting soiled or dirty clothes off, so that nothing is tight or confining. Keep in mind whether the patient has tubes in place, is paralyzed, or in pain. If your patient is confined to bed, hospital-type gowns are most appropriate. They are slit down the back for easy dressing and are loose-fitting to be pulled away from the body so the patient is not lying on wrinkled material, which can cause skin irritation. You can adapt any nightgown or pajama top by cutting it down the back and making fasteners with Velcro™ strips, snaps, or ties. Make several so you have some spares.

Gowns like this also can be purchased in many large department stores.

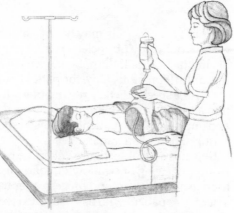

Fig. 16 Dressing with an IV line

To dress someone who has a problem with one arm, put that arm into the clothing first, and then clothe the unaffected arm. To remove the clothing, reverse the process: take the sleeve off the unaffected side first, then the affected side. To put a gown on a patient with an intravenous tube in his arm: gather up all tubing with the IV bottle and bring it through the armhole of the gown you are removing (figure 16); now bring all the tubing, and the bottle, through the new gown's sleeve before putting your patient's arm through. If the IV is connected to a pump, you will have to remove the tubing from the pump before you can get the gown on or off. Some hospital-type gowns come with snaps on the arms. (Read Chapter 5 on IVs and be sure you have been shown how to work with IVs before you do this.) If your patient can be disconnected from his IV for part of the day, that's the time to change your patient's clothes or bathe him.

There are many aids available to help the patient maintain his independence. Many patients work with specialists on this aspect of their care at the hospital and are well on their way to independent living. Specialists in a hospital's physical therapy or occupational therapy department help patients develop the skills they need to live and care for themselves.

Some devices need to be specially fitted to the patient and cannot be purchased in standard sizes. Other products can be found at a medical supply store. If you are having a problem locating a specific item, call your hospital and ask the occupational/ physical therapy department to direct you.

Eating

Maintaining the patient's nutritional health during illness and recuperation is very important. I will be covering basic nutrition and special requirements of the sick in Chapter 5.

Nourishment is of utmost importance at this time. Encourage eating, and if your patient refuses to eat, try to get to the bottom of the problem. Maybe he has an upset stomach, or is bloated and constipated, or has developed mouth sores, or simply finds foods unappealing. If you feel the problem is medical, notify your physician and explain the circumstances. Other factors often overlooked while we focus on the illness are: the patient may have ill-fitting dentures; he may be taking a medication that alters his sense of taste, or causes nausea or vomiting; the time schedule or portions for meals may be inappropriate; or he may be in pain.

Eating is not only a matter of survival, it's an important way of socializing. If the patient is confined to his room, perhaps you can bring the family in to eat with him sometimes; try to make it a party of sorts. Be sure to remove the tray as soon as the patient has finished and clean off the area. Often the hospitalized patient with the poorest appetite thrives once he returns home and can have his favorite foods prepared for him. Your goal should be to help your loved one receive the necessary nourishment and calories that are essential for him to maintain strength, energy, and rebuild tissues.

If your patient is able to get out of bed and eat with the rest of the family, encourage him to do so. Even if he has a special diet, there is no reason why he should not eat with the rest of the family. The family may have to make a few adjustments, but it's worth it. Be flexible and work around any obstacles, trying to follow the schedule the family had prior to this new set of circumstances. If the patient wears dentures, be sure he has them in place before coming to the table. If possible, have the patient dress for meals.

Take special dietary restrictions into consideration and try to make your patient's meals appetizing and appealing. The patient may need some help in eating. There are a number of eating aids available (figure 17). If the patient has trouble chewing or swallowing solid foods, purée the food in a blender or food processor, or use baby food. The stroke patient who has one-sided weakness should be propped in his chair with pillows on the affected side, if necessary. Never treat a stroke patient like a baby, even though he may act like one at meals. Stroke patients may drop food, drool, yell or moan, or bang on the table. They may be completely unaware of their behavior. Prepare other family members for this and try to make the patient feel as accepted as possible.

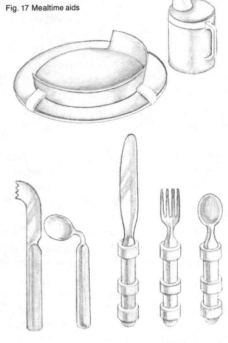

Fig. 17 Mealtime aids

The patient who eats in bed should be in a high sitting position, either by using pillows, a backrest, or by raising a hospital bed to the highest position. Give your patient an opportunity to use the bedpan or urinal before meals and have him wash his hands and face. A bedside tray is useful; be sure the tray is clean and presentation appealing. Hot foods should be hot; make sure beverages aren't too hot before you offer them. Do not forget to bring salt, pepper, and other condiments. Small, appetizing portions usually appeal to the sick patient who may need encouragement to eat in the first place. Sometimes small, frequent meals work better than the standard three meals a day.

The patient who must be fed should be elevated in a high sitting position. When you feed a patient, offer small portions of food placed on a fork or spoon. Give him time to chew and swallow before you offer another bite. Alternate choices of food and beverage. Never try to feed a patient food or beverages when he is lying down. If your patient must lie flat at all times, place the tray beside him. If he can turn on his side, let him do so. He will need your help to prepare and cut his food. Give him a flexible straw for beverages.

Never feed food or beverages to a comatose or unconscious patient; food or fluid could drain into his lungs, causing a life-threatening situation. Unconscious patients usually are fed with intravenous fluids or with a feeding tube. If you have a conscious patient on a feeding tube, check with your doctor to see whether anything may be taken orally.

Be sure you know how to perform the Heimlich maneuver, the emergency measure that helps to stop choking (see Chapter 16).

Rest and Sleep

The patient's sleep patterns probably have been disrupted during hospitalization because of illness, pain, hospital schedules, worry, or an uncomfortable bed. Now that your patient is home and in his own bed, there will not be nurses coming and going all hours of the night.

Due to his recent illness, and added demands on his energy because of the healing process, he may need more rest. See that these needs are met. Provide quiet times so your patient can rest during the day. You may have to limit visitors, telephone calls, and activities. The patient may be overzealous in attempts to get on with his life, and you should intervene if he overdoes it. If he had trouble sleeping during the night, he may need to catch up on some of that missed sleep during the day. Let the rest of the family know he is trying to get some much-needed rest and ask them to cooperate.

If your patient has trouble sleeping, try to avoid sleeping medications by using some natural methods first. A hot bath before going to bed often helps to promote sleepiness. Warmed milk or hot herbal tea can help, but avoid anything with caffeine before bedtime (including chocolate!). A back massage, a hot water bottle, or soft music will help to promote sleep. The patient's physician may allow the patient a drink of brandy or cognac before bedtime; but be sure you have the physician's permission to offer it. Techniques such as biofeedback, self-hypnosis, or guided imagery may also help to induce sleep. Many professionals train people in these methods; ask someone on the health care team for a recommendation.

Some patients may have been discharged from the hospital with sleeping medication. If so, speak with your patient's doctor to find out about the drug and its possible side effects. In most cases, you should not wake a sleeping patient to give him his sleeping pill. If he is sleeping at bedtime, save the sleeping pill and offer it to him if he wakes up. You probably should not give a sleeping pill after 4 A.M. (but check with your doctor). Remember that sleeping pills may be habit-forming and have a cumulative effect; they can lose some of their effectiveness after they have been taken for a long time. A patient who has problems with frequent urination at night (nocturia) may lose valuable sleep. Avoid offering fluids before bedtime, keep a bedpan or urinal at the bedside, and encourage the patient to empty his bladder before retiring.

Your patient may be sleeping a great deal during the day and unable to sleep at night. Try to get the patient back on a normal schedule by encouraging activities during the day so that he will be able to sleep at night. People often sleep out of boredom, or to escape problems or worries.

Wakefulness can be caused by any number of things. Is the temperature of the room comfortable? Is the room free from odors that may disturb or distract the patient? Is there too much light or noise in the room? These are all things that can easily be controlled yet are often overlooked. Some medications will cause sleeplessness, especially when mixed with other medications. Check to see if that may be a cause. The patient no doubt has fears and concerns about the expense of his illness, loss of work or salary, inconvenience to his family, and his prognosis. Talk to your patient, get up with him, or hold his hand. Maybe all he needs is to know that someone is there.

Pain is perhaps the greatest enemy of sleep. The patient in pain may not be able to sleep, no matter how exhausted he is. Try to find out what the source is and what, if anything, you can do to offer comfort. If he has pain medication offer it immediately, if he is entitled to it at that time. Ask your physician if you can repeat the dose if it fails to relieve the pain. The longer you wait, the more difficult it will be to control the pain. If no pain medication has been prescribed, or if the pain persists, notify the doctor. The doctor also should know if the patient has more than two wakeful nights in a row.

Sometimes the very sick or dying patient avoids sleep because he fears that he may not wake up. These fears are very real, and you should try to bring them out. The patient may not even know they exist. Try to talk it out, or enlist the help of a specialist. Just being there beside him may give him the comfort he needs. If it is appropriate, climb into bed with him, lie next to him, hold him, and comfort him until he falls asleep.

The care taker needs sleep too! You need your sleep probably more than ever before. Generally, if the patient is awake, you will be also. If this becomes a regular problem, you will need help. The patient will be able to catch up on missed sleep during the day, but you may have a household to run, children to feed, or a career to maintain. You cannot continue to go without sleep. If possible, share the "night shift" with another family member or relative.

You may have to consider bringing in a night nurse or nurse's aide, depending on your patient's needs. Non-professional sitters, some with a very basic medical background, can sit with patients and watch over them. Their services are not very expensive and they can be hired through most nursing agencies. If you are not sleeping at night because you are worried about your patient, you may wish to use a portable intercom system so that you can hear the patient if he needs you.

Daily Activities

A large part of your patient's day will be spent just getting through routine, especially if there is a great deal of medical attention. Don't fill the day with sickroom activities; make an effort to provide diversions and distractions.

If the patient has office work he can do, help him to feel useful again. Keep him up to date on daily news events; offer the newspaper, television, and take time to sit down and chat about what is going on. Ask his advice or opinion on something. Many of his roles have now been taken over by others and he may feel useless or left out. Include him in family decisions and activities. If possible, take him outside to sit or to go for a ride in the car.

Keep his mind active and don't let him focus on his illness. Get some games and include the whole family. If the patient is confined to bed, have the family gather around, rather than off in another room in the house, making him feel left out. If the patient is working on a strenous rehabilitation program, make a chart, and mark off goals as they are reached. For the elderly patient who might be forgetful or confused, provide a large calendar as well as a clock. Dress your patient daily, if possible, to keep up his morale and give him a better sense of day and night, time and place. Men and women should try knitting, needlepoint, or crochet to exercise hands and arms. Keep your patient supplied with interesting reading material. If you have a video recorder, bring in some new movies for the family to watch together. Keep your patient up to date on all the events he may have missed while in the hospital; but try not to burden him with little problems that can be handled without him. However, don't try to spare him from so much that he begins to feel left out.

Read him any greeting card that may have arrived and put some of them around his room to remind him of how much he is missed and loved. Encourage friends to visit; but be sensitive to your patient's needs for rest. Friends may hesitate to come around, either because of their own fears of illness or because they feel they should wait for your permission. Tell your visitors what to expect, so that they are not surprised when they see the patient. Accept the fact that some of your friends will not come to visit because of their own inability to face illness. Remember that many will rally around when the patient is in the hospital, and then forget that it is just as important to continue support on the long road to recovery.

Care Giver's Checklist

1. Encourage all the independence your patient can handle. Adapt clothing so he may dress himself; provide meals and eating utensils that make it possible to feed himself.

2. Socialization can brighten your patient's day. Try to include him at mealtimes and in family leisure activities. Encourage visitors, but make sure they are sensitive to any need for rest and quiet.

3. Keep your patient involved with life. Provide current magazines and newspapers; turn on the television or bring home the latest release from your video store. A hobby or some light paperwork from the office can keep up your patient's interest.

4. Make sure your patient gets plenty of rest. Try natural sleep inducers before using addictive sleeping medications. Get to the root of sleeplessness—it could be caused by stress and worry that can disappear if your patient gets an opportunity to talk about his fears.

5. Care givers need rest, too. Enlist the help of other family members, or a nursing agency sitter; don't exhaust yourself while trying to provide the best in home care.

5 Nutrition: Eating for Wellness!

Nutrition is the key to good health, disease prevention, and recovery from an illness or injury. Good nutrition can make the difference between restoring your patient's health, or prolonging the healing. To help you get your patient on her way to wellness through diet, study the nutrition basics listed below and adhere to any special diet or alternate feeding method prescribed for your loved one.

A patient who is sick or recuperating from an illness will have specific nutritional needs. If she has had surgery and has a healing wound, she may need to increase her protein intake to help in tissue repair. The patient who has suffered severe burns has lost a considerable amount of body fluids and electrolytes and will need to replace them. A diabetic who is ill will have to adjust her diet. Most patients will be helped with nutritional planning before discharge, working closely with the hospital dietitian or nutritionist.

The care taker and other family members should sit in on discussions about the patient's diet. Find out what foods will have to be prepared. Will there be any calorie, salt, sugar, or other restrictions? Can salt or sugar substitutes be used? Ask for a printed copy of the prescribed diet. Will you have to measure foods? Will you have to record your patient's intake? Write down any questions that come to mind—never feel that they may be stupid; they are not.

A Well-Balanced Diet

All nutrients are involved in maintaining a healthy body. *Carbohydrates* (sugar and starches) are the body's chief energy source. Carbohydrates are found in breads, cereals, and starches (pasta). Refined sugar, syrups, and other sweets are of no nutritional value and provide only calories. *Proteins* are needed for muscle building, maintaining body tissue, and to help enzymes in producing glucose. Protein foods are meat, poultry, fish, eggs, milk, and cheese. *Fats* provide energy, too. Some fatty foods are butter, cream, cheeses, and nuts.

If no diet was prescribed for your patient, she should be eating well-balanced meals with recommended daily servings from the following basic food groups:

Milk/Dairy Products (at least two servings daily): Milk, yogurt, ice cream, cottage cheese, cheeses. This group provides calcium-rich foods that aid in blood clotting, proper functioning of the heart and other muscles in the body, conduction of messages throughout the nervous system, and maintaining healthy bones and teeth.

Vegetables and Fruits (at least four servings daily): Dark green and yellow vegetables and citrus fruits. This group provides vitamin C to fight infection, strengthens blood vessel walls, and promotes tissue repair.

Bread/Cereal (four servings daily): Includes rice, spaghetti, noodles, corn meal. This group provides vitamin B and iron, which help nerve conduction and digestion along with strength and energy. Iron also prevents anemia.

Meat (two servings a day): Poultry, red meats, fish, eggs, dried peas and beans, soy extenders, and nuts. These are rich in protein, iron, niacin, and thiamine.

Fats and Oils (consult your dietitian for suggested daily intake): Cream, butter, margarine, oils, salad dressing. These provide mostly fat and have little nutritional value.

A well-balanced diet consists of selections from each food group along with fluids, vitamins, and minerals. Make a habit of reading food labels for nutrition information that can help your loved one heal.

Vitamins and minerals are essential to normal metabolic function, but are not synthesized in the body; therefore they must come from outside sources. There are two types of vitamins: water soluble, including B-complex and C vitamins; and fat soluble, vitamins A, D, and K. Vitamins promote wound healing, muscle building, blood clotting, eye strength, and strong bones and teeth. *Vitamin A* is found in whole milk, liver, yellow vegetables, eggs, and dark green vegetables. *Vitamin B* comes from liver, milk, eggs, nuts, mushrooms, breads, and cereals. *Vitamin C* foods include citrus fruits, cabbage, and strawberries. *Vitamin D* is in fish (tuna, salmon), milk, and margarine. *Vitamin E* comes from vegetable oils, whole grains, and cereals. *Vitamin K* foods are alfalfa sprouts and vegetables.

Foods high in *minerals* (zinc, iron, potassium, calcium) are milk, vegetables, oranges, seafood, and liver. *Folic acid* comes from leafy green vegetables and liver. Foods containing *niacin* are eggs, meat, liver, whole grains, breads, and cereals. *Fluids* are important, too; they move nutritional substances throughout the body, regulate body processes, and body temperature. The body cannot live without water. Everyone should have six to eight glasses of water or liquid daily, which can be derived from fruits and vegetables.

Special Diets

Your loved one may require a special diet for recuperation. Work closely with the health care team to make sure you're providing the best possible nutrition for your patient. If your patient can't, or won't, stick to the diet, the nutritionist may be able to suggest another plan. The following are standard special diets often prescribed for the sick or injured.

A *liquid diet* usually is recommended when the patient has been off foods for a long time; is unable to swallow solid food; or is having trouble keeping solid food down. When the digestive system has not worked in its usual fashion or is irritated, food is reintroduced orally in a slow progression from clear liquids to full liquids, soft foods, and finally a regular diet.

Clear liquids are any of the following: water, tea, gelatin, apple juice, broth, or ginger ale. When a patient has been vomiting or has had trouble keeping food down, begin with a clear liquid diet, and then progress as the patient's tolerance increases.

Full liquids are milk, soups, eggnog, ice cream, custard, or oatmeal. If the patient is losing large amounts of fluid from vomiting, diarrhea, severe burns, or a draining wound, fluids should be encouraged. At least six to eight large glasses a day are needed to maintain fluid balance. If your patient can't keep down fluids, notify the doctor. Fluids may be replaced intravenously (directly into a vein) if the condition exists a long time or the fluid loss is extensive. If your patient is unable to tolerate solid foods, she can be maintained with a well-balanced liquid diet. Food supplements may be prescribed by your doctor or nutritionist to add to the liquid diet to increase nutritional value or caloric intake.

When a patient has multiple episodes of severe vomiting or diarrhea, not only is she losing body fluid, but also valuable fluid electrolytes. These are charged particles or ions that help maintain fluid balance. Some common electrolytes are sodium, potassium, calcium, and chloride. Symptoms of fluid imbalance are mental confusion, muscle weakness, heart irregularities, coma, or paralysis. Electrolyte imbalance can be life-threatening and medical attention should be sought immediately.

When your patient's fluid intake is important, keep an accurate record of everything she takes into her body either by mouth or from a feeding tube (chart 1). Note what each item should be credited for, including foods that would be liquid at room temperature. These measurements usually are calculated in the metric system by using milliliters (ml) or cubic centimeters (cc), which are of equal value (1 ml = 1 cc). (See the Appendix for a table of metric measurements and their equivalents.)

A *soft diet* is prescribed when the patient is progressing from a liquid diet; has problems chewing solid food; has no teeth; has trouble swallowing; or has a partial obstruction in her digestive tract. Many foods fall into the soft food category and solid floods can be processed until soft. You can even take the meal you are planning to feed the rest of the family and put some of it through a blender for your patient. Save some of the natural juices or gravies to mix in for flavoring. Find out what her favorite foods are and blend them. Do not put the entire meal into the blender at once; process each dish separately.

A *bland diet* is soothing, mild in flavor, and void of seasonings. Some examples of foods for a bland diet are mashed potatoes, custard, or breads. A bland diet might be recommended for a patient with a stomach ulcer or intestinal disturbance, or a patient on cancer chemotherapy who has developed mouth sores and cannot tolerate spicy foods.

A *low sodium (low salt) diet* restricts the use of salt. A salt-restricted diet is prescribed for kidney problems; high blood pressure or cardiac problems; or edema (fluid retention). You can restrict salt by preparing foods without salt; using foods low in sodium; reading labels; or by using salt substitutes, if the doctor allows it. Foods high in sodium are seafood, bacon, some cheeses, and pork products.

Low cholesterol diets are free of fatty, lipid substances known as cholesterol. Avoid foods high in cholesterol, such as beef, pork, lamb, whole milk, cream, and some cheeses. This type of diet is for heart patients or patients at risk for heart disease; overweight or obese patients; or patients with elevated cholesterol or triglyceride levels. The American Heart Association offers a number of pamphlets with recipes for patients on a restricted cholesterol diet. You can write for them at the following address:

The American Heart Association
7320 Greenville Avenue
Dallas, TX 75231

In a *restricted calorie diet*, calories usually are confined to 1,000 to 1,500 calories per day. This type of special diet must be worked out carefully, often with the help of a nutritionist. According to the Food and Drug Administration, foods labeled or marketed as low calorie "must contain at least one-third of the calorie content of that of a similar food that has not been referred to as 'low calorie.' Foods that are labeled 'low calorie' must not contain more than 40 calories per serving." A restricted calorie diet may be prescribed for a diabetic, a patient with heart problems, or one who is overweight.

When preparing a calorie-restricted diet or high calorie diet (see below), the health care team will consider your patient's present and prior weight, height, physical condition, and the disease process. Even with specially designed diets, some patients will not do well. In this case, other treatments may have to be considered if diet alone cannot maintain the patient's health.

FLUID INTAKE SHEET

Date	Oral		Tube Feeding		Intravenous				
4/8/88	Amount	Type	Amount	Type	Amount Hung	Amount Infused	Rate	Type	Total
7 AM to 3 PM		Note: ml=cc							
7ᴬᴹ					500		100cc/hr	D₅W	
8ᴬᴹ	120 cc	juice							
9ᴬᴹ	300 cc	coffee / cereal	350 cc	Isocal					
10ᴬᴹ									
11ᴬᴹ	270	soup / juice				500			
12ᴺ					500		100cc/hr	D₅W	
1ᴾᴹ	120	ice cream				200			
2ᴾᴹ									
Total	810	➤	350	➤		700	➤		1860
3 PM to 11 PM									
3ᴾᴹ	120	water			300		100 cc/hr	D₅W	
4ᴾᴹ									
5ᴾᴹ						300			
6ᴾᴹ	390	soup /milk / jello			1000		100cc/hr	D₅W	
7ᴾᴹ									
8ᴾᴹ			300 cc	Isocal					
9ᴾᴹ	140	juice							
10ᴾᴹ						500			
Total	650	➤	300	➤		800	➤		1750
11 PM to 7 AM									
11ᴾᴹ			325 cc	Isocal	500		100cc/hr	D₅W	
12									
1ᴬᴹ	140	water							
2ᴬᴹ									
3ᴬᴹ						500			
4ᴬᴹ					1000		100cc/hr	D₅W	
5ᴬᴹ									
6ᴬᴹ	90	juice				300			
Total	230	➤	325	➤		800	➤		1355

Fluid Amounts/Approximate Measurements

4 oz. glass of juice	=120 ml	4 oz. serving of jello	=120 ml
6 oz. mug of coffee	=180 ml	4 oz. ice cream	=120 ml
5 oz. bowl of soup	=150 ml	3 oz. ice	= 90 ml

24° Hour Combined Total	4,965 cc

Chart 1

Never decide to place your patient on a high calorie or calorie restricted diet without consulting your physician.

A *high calorie diet* consists of a daily intake of at least 1,800 calories. This type of diet would be ordered for a patient who has lost a great deal of weight due to illness, treatment, or for psychological reasons such as severe depression. It is often difficult to get this type of patient to eat more food. In fact, a high calorie diet may overwhelm your patient and make it more difficult for her to eat.

With a patient who will not eat or who has appetite loss, you can begin by offering smaller portions of high calorie, nutritious foods. Supplement these feedings in between meals with a milk shake using eggs to add nutrients and calories. Ask your doctor or dietitian about commercial diet supplements (Isocal, Sustacal, Ensure). Often, a liquid is easier to take than solid food. Be sure whatever you have concocted is tasty as well as nutritious. Try it before offering it to your patient. Remember that "empty calorie" foods, such as candy bars, may increase caloric intake, but provide no real nutritional benefit.

In diets where weight is a concern, the only way to measure your patient's progress is by weighing her daily. Keep an accurate record of your patient's weight and be sure to take it with you when you visit the doctor. There are some metabolic conditions in which a patient takes in what seems to be adequate amounts of food, but still cannot maintain or gain weight. The patient who is being weighed daily should be weighed at the same time, preferably before breakfast. Be sure the patient wears similar amounts of clothing and remember to calculate weight the clothing may add. If your patient needs help standing on the scale, stay close by.

An extra-light patient who is easily carried can be weighed using the following technique: First weigh yourself; then get on the scale while holding the patient; now subtract your weight from the total and you have the patient's weight. (Example: You weigh 175 pounds; the combination weight is 270 pounds; $270 - 175 = 95$ pounds, the patient's weight.) If you are afraid of leaving your patient alone on the scale, get on with her and use the above equation to determine the weight. A common bathroom scale is sufficient; check to see that it's calibrated accurately. A patient who is bedridden or unable to stand cannot be weighed at home; hospital bedscales aren't feasible for home use.

U.S. hospitals routinely use the metric system and your patient's weight may have been calculated in kilograms, the basic metric unit of mass and weight. One kilogram is equal to 2.2 pounds. You can convert from pounds to kilograms by dividing the weight in pounds by 2.2. (Example: 121 pounds $\div 2.2 = 55$ kilograms; to convert from kilograms to pounds, simply multiply the weight in kilograms by 2.2. See the Appendix for metric conversion tables.)

The *high protein diet* contains added amounts of protein from egg whites, meats, milk, and cheeses. A high protein diet is recommended for a patient with severe burns, healing wounds, bedsores, or if bed rest is required.

High fiber diets offer increased amounts of fiber or foods providing bulk that push other foods through the intestines. Foods containing fiber or roughage are fruits with skins, raw vegetables, breads, cereals, and other grain products. Such a diet is prescribed for a patient with diverticulosis (an intestinal condition making digestion difficult); a patient confined to bed who has a tendency toward constipation; or one with other bowel disorders. Stay away from high-fiber foods if your patient has severe intestinal or bowel disorders, diarrhea, or an ostomy. Check with your doctor before offering increased roughage, which also is available in commercial products.

A special ***diabetic diet*** is vital to the health of a diabetic patient. Illness can place additional stress on management of diabetes and you may have to make adjustments in your loved one's diabetic diet. For complete information about nutrition for diabetics, see Chapter 14.

Alternate Nutrition Routes

All patients will not be able to receive adequate nutrition orally; some must be fed by alternate routes. Until recently, some of these feeding techniques were not seen in the home. If a patient had special needs, such as intravenous feedings, she was placed in the hospital and had to stay there until she no longer required special feedings. Now, because of rising health care costs, new technology, and home service companies that specialize in this area, patients and their families are being trained to handle this treatment at home.

I will explain each procedure in some detail, with the assumption that you have been trained by someone on the health care team. *Do not attempt any of these procedures until you have been trained and have performed them in the presence of a health care professional.* The basic information below is intended as a written reference for procedures you have been shown; if these steps differ from what you were taught, continue to do the procedure as instructed by your health care team. If this section, or any other part of the book, provokes thoughts or questions, confer with your physician or health care team.

Before continuing, I want to stress one more important point: whenever you are using needles and syringes, they should be stored in a safe place, or locked away. Because of the threat of AIDS, the disposal of needles and syringes has been revised in the past few years. After using, they should be placed in an impenetrable needle container. Consult with the health care team about proper disposal of needles and syringes. Some solutions are considered contaminated waste and should not be flushed down the toilet or into your sewer system. Find out how you should dispose of your patient's supplies.

If you stick yourself with a used needle, wash the wound immediately in cold water with disinfectant soap and contact your physician. Some agents should not touch your skin and you should wear protective gloves when working with them. Find out what to do if you spill these on yourself.

Intravenous Therapy (IV)

Intravenous feeding is a centuries-old concept, but it was not widely used until the 1920s. Valuable nutrients and fluids are infused into the patient through a cannula or tube placed into one of the body's large veins. The hand or lower arm usually are used, but in some cases the IV must be placed elsewhere.

Intravenous therapy is a safe and proven treatment. After you have been trained and have had some supervised experience, you should feel quite comfortable caring for your patient at home. Know that you have the support of the health care team. By administering IV therapy at home, you can have your loved one with you, whereas patients previously were forced to stay in the hospital for the sole purpose of intravenous therapy.

IV solutions consist of a number of substances, usually with a water base. Some of the additives may be salt (sodium), sugar (glucose/dextrose), electrolytes, vitamins, or medications. Generally, a patient requiring IV care will be hospitalized until her illness or disease is stabilized. When your loved one no longer needs acute hospital care, she may be discharged with an IV line in place. Intravenous therapy may be recommended at home for a patient who needs antibiotics over a long time; a patient who cannot receive nutrition orally; or for pain control and anti-cancer or heart treatments.

If your patient will be going home with an IV, remember that home management of IV therapy is overseen by your physician, an IV nurse (usually certified in IV therapy), and possibly a home care company or special department within your hospital. The Visiting Nurse Association in your area may also take care of patients on home IV therapy.

Insurance coverage for this will vary; make sure you or the hospital staff check with your insurance carrier. Medicare will not cover some home IV therapy. Since a registered nurse also will be involved, be sure those services are covered.

Your patient will have had the IV inserted in the hospital or an IV nurse will come to your home and insert it. The place where the needle or catheter is inserted should be kept covered, dry, and clean. The needle site covering is called a dressing. Different hospitals, nurses, and doctors use various methods to protect the IV entry site. Usually, a gauze pad with an antiseptic solution is taped over the needle site; then the IV tubing is secured so it will not slip out.

Your only responsibility may be to make sure the dressing stays dry, clean, and in place. The IV nurse will visit regularly to oversee problems. The nurse will change the IV site and dressing to prevent against infection and phlebitis (inflammation of a vein). The nurse or the home care team should be available on a 24-hour basis in case problems arise.

If possible, the IV should not be placed directly over a joint. Also, if the patient is right-handed, ask that the IV be placed in the left arm, or vice versa. If your loved one is restless or confused and apt to pull out the IV, restraints should be considered. If your patient is to be restrained, have the nurse show you how. Don't put a restraint directly over the IV site; it will constrict the flow.

The IV will be used on a continuous or intermittent basis. Most equipment will be provided by the home care company. Ask what supplies you should have on hand and where to find them. Your job may be only to oversee supplies and be sure you do not run out.

A continuous IV means the solution is infusing into the patient at all times. An intermittent IV is used only when needed to administer medication or solutions. If your patient is on intermittent IV therapy, she probably will have a needle/catheter commonly called a heparin lock (figure 18). It's a special kind of needle and tubing with a rubber cap on the end that is reusable because it seals itself after each needle puncture. The device is known as a heparin lock because, after each use of the IV, heparin (an anti-clotting agent) is flushed into the catheter to prevent blood from clotting in the IV tubing and needle.

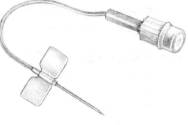

Fig. 18 Heparin lock

Since it is intermittent, the needle/catheter remains intact, but the patient is disconnected from the rest of the IV when she does not require medication. Patients who use this type of therapy may be receiving antibiotic therapy or other drugs required only at certain intervals.

Equipment for IV Therapy

Here is a list of the important items you will need on hand if your patient is on intravenous therapy:

Alcohol sponges: These are used for many aspects of IV care, primarily for cleansing and killing bacteria on the skin.

IV solutions: The solution to be infused into the patient should be sealed with a metal cap, rubber seal, or plastic cover, and the bag or bottle of solution should be clear and free of sediment (if not, *don't* use the solution). Find out how solutions should be stored. Do they need refrigeration? Can they be exposed to light? Check the expiration date on the label. The bag or bottle should have a label showing the type of solution, any medications that have been added, and any other pertinent information. If the label is missing, do not administer the solution and notify the health care team.

IV pole: This is a metal or aluminium pole with a piece across the top to attach the bottle/bag. The pole is adjustable, like a telescope, so you can change it to different heights. Some patients on intermittent IV therapy use just a picture hook or nail in the wall to hold the bag.

IV tubing: The IV tubing is sterile and should arrive in a sealed package; do not use it if it does not. This tubing runs from the patient's IV site to the IV solution.

Volume control set: A calibrated chamber for the medication or solution. The volume control setup helps to deliver precise amounts of fluid, and shuts off when the fluid is delivered, preventing air from entering the IV tubing.

Insertion needles: The winged or butterfly needle is attached to a short tubing used for IV therapy. The needle comes in various widths and the size depends on the condition of the patient's veins, as well as the type of solution used. The larger the number size on the needle, the smaller the needle.

Inside-the-needle catheter: This device (angiocatheter) has a plastic tube (catheter) covering the needle. The catheter and needle are threaded into the vein, the needle is removed, and only the small plastic tubing remains. Many home care professionals feel this type of device stays in place longer and is more comfortable.

Adapter plugs: Male and female adapter plugs serve many purposes. They should be in sealed, sterile packages; again, do not use them if they arrive unsealed.

Antiseptic solutions or jellies: These medications are applied to the skin to kill bacteria (Betadine, Bacitracin, Neosporin).

Administering IV Therapy

If your loved one has an IV, keep the work area clean. You can use 70% isopropyl alcohol or plain water to clean the work area; let it air dry. Choose a spot with good lighting, minimal "people traffic" and distraction, and free of drafts.

Keep all your supplies in one place, safely out of reach of children. Before you start any procedure, always wash your hands with soap and water. Gather all supplies; makes lists if it's helpful.

Apart from making sure the IV dressing is dry and intact, you may be participating in the administration of IV solutions. In most cases, the IV nurse who comes to your home to insert the IV, or to change the insertion site, will not be there whenever a medication or solution is given; it's not practical, feasible, or cost-effective. However, if the infusion requires medical monitoring, the nurse will stay throughout the infusion. Ask the nurse or a member of the health care team to teach you procedures, safeguards, and complications of IV therapy. Never undertake a new procedure without instruction. The nurse or home care company should provide a telephone number that you can call at any hour with emergencies, problems, or questions. In most cases, a nurse will come to your home if there is a problem. If you are unable to reach someone and feel you have an emergency, call your physician or take your patient to the local emergency room.

Before administering any IV solution, make sure the IV insertion site is intact and the needle in place. One way to check is to take the bottle or bag off the IV pole and lower it below the level of the patient's heart (the IV works on gravity principles). If the line is intact, you should get a slow pinkish return (blood) indicating the needle is in the patient's vein. Occasionally, you may not get this pinkish return, but it does not necessarily mean that the needle is out of place. Sometimes when the needle is in a very small vein, a blood return is not possible.

The dressing should be dry and the area around it should show no signs of swelling or redness. If the dressing appears to be lifting, gently reinforce it with some tape. If your patient complains of pain or burning, it is often an indication that there may be a problem with needle placement. Some medications burn when infusing; find out if your patient can expect some discomfort. If the dressing gets wet, call your IV therpist. Sometimes the dressing is wet because the needle has slipped out of the vein and IV fluid is going directly into the tissues. Another cause may be that one of the connection points is loose and requires tightening.

To hang an IV solution, first check the label to be sure you have the proper bag or bottle. Then, with the bottle upright, remove the cap and the inner disk, if present. Place the bottle on a sturdy, flat surface and wipe the top of the bottle with an alcohol sponge. Shut off the flow clamp by sliding it down so no solution or air can run into the tubing while you have it disconnected.

Take down the used bottle/bag and place it upright on a flat surface. Remove the administration tubing spike and insert it into the new bottle, using caution not to contaminate it with your hands. Hang the bottle on the IV pole, unclamp, and adjust the flow rate. If you are administering a new IV, an intermittent IV, or replacing tubing, after you hang up the bottle/bag, squeeze the drip chamber and fill it half full. Let the solution run through the tubing and re-clamp. Attach the IV tubing as you have been instructed, unclamp, and adjust the flow rate.

It is important to keep a close watch on each bottle so that you are prepared when it finishes. If not, the last of the solution will run down the tubing with nothing but air behind it. If a bottle is allowed to run dry before you have a chance to change it, the air will not be a problem, but there will be a stasis, or clotting, of blood at the insertion site. When this happens, the IV site usually is lost and the nurse will need to start a new one. This is something you want to avoid at all costs.

Mark the bottle with different time intervals, depending on the flow rate, so you have some idea when the next bottle is due. Set an alarm clock or timer to remind you. If she is alert, your patient will be able to help remind you. The danger of air in the line has been somewhat exaggerated through suspense novels and films. A patient will not be harmed by a little air or air bubbles in the IV line; it would take a syringe full of air injected under pressure to cause harm.

Adjusting the Flow Rate

If your patient receives too much fluid over a short period of time, it can put undue stress on the heart; this is particularly dangerous for someone with heart problems, high blood pressure, kidney disease, or edema. That's why adjusting the IV flow is so important.

The flow rate clamp on the IV tubing controls the rate at which the fluid infuses. The rate coincides with the amount of fluid and the period of time the physician wishes the patient to receive the fluid. Factors influencing this are the patient's age, weight, height, and physical condition. The small, frail, elderly patient does not receive the same amount as a large, obese man in his thirties. The doctor usually orders an IV by the amount of cc/mls infused over a specific time period. Most IV bottles come in 500 cc or 1,000 cc sizes. If the doctor is concerned about the accuracy of the amount received, he or she may order the IV to have a volume control set to deliver precise amounts (figure 19).

The doctor or nurse will calculate flow rates for these solutions, but it's helpful to know how this number is derived. Remember that 1 milliliter (ml) equals 1 cubic centimeter (cc). To calculate flow rate:

1. $\dfrac{\text{total amount of solution}}{\text{number of hours}}$ = the number of cc/hour

2. $\dfrac{\text{cc/hour}}{60}$ = the number of cc/minute

3. cc/minute $\times$ number of drops/cc on IV tubing label
= number of drops/minute

Each package of IV tubing will be labeled telling you how many drops you will receive per cc.

Example: Your doctor has ordered your patient's IV to be 1,000 cc over eight hours. You need to know how many cc that will be per hour, and the solution set's number of drops per cc. In this example, your solution set will administer 15 drops per cc.

1. $\dfrac{\text{total amount of solution}}{\text{number of hours}} \quad \dfrac{1{,}000\ \text{cc}}{8} = 125\ \text{cc/hour}$

2. $\dfrac{\text{cc/hour}}{60} \quad \dfrac{125\ \text{cc/hour}}{60} = 2.08\ \text{cc/minute}$

3. cc/minute $\times$ drops/cc on package $\quad 2.08 \times 15$
= 31.20 drops/minute
Round it out to 30/31 drops per minute. Label your bottle before you hang it up (figure 20).

Once you have the correct number of drops per minute, use a watch with a second hand to time the drops going into the chamber. Make adjustments with the flow clamp. After the rate is set, it's a good idea to tape the clamp in position.

If the IV is running behind schedule, don't increase the flow rate to catch up. Consult with the doctor or home care professional. Also check your patient's position; sometimes it can affect the flow rate.

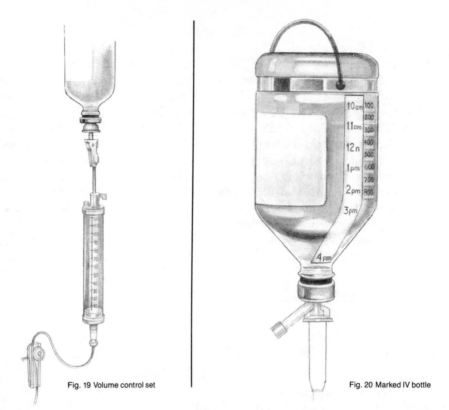

Fig. 19 Volume control set

Fig. 20 Marked IV bottle

Infusion Pumps

Infusion pumps are designed to automatically deliver the precise amount of fluid ordered. Different types of pumps are available; some even have built-in alarm systems that sound off when air is in the line, when the infusion has finished, or if there's some kind of mechanical failure. The type of pump recommended for your patient will depend on the volume and rate needed and venous access. Each pump operates differently and usually requires a special type of IV tubing. These pumps are electrical and can be battery operated so a power failure should be no trouble. The pumps usually require a three-pronged plug outlet. If your home doesn't have suitable outlets, you can get adapters at the hardware store. Read the instruction manual and discuss the operation with a member of the health care team before attempting to use a pump.

Heparin Lock

If your patient is on intermittent IV therapy, you may be responsible for injecting the catheter with heparin, an anti-clotting agent, after each dose of medication. Be sure you do this procedure each time you finish infusing something into a vein. Your doctor will prescribe the type and amount of heparin to use.

The heparin will come prepared in the syringe, or you will be provided with syringes and medication to prepare at home. If you are preparing the heparin injection, you will need: syringes, needles, alcohol sponges, and heparin. You can obtain all of these supplies from your pharmacy or home care company. (See Chapter 8 for information about preparing syringes.)

Use a clean, well-lit work area. Wash your hands and take out all of your equipment. Clean the top of the heparin bottle with a fresh alcohol sponge. Look at the label to make sure this is the medication your doctor ordered. Also check the expiration date; all medications should be labeled with an expiration date, and never use one if the date has expired.

Take out your syringe and attach the needle, if it has not come with the needle already attached. Hold the syringe up to eye level and draw back the same amount of air as of required medication. For example, if you need 1 cc of heparin, pull back 1 cc of air. Inject the air into the bottle of heparin, invert the bottle, and draw out the prescribed amount of medication. It might be helpful if you pull the plunger of the syringe a little past the amount you need and then slowly inject the medication back into the bottle until you have reached the desired amount. Take out the syringe and recap the needle. Be careful not to contaminate any part of the needle or syringe that will touch the patient or the IV. If you're unsure about contamination, always discard and replace the contaminated portion.

Tiny air bubbles can be removed by gently flicking the side of the syringe with your finger. Again, double check the dose of medication in the syringe to see that you have drawn up the correct amount.

With an alcohol sponge, clean off the rubber stopper attached to the patient's arm. Before injecting the heparin, gently push out a tiny drop of medication through the needle to be sure all the air has been removed. Recheck the medication dose. Now inject the medication slowly into the patient's catheter. Your patient may complain of a slight burning or stinging; this is normal, and will subside in a few minutes. If you have any problem injecting the heparin, stop the procedure and notify the nurse or physician right away.

If your patient is receiving more medication through an IV, you probably will be told to flush the line with saline between medications to avoid mixing them in the line. Remember that the heparin injection is always your last step in this process.

Problems and Complications

If the IV is not running, the most common reason is because it has slipped out of the vein. If this happens, the nurse probably will have to remove the IV. The nurse may have shown you how to remove the IV, but never take this step on your own. It's best to clamp the IV tubing and call immediately for help.

Some other reasons for the IV not running are: the level of the IV pole is too low; there is blood or air in the IV line; the patient is lying on the tubing and blocking the line; the line is clamped; the pump has malfunctioned; or the dressing is taped too tight, impairing the flow. Be sure the tubing is clear of the patient and that it does not become twisted. Is the power switched on, the pump plugged in, or the battery charged? The problem often is some forgotten minor step. After you have checked all possible oversights, call for help. The longer you wait, the less likely that the IV will be saved.

If the IV needs to be restarted, most nurses guarantee they will restart it before the next scheduled medication dose. Ask your physician whether an IV that comes out during the night must be restarted before morning. If your loved one is on IV pain medication or antibiotics, it's a good idea to have oral or injectable doses on hand if the IV fails.

If you find the IV solution has run out and there is blood backing up the line, change the tubing completely and start with a fresh bottle. After changing the tubing, you may find the IV still will not run since blood probably has clotted the catheter. If the IV catheter/needle falls out completely, leave it out. Apply pressure to the needle site with a sterile gauze pad until the bleeding stops. You may find that the patient on anticoagulants, chemotherapy, or with low blood counts or clotting problems will take longer to stop bleeding. You may want to apply a pressure dressing by putting two or three gauze sponges directly over the needle site and wrapping them tightly with tape. Keep this on for 15 to 20 minutes, or until the bleeding stops.

Some common side effects of IV therapy are infiltration, phlebitis, allergic reaction, and infection. **Infiltration** occurs when the IV/catheter has slipped out of the vein and the fluid leaks into the tissues, causing inflammation and irritation. This can be serious depending on the type of IV fluid. Find out what is being infused into your patient, what will happen if it leaks, and what to do if this occurs.

Infiltration does not happen often and usually occurs when the patient is careless and knocks her arm or pulls on the tubing. Safeguard against this! It may be necessary to immobilize the area with an arm board, a flat board placed under the insertion site and secured with tape, thus limiting movement. If the infiltration is recent (within the last 30 minutes), apply an ice bag, then follow with warm, wet compresses. If you failed to catch early infiltration, apply only the warm compresses, not ice. To prepare a warm compress, take a small towel, run it under hot water (not so hot that it burns the patient), and squeeze out the excess. Apply directly to the infiltrated area. You can put some plastic wrap over the towel to help retain the heat. The heat helps to increase circulation and limit tissue damage; the ice discourages swelling. Elevating the extremity also will help. Within 24 hours, most of the swelling and inflammation should disappear.

Phlebitis is an inflamed or irritated condition of the vein caused by prolonged use of IV therapy, irritating medications or solutions, or injury to the vein itself. Signs of phlebitis are increased swelling and pain; redness or a red line along the course of the vein; the area feels warm to the touch; or the vein feels hardened. Usually, two or more of these symptoms will occur. The patient also may have a fever. If you note any of these, notify your physician at once. Do not massage the area.

An **allergy** to medication usually will occur quickly, not long after the medication begins to infuse. In some cases, the patient may have received the same drug previously and had no problems. The best safeguard against allergic reactions is to be sure your patient has no known allergies to the drug. The chances of your patient having an allergic reaction are limited, but the possibility always exists. Watch for itching; a red line along the vein; skin rashes or hives; a sudden warm feeling; or shortness of breath. If any unusual effects occur, *notify the physician immediately and ask for instructions.* You may be told to shut off the infusion, or to substitute a bottle/bag of plain solution for the medication. The object is to stop the reaction while keeping your patient's IV open. If it is completely shut off, the IV will most likely clot and have to be removed. In the case of a life-threatening reaction, the doctor or rescue squad may wish to have IV access for an antidote. In extreme circumstances, the doctor may give you a medication antidote to have on hand in case of an allergic reaction.

Sometimes the IV patient can develop an **infection** at the IV site. It may remain as a local infection or spread throughout the body. This can be caused by poor technique when caring for the IV and needle insertion site; exposure to bacteria; or prolonged use of IV therapy. Some signs and symptoms of infection are elevated body temperature; swelling or redness at the IV site; increased tenderness or pain in the area; or generalized weakness. Call your physician at the first signs of infection. Assign one family member to care for the IV patient to decrease risk of infection.

Living with an IV

If they are allowed to get out of bed, most patients should be encouraged to be up and about. However, walking with an IV and all of the accessories can be cumbersome. Your patient may need your help, especially if she is weak. Have her walk with the pole on the side of the arm without the IV, pushing with the unused arm. Be sure that the height of the pole has been adjusted to clear the doorway. If you have wall-to-wall carpeting, it can be difficult to walk pushing the IV pole. If it won't roll at all, you will have to carry the IV solution at a level higher than the patient. The same is true for going up and down stairs. Some people keep two IV poles in a two-story house. If the patient is using an infusion pump, she will almost certainly need your help. Most of these pumps hang on the IV pole and run on batteries, so they will run even when unplugged.

With the doctor's permission, your patient may bathe. Be sure the patient has the IV site covered with plastic to keep it dry. A tub bath is probably easier and safer than a shower. Put the pole beside the tub, taking care to prevent the tubing from falling into the tub. Unplug any pumps while bathing. If your patient has intermittent infusions, save these activities for when she is disconnected from the IV.

Removing the IV

Never remove an IV line without specific instructions from your physician. If you are told to remove the IV, use these general guidelines along with any specific steps recommended by your doctor. Wash your hands before you begin.

1. Shut off the IV flow.
2. Prepare a sterile gauze sponge to place directly over the needle site after the needle is removed.
3. Gently lift all tape covering the needle site.
4. Pull the needle/catheter straight back out of the vein in one quick motion.
5. Apply firm pressure for two minutes with the gauze sponge.
6. Put a bandage or pressure dressing over the needle site.

Tube Feedings

When your loved one cannot take foods by mouth for medical reasons, a tube can be placed directly into the stomach to allow the feeding of liquid nutrients. One common method is by the use of a *nasogastric tube*—a long thin, tube passed through the patient's nose, along the gastrointestinal tract, and into the stomach. Insertion of this tube can be done by a registered nurse or a doctor in the hospital or home. It is a fairly easy procedure, causing only slight discomfort.

You can be trained to manage the patient at home on this therapy. You will need liquid nutrients; an irrigating solution; an irrigating container and syringe; and some non-allergic tape. This equipment can be found at a pharmacy or medical supply store.

The nutrients usually are supplied by commercial companies and ordered for the individual patient's needs by the doctor or nutritionist. They contain all of the essential nutritional elements. The solutions or supplements should be administered at room temperature. If they are cold or administered too rapidly, the patient may experience diarrhea, cramps, excess gas, or even nausea and vomiting. Note how each solution should be stored and if there is an expiration date. Pay close attention to your supply; don't allow yourself to run out. Watch for any adverse effects and report them immediately. A nutritionist probably will be working closely with you and your patient to follow progress and make adjustments in the solution based on the patient's tolerance and weight.

When a patient is on tube feedings, you may need to record everything that goes in and out of the patient on your intake and output sheet (see Chapter 9). To care for the patient with a nasogastric tube, special attention should be given to the patient's mouth. She probably will not be allowed to take anything by mouth and her mouth may be quite dry. Offer ice chips to suck on, or if your patient is comatose, clean her mouth with a lemon/glycerin swab. Use a damp gauze sponge to clean and moisten the inside of the mouth. The alert patient should be allowed to brush her teeth and gargle with mouthwash. If her lips are dry, apply petroleum jelly or lip balm.

The tube usually is kept in place by a small piece of tape attached to the patient's nose. Use non-allergic tape to limit skin irritation. Due to perspiration, some patients have problems getting the tape to adhere; if so, try another type. The tape holding the tube should be changed regularly, but be careful not to displace the tube. Whenever you change the tape or find it loose, check for proper placement of the tube. Clean the area with warm water, try to remove any excess adhesive, dry throughly, and reapply the tape to the tube and nose.

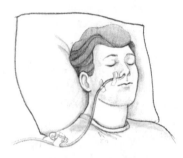

Fig. 21 Nasogastric tube

When the nasogastric tube is not being used, you will have a clamp or cap to keep gastric contents from leaking out. Apply it to different places along the tube each time so that one area is not allowed to wear. If you loop an elastic band through the tube, or add a piece of tape, it will provide a nice device to attach a safety pin to so you can fasten the excess tube to the patient's shirt (figure 21). There should be eight to 10 inches of excess tube. Securing the tube will prevent pulling or tugging on the tube when the patient moves. Be careful not to puncture tubes with safety pins or scissors.

When you adminster solutions of any kind into the tube, check to see if the tube is properly placed in the patient's stomach and has not slipped out into another area. To do this, take the large irrigating syringe and attach it to the end of the nasogastric tube, unclamp the tube, and pull back gently on the syringe until you obtain gastric contents. The color will be light yellow. If you are unable to obtain anything, chances are the tip of the tube is pressed up against the side of the patient's stomach and blocking passage of fluid. Turn the patient on her left side and try again. If you still get nothing, move the tube one to two inches into the stomach and try again. When you are concerned about placement, do not give the feeding; call your nurse or physician. *If the tube is not in the stomach it is dangerous to proceed.* A tube that is pulled out or falls out does not constitute a medical emergency, but the doctor or home care professional should be notified.

If you are sure of placement, you can administer fluids through the tube. This is done either by using gravity (attaching the irrigating syringe or bag to the tip of the tube, pouring fluids into the syringe, and letting the solution drain into the stomach) or with an infusion pump that automatically pumps in the fluids. Always put in some plain water (room temperature) after the feeding to rinse out the tube.

A **gastrostomy tube** is inserted directly into the stomach through the abdomen. The gastrostomy tube usually is held in place by a few surgical sutures and is less likely to slip out than the nasogastric tube. If you see leakage around the tube, clean the skin immediately with a damp cloth. Gastric

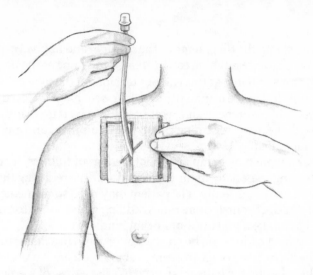

Fig. 22 Placing sponges around tube

juices are quite acidic and can irritate or cause skin breakdown. Let your doctor know if this is happening. During the patient's daily bath, clean the area around the tube with warm water or a little hydrogen peroxide. Be sure to remove any crust that may have formed around the tube.

The gastrostomy tube is an alternative to intravenous and nasogastric feedings. Its advantages are that the patient can do the feeding herself; there is less risk of infection than with IV therapy; and the tube can remain inserted over long periods of time. The tube may be removed for patient comfort and mobility, and reinserted for feedings. There is an adapter with a cap to put on the patient when the tube is taken out. When the tube (or TPN catheter, as above) is in use, cut some small sponges four inches square with a slit halfway to the middle and apply each one in opposing directions around the tube (figure 22). This will help keep the skin clean and dry.

Feeding formulas vary. There are commercially available products or a nutritionist may prepare a special formula for your patient. After they are opened, most must be refrigerated and are not good after 24 hours. If the patient is allowed liquefied solid foods, they will help promote normal bowel function. These feedings can be given either by the gravity-drip method or by use of a commercial feeding administration set.

To give a feeding, have the patient sit or elevate her bed to a sitting position. This will promote digestion and make the flow of solutions into the stomach easier. Keep the tube clamped and attach the feeding syringe to the end of the tube; this will reduce the amount of air going into the stomach. Always make sure the tube is open by inserting a small amount of water first. Release the clamp, and if the water flows freely, the tube is open and you can proceed. If it does not, notify your nurse or doctor. Pour the food into the syringe, holding it slightly tilted so air bubbles can escape. Keep adding the remaining solution to prevent air from entering the stomach. Raise the syringe to increase the flow rate, or lower it to decrease the rate. The feeding should be done over a 20-minute period. When you have finished, put a small amount of water (about 30 cc) into the tube. This will help remove any particles or excess remains of the feeding and keep the tube open. If your patient's intake is being monitored, record the total on your chart. After the feeding, your patient should remain in a sitting position for 30 minutes to enhance digestion.

Now clamp the tube, remove the syringe, and apply a cap on the end of the tube, if you have one. Any excess tubing can be treated the same as the nasogastric tube (figure 21). Do not allow the tube to hang, as this will put tension on the tube or sutures, possibly even allowing it to drop out. If you are using a formula bag, see that it is closed between feedings to avoid contamination. Most of the feeding equipment can be reused and cleaned in the dishwasher. Check with the nurse regarding care of the equipment and any problems that you should look for in your patient.

Your patient may complain about feelings of fullness, increased gas, belching, or diarrhea after a feeding, especially in the first few days. Try reducing the amount of each feeding and offer them more frequently. The patient may need some medication for diarrhea, but discuss this with the doctor first. Sometimes, adding water to the formula will help, but remember to record it as intake if you are monitoring fluids.

Most medications can be crushed or ordered in a liquid form so that they pass easily down the nasogastric or gastrostomy tube. If you are having problems getting substances down the tube and the patient is forced to miss a dose of medication, report this to the doctor. He or she may wish to order an alternate approach. Do not try to put whole pills or even crushed pills directly into the feeding tube; mix the medication with a little water or formula first. Always rinse the tubing after administering medication to be sure all of it has infused into the patient. Any water infused into the patient must be recorded as intake.

Do not forget mouth care and oral hygiene. Your patient probably is not allowed anything by mouth, and her mouth will be quite dry. If she is unconscious, offer oral care every four hours. The incontinent, unconscious patient will require extra care if she is having problems with diarrhea because of the feedings. Always report diarrhea to the health care team; it usually indicates feeding intolerance and can cause severe dehydration if allowed to continue. Constipation may be a consideration, although it is seen less frequently. This can be managed by manipulating the feeding formula.

Clysis Feedings

With the evolution of modern technology and advances in providing nutrition to the patient who cannot take food orally, the use of clysis therapy has all but been abandoned. I want to mention how it is done for the few families that may have a patient on clysis feedings.

A clysis feeding is the delivery of fluids and nutrients to the body by using a small needle placed in the subcutaneous layer of the patient's skin, usually the thigh. A solution is delivered by slow infusion. This method can supplement a patient's poor oral intake, or give the dying or unconscious patient just enough fluid to keep her hydrated and comfortable.

Make sure the needle is secure. You or the nurse may be responsible for providing a fresh dressing over this site daily. The needle is changed as necessary, or every 72 hours. Reinserting the needle is an easy procedure and relatively painless; ask the doctor if you may be trained to do it.

The infusion must run very slowly, since the subcutaneous tissues cannot handle the increased amounts of fluid that a vein can. To maintain this slow infusion, the patient probably will have an infusion pump or a volume control infusion set. The infusion is much like that of an IV, with the solution hanging from a pole with IV tubing attached.

Watch for increased swelling in the area; redness; fever; tenderness; or warmth. Report any of these symptoms to the doctor.

Total Parenteral Nutrition (TPN)

Total parenteral nutrition (hyperalimentation) is the administration of a solution of dextrose (sugar), proteins, electrolytes, vitamins, and minerals usually into a central vein that goes directly into the superior vena cava in the heart. This is delivered by the insertion of a special catheter or disk device into the upper chest. This very sophisticated type of nutrition therapy may be used by a patient with chronic bowel disease; a burn patient; a patient with cancer or kidney problems; an AIDS patient; or a severely anorectic patient.

(Another popular method of providing long-term venous access is the use of internal ports surgically implanted under the superficial skin layer. A special needle is inserted whenever intravenous access is needed. Consult with your doctor or home health team about care for a patient with an internal port.)

Sending a patient home on TPN therapy is not uncommon today. To be discharged home, the patient must be stable; she must have tolerated the therapy well in the hospital; she should be gaining weight; and the patient and her family must be willing to undertake this complex therapy at home.

The patient at home on TPN therapy is followed closely by the physician and home care team. She will be monitored by lab studies, attention will be paid both to weight gain and overall progress. Before she leaves the hospital, you should have a general understanding of TPN therapy; know about the various solutions and preparations your patient will be receiving; the infusion schedule; sterile technique (see Chapter 3); care of the catheter and dressing; and any complications that may occur.

This therapy requires special equipment that you should have on hand before the patient comes home. Have the staff help you prepare a list of supplies, where you will get them, and how often you will need to reorder. Many home care companies specialize in this type of therapy and will provide just about all the service and supplies you need.

This therapy is expensive and in most cases will be covered by your insurance, Medicare, or Medicaid. Be sure you know what areas will be covered. Will your policy pay for nursing charges? Premixed solutions? Infusion pumps? Find out before your loved one comes home.

A home health care company usually will check your insurance coverage before starting therapy. The company will provide all necessary supplies; TPN solutions; regular deliveries; and nursing assistance. The nurses reinforce hospital teaching and sometimes will meet the patient in the hospital to bring continuity of care into the home. In most cases, these nurses are not provided on a 24-hour basis, but will come into the home to assist the patient and her family until they are able to take over their own independent program. The nurse will make regular visits to check on the patient's progress and usually is available for emergencies, problem solving, and questions.

Often, this type of therapy is started before the patient retires for the evening and ended in the morning. This helps the patient lead as normal a life as possible. The patient requiring TPN may be in general good health and allowed to pursue her usual activities.

In some cases, the therapy will be continuous and require constant attention. Depending on your patient's needs, you will have to adapt schedules accordingly. Even if the patient will be administering her own treatments, it is important that you sit in on the teaching sessions, too.

Caring for the TPN Catheter Dressing

The frequency of dressing changes will vary from doctor to doctor and hospital to hospital. During the first month, it's generally recommended that the dressing be changed three times a week, or more often if it gets wet, soiled, or is lifting up. Doctors are cautious with a newly inserted catheter. After the catheter has been in place for a month without problems, your doctor may become less cautious and even switch from sterile dressing changes to clean technique. However, some physicians feel the procedure should always be done under sterile conditions. Consult with your home care team on this issue.

Most hospitals use a dressing catheter kit, which includes all the basic supplies: Betadine (providone-iodine) swabs or ointment; a dressing; alcohol swabs; and sterile gloves and face mask, if required. Non-allergic tape is recommended to cut down on skin irritation.

To begin, clean a smooth, flat surface with isopropyl alcohol and let it dry. Gather your supplies and wash your hands. If you are using sterile gloves, don't touch anything unsterile after they are applied. Prepare all your supplies on a sterile field, either a sterile towel or the sterile wrapper from your

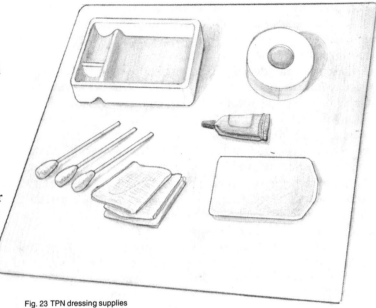

Fig. 23 TPN dressing supplies

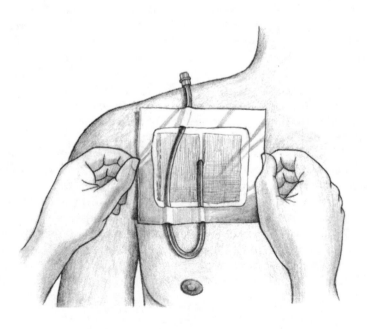

Fig. 24 Coiling a TPN catheter

dressing kit (figure 23). If your patient is alert and can help, she may be able to open the packages and hand you additional supplies. The patient often is taught to change her own dressing and should follow the same procedures. If she does her own dressing changes, a mirror is helpful.

Remove the patient's dressing and dispose of it. Don't pull at the tube or touch the area with your hands. Inspect the site for swelling, redness, or drainage. If there is any, report this immediately following the dressing change.

Clean the site with alcohol swabs or a recommended cleansing solution. Start from the inside, working in a circular, clockwise motion out to three inches in diameter around the exit site. Repeat as many times as you have been told, discarding each swab after a single use. If the patient complains of pain or tenderness, it may indicate a problem you should report. Allow the area to air dry. If your doctor wants you to use an antibacterial jelly, put some on sterile gauze and apply directly over the catheter exit site. (Some doctors prefer a dry sterile dressing.)

Apply the gauze dressing and then a plastic or occlusive dressing. Some doctors recommend tincture of Benzoin around the outer edges; this cuts down on skin irritation and helps the adhesive to stick. Do not apply large amounts of tape, which only irritates the skin.

The catheter should be coiled near the chest area and taped in place (figure 24). Never use scissors around the catheter. If it is cut, there will be copious bleeding and a life-threatening emergency. You should have a special clamp to deal with such a crisis. Immediately apply the clamp just above the cut and call the doctor. Clamping the catheter should stop the bleeding. Keep this clamp close at hand and carry it with the patient wherever she goes.

Irrigating the TPN Catheter

To keep the catheter open and free from blood clots, it must be flushed with heparin (an anticoagulant) each time it's used. Most catheters have a plastic cap with a rubber stopper on the end where you inject the heparin or any other medication that may be ordered. Some catheters have two plugs capping off two catheter tips placed in the patient; this is a double lumen or Y-type catheter. These may be placed in patients who need two medications or solutions infused simultaneously. *Ask your home care team for specific instructions on irrigating the TPN catheter and changing the catheter tips.* After injecting a solution or medication, you also may be asked to flush the catheter with a saline solution. This is done to thoroughly clean the catheter, since some medications are not compatible with others. The heparin injection is always the last step.

The frequency for changing the catheter caps will vary from doctor to doctor; generally it's done three to four times a week, or whenever the dressing is changed. Some doctors recommend that a new catheter cap be used each time you start a new infusion.

Bathing for TPN Patients

Most TPN patients will be allowed to bathe. Some doctors will not allow the catheter dressing to become wet; others will allow the patient to take the dressing off and take a full bath or shower. Any catheter dressing that becomes wet should be changed as soon as possible. If the dressing is dry, but the edges are just lifting up, you can add some tape to the lifting edge.

Administering the TPN Solution

The TPN solution meets your patient's total nutritional needs; she probably won't express hunger. The infusion will be given either continuously or at bedtime over a 10- to 12-hour period. An infusion pump is almost always used because of the importance of delivering precise amounts of solution over a specific period of time. The pump can be calibrated to deliver exact amounts and has a built-in alarm to notify the care taker and patient if there is a problem. This is especially reassuring if the patient or care taker is sleeping during the infusion. You should have instructions in pump operation and feel comfortable using it. The infusion rate is precise; *never speed up the rate if the infusion is running behind schedule.* If you have problems maintaining the prescribed rate, report them immediately to the health care team. You may wish to mark your solution bottle with time increments so you can tell at a glance if the solution is on schedule.

Take the solution out of the refrigerator at least two hours before the infusion so it adjusts to room temperature. Inspect the solution to be sure it is clear and free of sediment, and that the bottle is sealed. Do not use it if you feel the bottle/bag has been contaminated.

Some solutions come pre-mixed; others will have to have substances added. Insulin is one medication that may have to be added. Your patient may be taught how to test her urine for sugar. Lipids (fats) often are added to TPN solution or given separately. Lipids are very thick and can cause administration problems, so be sure you have special instructions if your patient needs lipids. Medications (vitamins, heparin) are added at the time of administration because they are not stable over a long time. They usually are added with a syringe directly into the bottle/bag. Never add substances to the TPN solution without instructions, and be sure to double-check labels and doses of additives.

Your home care team will give you specific instructions on administering TPN solutions. Before starting, have your solution and supplies at the bedside. Inspect the tubing for any cracks or contamination. If you feel uncomfortable doing this procedure alone, ask for help—that's why you have the home care team.

Remember to note the time the infusion begins and ends. Some doctors like the infusion to be slowed about an hour before it ends to cut down on hypoglycemia (decreased blood sugar), which occurs when the patient comes off the infusion too fast. This is not the case with all patients. Have your saline and heparin syringes ready when the infusion has ended. Flush with saline, then heparin.

To insure a restful night for your patient, have her urinate before she begins the infusion. Keep a urinal or bedpan at the bedside. Your patient will be receiving extra fluids that cause increased urination, and she may have to get up to go to the bathroom while connected to the pump. This is difficult, but not impossible. Provide a soft, dim light so the patient can look at the progress of the infusion during the night.

Common Complications with TPN Therapy

The best advice I can offer is that proper training and good technique will limit many of the complications that can occur. Most can be solved by a telephone call to your physician or TPN therapist. Some, however, are life-threatening emergencies and your actions could save the patient. Here are some common complications; ask your home care team for specific instructions on handling these situations:

Air embolism occurs when air goes directly into the line. This is far more serious than when air enters a traditional IV. Air embolism can happen if the IV tubing becomes disconnected. The best way to prevent this is by locking the tubing into the IV catheter, instead of using a needle through the injection cap. Air embolism also can occur if the catheter cap, the syringe, or tubing is removed without the catheter being clamped, or if there are undetected holes in the tubing. Some symptoms of air embolism are chest pain, difficulty in breathing, or excess coughing. If this happens, clamp the patient's catheter above the suspected leak. Have your patient lie on her left side with her head down, and call the doctor immediately. You can help prevent this by applying tape to all connection sites. Always clamp the patient's catheter whenever entry is made.

When any foreign body is placed in a patient, she is at an increased risk for **infection**. The longer the tube is in place, the greater the risk. Infection can be caused by poor cleansing technique, contaminated equipment, or simply as a result of the body rejecting the catheter. Some signs of infection are: swelling; redness; tenderness around the catheter insertion site; excess drainage at the catheter site; temperature above 100° F; chills; weakness; or sweating. If any of these occur, call your doctor.

A **catheter break** can happen from frequent manipulation (although rarely) or by a traumatic injury to the catheter. If this occurs, immediately clamp the catheter above the break and notify the doctor. Prompt attention may allow the doctor to salvage the line and avoid inserting a new one.

Catheter clot occurs when the catheter has not been flushed with heparin or the infusion has been allowed to stop over a period of time. You will recognize this problem if the solution will not run through the tubing, or if an injection will not go into the tubing. Clamp the catheter and call your doctor.

Two possible complications are **hyperglycemia** and **hypoglycemia**. Hyperglycemia (increased sugar) can occur when the solutions are infused too quickly; there is too little insulin in the solution; or if the patient has an infection.

Symptoms of hyperglycemia are: nausea, weakness, thirst, headache, vomiting, diarrhea, confusion, and change in mental alertness. Notify your doctor if any of these occur. You may be told to alter the infusion rate or add insulin to the solution. This complication is prevented by having the patient check her urine regularly for sugar and by regular blood tests for sugar levels.

Hypoglycemia (decreased blood sugar) occurs if the patient is taken off TPN too abruptly, or if there is too much insulin in the solution. Signs of hypoglycemia are sweating, headache, blurred vision, lightheadedness or shaky feeling, heart palpitations, muscle weakness, increased confusion or restlessness. Call your doctor immediately. You may have to adjust the infusion rate, or decrease the amount of insulin in the infusion. If you suspect hypoglycemia, you can offer the patient a glass of orange juice with two teaspoons of sugar in it (if the patient is allowed to take liquids orally), or even offer some hard candy to quickly raise the sugar level.

Fluid excess may occur if the patient receives too much solution in too short a time, or if the patient is prone to fluid retention. If you note increased fluid or puffiness (edema) in any of the extremities (puffy eyelids, abnormal weight gain, swollen abdomen, or a "gurgly" sound as the patient breathes) stop administering the fluid, clamp the catheter, flush with heparin, and call the doctor.

It is possible for the **catheter line to become disconnected in the patient**. You would notice puffiness or swelling in or near the area where the catheter is placed. Your patient may complain of burning around the area, or the dressing may be wet with fluid seeping around it. If you feel this may be a problem, shut off the solution, clamp the patient, and notify the physician immediately. This is not life-threatening, but the solution or medication can irritate the skin. The doctor probably will want to see the patient and will need to take X-rays to determine placement. All catheters are made of a special substance so they can be seen on an X-ray.

Your patient's nutritional health will be regularly assessed by weighing her and checking different blood levels. If she is confined to bed, there are a number of different laboratory services that will make house calls. If the doctor allows it, the blood can be drawn out of the catheter line, thereby avoiding an added puncture. Check with your local lab to see if a trained technician will draw blood from that type of line. Some labs will want payment upon each visit; others will bill your insurance company, which is preferable. Ask about billing procedures. The lab probably will give the results directly to your physician. Some may give you the results if you request them, but others may refuse to do so. Different tests take different periods of time. Unless a test is ordered "stat" (must be done immediately), it will be done on a routine basis.

Most of the solutions will have to be refrigerated and a week's supply usually is delivered at once. Since the containers are quite bulky, your refrigerator may not be large enough to store the solutions with your food. You may need a separate refrigerator for the TPN solutions. Discuss this with your health care team; some insurance and home health care companies will supply a refrigerator, or you may buy one and be reimbursed for it.

Most hospitals have nutritional support teams that specialize in the care of TPN patients and work closely with your private physician, the surgeon who placed the line, and the rest of the health care team. Find out who you should call for problems. Will someone be available 24 hours a day? It is a good idea to keep your own report of your patient's progress including daily weight; patient tolerance and response to therapy; amount of solution infused; medications and solution additives; and any other pertinent information. Report problems as soon as they occur and follow guidelines established for your patient.

Psychological responses to TPN therapy vary from patient to patient. For some, this therapy is temporary; others may require it for the rest of their lives. It will be a difficult adjustment under most circumstances, both for the patient and her family. Your loved one may feel different—physically and socially—and there may be anxieties during the adjustment to TPN therapy.

The first week or so after discharge will be stressful for all concerned. You won't be left to fend for yourself; there will be much professional support if problems arise. In time, you will adapt and TPN therapy will be a part of everyday life.

Ask your health care team for information about support groups. For a bi-monthly newsletter available free to TPN patients, contact:

Oley Foundation
214 Hun Memorial Building
Albany Medical Center
Albany, NY 12208

If your TPN patient will be going out on her own, it is a good idea to carry appropriate medical information or wear a bracelet or medallion indicating her condition. If your loved one is in good health, it's possible to travel while on TPN therapy. Most home care companies have a national network for TPN patients who travel.

Care Giver's Checklist

1. Nutrition is the key to good health; recuperation and recovery can depend on your patient's diet.

2. Ask the health care team for a written nutritional plan. Find out whether you must keep intake and output records.

3. Your patient may require a special diet. Find out if the illness, injury, or treatment causes nutritional deficiencies, and whether supplements could combat complications.

4. Intravenous therapy, tube feedings, and total parenteral nutrition require specific care and strict attention to procedures. Do not attempt any of these therapies in the home without instructions from the health care team.

5. If your loved one needs sophisticated nutrition therapy, find out what complications you can expect. You'll be able to notify the health care team immediately if you observe problems.

Assessing Vital Functions

6

In your role as care taker, you must tend to the patient's immediate physical needs while also watching for some of the more subtle problems that may emerge. This chapter provides you with some of the tools and knowledge you'll need to accurately observe and follow your patient's condition. Only your patient's physician is qualified to determine the meaning of certain signs and symptoms. Something that may seem unimportant to you may be of major significance, so observe your patient carefully. Look at the condition of her skin when you bathe her; note the color, texture, and temperature. Are there reddened or painful areas? Do you find drainage, blood, or unusual odors? Your role is to observe and report these signs; it's the doctor's job to interpret them.

The Vital Signs

The four vital signs are pulse, temperature, respiration, and blood pressure. Vital signs are important indicators of the patient's condition, and can serve as early warning signs of things to come. Everyone's base line or "normal" vital signs differ. Get to know your patient's base line and use it as a reference point. Ask your doctor or nurse what your patient's base line was in the hospital, and what it should be now.

While your patient is still in the hospital, ask whether you should check vital signs at home. This data could be important if your patient has a history of high blood pressure, has been known to run fevers, is prone to infections, has certain heart conditions, or if she is taking certain medications. Some patients may not need their vital signs monitored at home. If you are going to follow your patient's vital signs, you will need to be consistent. A daily record is important as a reference point (chart 2). The numbers may not represent anything significant to you, but they can mean quite a lot to the doctor. Ask how often readings should be taken. If it will be daily, it's a good idea to take them at the same time each day.

VITAL SIGNS

Date & Time	Temperature (Route)	Pulse	Respirations	Blood Pressure	Observations
4/4/88 10 AM	98^6 orally	60	22	110/70	Good day, no complaints
4/5/88 10 AM	98^8 orally	68	24	110/68	
4/6/88 10 AM	102^4 orally / 103 rectally	84 / 80	28 / 24	112/72 / 110/68	Aspirin given for fever.
4/6/88 12 N	99^6 orally	70	24	110/64	Temp to normal at 3pm.

Chart 2

Pulse. As the heart pumps blood, it expands, generating a wave of blood through the arteries. This wave is known as the pulse. The heart normally beats about 70 times a minute, sending blood circulating throughout the body. The heart will pump faster or slower in response to certain conditions. For example, strenuous exercise makes the heart speed up, increasing the pulse rate. The patient who is bleeding or who has lost a lot of blood will initially have a rapid pulse rate as the heart tries to compensate for this loss of blood volume. Unless the blood is replaced, the heart and pulse will become slow and weak.

The easiest place to find your patient's pulse is over the artery on the back of the wrist (radial pulse). (For other areas where a pulse can be felt, see figure 25). To take your patient's pulse, have her sit up. Place your first two fingers (never your thumb—you'll get a false reading) gently over her pulse area. Do you feel the beat? It's not always easy to find the pulse, especially in obese patients. If you don't find it in one wrist, try the other. Don't press too hard, or you won't be able to feel it at all. If you're still having trouble, don't worry—I'm sure your patient has a pulse! Have the nurse or doctor show you how to find your patient's pulse. You can even mark the area with a felt pen so you can easily find it the next time.

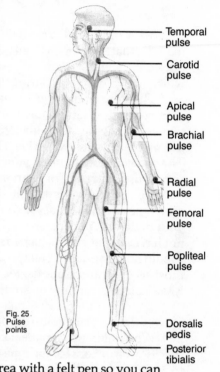

Fig. 25. Pulse points

Temporal pulse

Carotid pulse

Apical pulse

Brachial pulse

Radial pulse

Femoral pulse

Popliteal pulse

Dorsalis pedis

Posterior tibialis

To count the rate, you will need a watch with a second hand. Count each beat over a period of 15 seconds and multiply the number of beats by four. If, for example, in 15 seconds you count 20 beats, multiply 20 by four; your patient has a pulse rate of 80 beats per minute. Normal pulse rate will vary from one person to another. A healthy, athletic man may have a resting pulse rate of 50, whereas a frail, elderly patient's pulse rate may be 68. The normal range for a resting adult is 60 to 90 beats per minute. Women have slightly faster pulses than men, and infants and children have the fastest pulse rates.

Another thing to be aware of when checking the pulse is the rhythm. Is the beat consistent and even? Does it feel strong and forceful, or weak? Do you feel a few regular beats and then a few beats not in the same rhythm? Some patients have an unusual rhythm; they may have had it all their lives, and there may be no cause for concern. If you notice a sudden change in your patient's pulse rate or rhythm, tell the doctor.

The apical pulse is a pulse rate measured at the apex of the heart. This is a more accurate measure of the heart rate. Sometimes, you will be required to take an apical pulse before you give certain medications. To take an apical pulse, you will need a stethoscope and a watch with a second hand. The patient must lie flat in bed with her chest exposed. Place the bottom of your stethoscope slightly to the left of the middle of your patient's chest, almost directly over her heart. Place the ear portion of the stethoscope in your ears. Do you hear the heartbeat? Move the stethoscope to the point at which you hear the loudest beating. Now count the beats for a full 60 seconds; this is the apical pulse rate.

Temperature. Normal body temperature is 98.6° F (37° C). Fever is an increase in normal body temperature. Americans traditionally use the Fahrenheit scale, but many physicians have converted to centigrade. (See the conversion chart in the Appendix.) Some people may fluctuate within this general range of temperature; there can be differences of a degree or two throughout the day. Most people have a lower temperature early in the morning, which may rise slightly during the day and decrease at night.

There are many types of thermometers: standard oral and rectal glass mercury thermometers, disposable paper thermometers, and electronic digital ones. Which type should you use? A digital thermometer may be easier to read than a mercury glass one, but a glass thermometer is less expensive. Disposable thermometers tend to eliminate cross-infection. The choice is yours, unless your doctor recommends a specific type. Check to see if you should use centigrade or Fahrenheit.

Do you take your patient's temperature by mouth (orally), by rectum (rectally), or under the armpit (axillary)? You and your physician will have to decide which is best for your patient. A patient who is prone to seizures or who has a feeding tube in her nose should not have an oral reading; a patient who has hemorrhoids or who has had recent anal surgery should not have a rectal temperature reading. A temperature taken rectally is considered the most accurate and is one degree higher than a temperature taken orally; the axillary method is the least accurate and one to two degrees below a temperature taken orally.

How to Take a Temperature

When taking your patient's temperature, follow the general guidelines in addition to specific instructions for the type of reading you're taking. If you are keeping a record, be sure to note the method used.

1. Wash your hands.
2. If the thermometer has been soaking in disinfectant, rinse it off in *cold* water. (Hot water can cause the mercury to expand and break the thermometer.)
3. Shake down the thermometer, using a few quick snaps of your wrist, until it reads 95° F (or 35° C).

Oral Reading
4. Be sure you're using an oral thermometer.
5. Place the bulb under the patient's tongue, and close her mouth gently over it.
6. Keep the thermometer in place for eight to ten minutes.
7. Read the thermometer at eye level, shake it down, and disinfect it. Never use an oral thermometer for rectal temperature. Do not take an oral temperature just after the patient has been smoking, or has had cold or hot food or drink.

Rectal Reading
4. Be sure you're using a rectal thermometer. Never use an oral thermometer to take a rectal temperature.
5. Have your patient turn on her side, keeping her covered for privacy.
6. Lubricate the thermometer with some lubricating jelly (only a small amount is necessary).
7. Spread your patient's buttocks and gently insert the thermometer about 1½ inches into the rectum. (Stool in the rectum may increase the temperature.)

8. Hold the thermometer in place for three minutes. (Never leave a comatose or confused patient unattended.)
9. Carefully remove the thermometer, wipe it clean with a tissue, read, shake it down, and disinfect it.

Axillary Reading
4. Use an oral thermometer. Have the patient lie flat on her back, with her armpit exposed.
5. With a tissue, wipe off perspiration in the armpit.
6. Place the thermometer in the axilla (armpit) and have the patient keep her arm down for eight to ten minutes.
7. Dry the thermometer, read it, shake it down, and disinfect it.

Fever is almost always an indication of infection. Other factors also may contribute to a fever by interfering with the body's thermoregulatory system, its natural thermostat.

Fever may be caused by an infected wound; pneumonia; tissue damage resulting from a heart attack; and some neurological disorders. Report any fever to the doctor; it may represent other problems that he or she can identify.

When fever occurs, the entire body is mobilized into action. In the body's effort to compensate, the heart rate or pulse rate may speed up, the blood pressure may drop, and respirations may increase. There are increased oxygen requirements, and if a high fever is not treated, the patient's brain will not receive enough oxygen. This is why fevers should be treated as soon as possible. In the early stages of a fever, the patient may feel warm to the touch, her face may be reddened or flushed, her pulse may quicken, she may feel chills, or be confused.

At the first sign of fever, call the health care team and ask when to take anti-fever measures. Generally, they should begin when the temperature is 101° F or higher. As soon as you see that the temperature is increasing, take your patient's temperature every hour. Ask the doctor whether you should give the patient aspirin or non-aspirin acetaminophen; do not offer aspirin automatically without first checking with the doctor. The patient may be on certain medications that should not be taken with aspirin.

Continue to check the patient's temperature every hour; if the fever is down, you can decrease this to every two hours, and then every four hours, until it returns to normal. Continue to measure pulse, respirations, and blood pressure during this period, if advised by the physician. Meanwhile, it's important to offer more fluids, unless they are forbidden for other medical reasons. Offer any cool liquid your patient will drink. Keep her warm, but don't pile on the blankets.

Another anti-fever measure for high fevers is a tepid (moderately warm) sponge bath, 80° to 90° F (26° to 34° C; see Bathing in Chapter 3). Keep the water temperature at the high range, since it will cool as you bathe the patient. (You can add rubbing alcohol if you have the doctor's permission—a solution of half water and half 70% isopropyl alcohol.) Be sure the room is warm and free of drafts. Use several washcloths, wrung out, and placed in the following areas: under each armpit, over the groin, on the forehead, and on the inner elbows and knees. Bathe each part of the patient's body for about five minutes. Replace the cloths as they become warm.

This procedure will not be comfortable for the patient, but it can be very effective in reducing fever. It should not be done without the doctor's permission. If the patient is allowed aspirin or Tylenol, give two before starting the treatment, as long as the patient has not had any within the last three to four hours.

There can be some serious side effects to this treatment, so check the patient's temperature, pulse, and respirations every ten minutes. Stop the bath and call the doctor immediately if the patient shows any of these symptoms: severe chills or uncontrollable shivering, purple lips, or abrupt changes in vital signs.

If the temperature does not fall after 30 minutes, call the doctor. End the bath when the patient's temperature has dropped to one or two degrees above normal; the temperature will drop the rest of the way on its own. Be sure to pat each area dry; avoid rubbing. Make sure the patient is dry and comfortable, dress her in fresh pajamas, and cover her with a light blanket. In severe cases, especially in patients who have frequent fevers, you may need an electric cooling blanket, which can be rented from a medical supply store. You will need training to use a cooling blanket, and you should not use one without the doctor's permission. This blanket can effectively lower the patient's temperature, but you have to be careful that her temperature isn't lowered too dramatically.

Often, when fever occurs, the doctor needs to investigate its cause. Typically, he or she suspects the source of the infection and orders a test to confirm this suspicion. In other cases, the cause is determined by process of elimination. Common infection sites are the urine, the blood, wound or catheter site, the sputum, or a foreign body (drain or tube) inside the patient.

To identify the source of infection, the doctor will take a sample of the urine, blood, pus, or sputum and send it to the lab. Once the source and the organism are known, generally within 48 hours, the doctor will know which antibiotic to use. One major reason you should never start your own antibiotic regimen is that you can distort the results of the test. Once the patient has begun to take antibiotics, her fever will subside and she will begin to feel better.

Respiration.   Every breath your patient takes—its quality, depth, rate, and pattern—can tell you something about your patient's condition.

When you measure respiration, you are measuring the number of breaths per minute in which your patient takes in air (inspiration) and lets it out (expiration). To measure this, place one hand on your patient's chest and time how often her chest rises up in 30 seconds. Then multiply that number by two and you will have the patient's respiration rate. Sometimes, your patient will become self-conscious and the rate will be affected. Another way to measure respiration rate is just by watching your patient's chest rise; you can time it by the same method. A normal respiration rate is 12 to 18 breaths per minute at rest. You should be listening, too. Do you hear any wheezing or a gurgly sound? Breathing should be quiet, and if you hear anything as your patient breathes, she may be having respiratory difficulty. Does she seem to be gasping for breath? Has her color changed? Is she short of breath after slight exertion?

Patients who may be prone to respiratory difficulties are chronic pulmonary patients, asthmatics, patients who have fluid collecting in their lungs, patients who are allergic to certain medications, and the dying. If your patient is prone to breathing problems, should you have oxygen in the home? Talk this over with your doctor.

If your patient seems anxious; if her nostrils are flaring; if her respiration rate is greatly increased or decreased; if her color is a dusky gray; or if she appears to be struggling to get air, she is showing signs of respiratory problems or may already be in real distress. If you feel your patient needs emergency attention, call your local rescue squad.

Blood pressure.   Blood pressure is a measure of the pressure of blood as it circulates through the arteries. The peak of this cycle is called the systolic pressure. This is the force exerted by the heart and the highest degree of resistance against the arterial walls. The systolic is the top number in a blood pressure chart. The bottom number is the diastolic, which is the point of the greatest cardiac relaxation. Blood pressure is measured in millimeters of mercury and is written as a fraction; for example 120/80 is 120 for systolic, 80 for diastolic.

The systolic blood pressure rises during activity or excitement and falls during sleep. In the normal, relaxed adult, this number should be between 110 mm and 145 mm of mercury. The diastolic depends on the elasticity of the arteries and should not fluctuate under normal conditions. This number should be between 60 mm and 90 mm of mercury.

Blood pressure is measured with a sphygmomanometer. There are many different ones, some quite sophisticated. Choose one that suits your needs if your doctor wants your patient's blood pressure monitored at home. They can be bought at most pharmacies and medical supply stores. Check to see if this is covered by your insurance. If your insurance company does not cover the purchase, keep the receipt; you may be able to deduct the cost from your taxes as a medical expense.

The sphygmomanometer consists of an inflatable cuff that fits around the patient's arm and the mercury meter that measures the patient's blood pressure. You also will need a stethoscope. Take your patient's blood pressure each day at approximately the same time, after she has been resting for a short period. The patient should be sitting or lying (or follow physician's orders; sometimes, the doctor will need blood pressure readings taken with the patient in different positions). Try to use the same arm every time; often blood pressures are different in each arm. Use the arm on the opposite side of an IV line, a dialysis shunt, an arm injury, or a radial mastectomy.

Place the cuff around your patient's upper arm. The bottom portion of the cuff should be resting just above the elbow. Now place the meter in front of you at eye level. Be sure to connect all the tubing, which should hang down at the inside of the patient's elbow. Place the stethoscope in the middle of the bend in the elbow, below the inflatable cuff. Inflate the cuff with the rubber bulb. It may be a bit awkward at first as you must manage this with one hand while your other hand holds the stethoscope in place. Pump up the cuff until you no longer hear the pulse beat. Try to do this as fast as possible, as the cuff becomes uncomfortable. Now begin to deflate the cuff slowly, listening carefully for the first pulse beat. When you hear it, check the meter; the first beat you hear will be the systolic or the top number. Continue deflating the cuff until you no longer hear that pulse beat and check the meter again; this is the diastolic or the bottom number. For example, if the mercury on the meter was at 170 when you heard the first sound, that is the systolic; if the last sound was heard when the mercury measured 100, that is the diastolic. Your patient's blood pressure would be 170/100. If you're not sure, wait a few minutes and try again.

Sometimes you'll have problems hearing it in one arm, so try the other. If you are still unsuccesful, have the doctor or nurse check it. Some people's blood pressures, especially in dying patients, are more difficult to hear. But in most, you will hear an unmistakable strong sound. The standard cuff may not fit the arms of very large or very small patients and an incorrectly fitted cuff may give a false reading. Larger and smaller cuffs are available.

If you are having problems getting a blood pressure reading, check to see if your are making any of these common mistakes.

1. The cuff is too loose.
2. The cuff is not big enough, or is too narrow for the patient.
3. The stethoscope is not placed correctly.
4. The stethoscope diaphragm (the circular area on the bottom) is loose.
5. The cuff was deflated too slowly or too quickly.
6. The cuff is not pumped up high enough, thereby missing the correct top number (systolic).
7. The mercury meter is tilted; it should be placed on a flat, sturdy surface and read at eye level.

Various factors can influence blood pressure: stress, anxiety, weight, certain medications or diets, exercise, and some medical conditions. A drop or rise in blood pressure by 10 to 20 mm in a patient who has had no history of fluctuation should be brought to the doctor's attention.

Hypertension is a persistent elevation above 140/90. An increase in the diastolic (bottom number) is especially significant, as this shows the pressure is elevated even during the heart's resting phase. Hypertension usually is managed through diet and medication. The signs and impending problems are a severe headache and blurred vision. Some patients may experience no symptoms at all (hence the name "the silent killer"). If high blood pressure is untreated, it can lead to strokes, cardiac and kidney problems, and massive brain hemorrhage. If your patient is being treated for high blood pressure, she is still at risk for these problems and close attention should be paid to her blood pressure. In most instances your doctor will want it monitored on a regular basis. Report any changes when they occur. Keep an accurate record so you have a basis of comparison from reading to reading.

Hypotension is a blood pressure of 95/60 or lower. However, the patient with blood pressure around 200/110 may be considered hypotensive if her pressure drops to about 150/100. Conditions that may decrease blood pressure include excessive loss of blood, severe vomiting or diarrhea, a heart attack, dehydration, and some medications. Hypotension is generally considered serious and medical help should be obtained. A hypotensive patient may experience dizziness, a sudden drop or increase in pulse rate, and cold and clammy skin. The blood pressure may drop off slowly or quite suddenly, depending on the cause.

Blood pressure normally fluctuates with changes in position, exercise, and emotion. Learn how to take an accurate blood pressure reading, recognize the symptoms that your patient may be experiencing, and report them immediately to your physician. Be aware of any special blood pressure medications your patient may be taking and their side effects. For more information, write:

American Heart Association
7320 Greenville Avenue
Dallas, TX 75231

Objective and Subjective Assessment

Objective assessment is the evaluation of the patient's condition by physical means of diagnosis. For example, if the patient has a lump you can see or feel, this is an objective assessment.

A subjective assessment is a condition that may not be visible, but may be felt by the patient or presumed by the observer. For example, if your patient cannot speak, you may realize she has stomach pain after you see that she is groaning in her sleep and holding her stomach.

These two types of assessment are important in learning about your patient's condition. Often, establishing the patient's problem is like putting together the pieces of a jigsaw puzzle. You may be the one to supply that missing piece—an important reason why reporting is so vital. The information gathered is accumulated from many sources: listening, touching, observing, and communicating. Even in this world of modern medical technology, the human touch is essential.

Touching.　　Touch is an important tool to help evaluate the condition of your patient. Does your patient's skin feel warm, or is it cold or clammy? Does she experience pain or tenderness when you touch a certain area? Do you feel a lump that was not there before?

While you can't treat these symptoms yourself, there are some things you can do. For example, if the patient feels warm, take hertemperature. Or if the patient is complaining of pain or fullness in her abdomen, does her abdomen feel bloated or hard? When was the last time she moved her bowels? Could she be constipated? You shouldn't be diagnosing conditions at this time; you're still gathering information. If your patient feels warm, call the doctor only after you take the patient's temperature and determine she has a fever. Then the doctor can advise you based on the information you offer.

Listening and Communicating.　　Communication is probably the most important tool you have to help you to understand and assess your patient's condition. You must *listen* to your patient as well—not only to what she is saying, but to what she is not saying. This can be difficult, but you have an advantage over most doctors and nurses: you know what the patient was like before she became ill. You know how she reacts to certain circumstances, and you are someone she loves and trusts. When the doctor or nurse sees the patient for the first time, he or she does not know the patient personally. The doctor may know a lot about the patient's medical condition, but nothing about who she is and how she may feel. One very important way of helping your patient through her illness is by keeping the lines of communication open.

Apart from the human need to communicate, there also is the medical need. If the doctor doesn't know the patient is in pain, or isn't eating, he or she can do very little about it. In the hospital, nurses bridge that gap between the patient and the doctor. In the home, you will take on that role.

What the patient is not saying is as important as what she is saying. Perhaps the patient is having chest pain, but has told no one about it. This could be her way of denying that the pain exists, for fear of what it may represent. Is she sleeping poorly? Does her facial expression tell you anything? Does she try to carry on as if everything is OK, but has trouble doing so because of the pain? All are subtle forms of silent communication, and if you aren't careful, they may go unnoticed. To open the lines of communication with your patient, follow up on certain remarks she may make. For example, she may say, "You know when my friend George died from his heart attack, he had pain in his right arm, not his chest." This could alert you to the possibility that there may be a reason behind her remark. You could respond with "Yes, why do you mention it?" Often, there is so much going on during the day, there never seems to be time to sit down and talk. Try to take the time. Ask leading questions, repeat or pick up on what your patient is saying, and be sensitive to her needs and concerns.

The patient who is unable to communicate will require extra attention. You must be especially keen and alert here. Does her usual quiet sleep pattern suddenly appear restless and disturbed? Is there a lot of moaning and groaning? Does she cry out when being turned or moved? Do you notice appetite changes? The fact that the patient isn't able to tell you makes it all the more difficult. Be aware of these subtle forms of communication, and report them to your physician as they occur.

Diagnostic Studies. A diagnosis is made using any number of tests and procedures to determine the cause of the patient's problem. Diagnosis may be made by laboratory analysis of blood, urine, sputum, pus, and other body fluids; X-rays; surgery; physical assessment; or biopsies.

The type of test or procedure is determined by the problem or group of problems based on physical examination and symptoms. The doctor usually has a good idea of what the problem may be, but wants to be absolutely sure. Definitive confirmation may be done by running a series of tests on the patient. Some of these may require special preparations prior to the test such as an enema, a laxative, or fasting the night before.

It is important that you know what special preparations may be required for a diagnostic test your patient needs. If you are not given instructions, ask for them. The fact that you were not told doesn't necessarily mean there is no special preparation. If you have a problem or feel you were not able to carry out instructions as directed, report it before the test. This may save you and the hospital staff time and effort. If your patient will be receiving any medications, ask what they are to be sure she has no known allergies to them. If your patient has any special needs, such as special transportation, be sure to let the staff know; perhaps this can be taken into consideration when scheduling the patient for the test. Ask about the procedure, how long it will take, and what will be involved.

If the lab needs samples or specimens, you may be able to collect them from the patient yourself and deliver them to the appropriate place. This would spare having to transport the patient. Find out if you need to have special containers to collect the specimens. If you are obtaining specimens on your own, be sure to follow guidelines to avoid contamination.

The length of time it takes to get a report will vary. In order to allay your fears, ask what the expected amount of time will be; if it takes longer, there's generally no reason to panic. You won't be able to interpret results of lab tests, biopsies, and other procedures, so be sure you have them explained.

Most times, you will not be responsible for selecting a lab service; the health care team or social worker will arrange this. There are many laboratory services available that make house calls. You can ask your social worker or physician about them, or look under laboratories in the telephone directory. It's important to determine whether your insurance company will cover tests conducted in the home. If not, this service can be much more expensive than going to your physician or hospital. Find out about the setup of the lab: Will the lab bill your insurance company or Medicare directly, or will you have to pay out of pocket first? What will the charges be? Can the lab accommodate your needs and do emergency work in a timely fashion? Have reports been reliable? Do technicians come when they say they will? If your patient has a special type of catheter, does the lab have personnel trained to draw blood from that catheter? Most labs are efficient and reliable. If you are not happy with a lab's service, speak to the director. If you are dissatisfied and not able to work out the problems, find another lab.

Care Giver's Checklist

1. Your patient's vital signs are pulse, temperature, breathing, and blood pressure. Find out whether vital signs must be monitored daily; if so, keep records for the physician.
2. Document your need for special equipment (thermometers, stethoscope); you may be eligible for insurance reimbursement or tax breaks.
3. Establish your patient's vital signs base line and watch for signs of distress, which should be reported to your physician immediately.
4. Touching, talking, and listening are important tools in caring for the sick. A casual remark or fleeting grimace can tell you a lot about your loved one's condition.
5. Laboratory studies are valuable diagnostic tools. Find out as much as possible about tests planned for your patient so you will know how to prepare for them, and what to expect.

7 Hazards of Bed Rest

The human body is a complex piece of machinery created to be mobile and active. When disease forces the body to stop moving, problems arise. Just as an unused piece of machinery may shut down, an inactive body will become sluggish or even refuse to work.

A patient confined to bed, even for a few days, may develop complications from sudden inactivity. Her lungs may accumulate fluid, her joints may stiffen or lock, and her skin may become irritated. Other complications of bed rest are constipation; kidney stones; bladder and urinary problems; loss of phosphorus, sulfur, sodium, and potassium; decreased tolerance for exercise; and mental depression or boredom. Some of these problems can be prevented and corrected; others, if not treated, could cause permanent damage.

Bed Rest and the Respiratory System

Our lungs and pulmonary systems work best when we are standing. When your patient is confined to bed, her lung capacity is diminished. The lungs cannot fully expand, fluids sit dormant in the lungs due to lack of movement, and the circulatory system becomes sluggish.

Lung and respiratory problems can be prevented. If your loved one is at risk, be sure to consider her prior health; length of illness; how long she will be confined to bed; her age; whether she is overweight or a smoker; if she is allowed to get up at all; her nutritional health; plus any previous respiratory problems.

Some signs of respiratory problems are shortness of breath; difficulty in breathing; gasping for air; inability to breathe lying down; wheezing, gurgling, or raspy sounds; fever; increased pulse rate; chest pains; coughing; increased amounts of sputum; anxiety and restlessness; mental confusion; or loss of appetite. Report your observations to the doctor. If your patient seems to be having trouble breathing, it could be a medical emergency and you should act immediately.

Anyone confined to bed should be encouraged to turn and move around, get up into a chair, or turn from side to side in bed. Movement and exercise are essential. If your patient isn't able to do this on her own, it will have to be done for her. Such a patient should be turned and repositioned at least every two to four hours around the clock. Confer with the health team about what's best for you and your patient. If your patient is allowed to get up, encourage her. If she can walk, all the better. Be a nag or drill sergeant if you have to because you will be doing much to prevent serious lung complications such as pneumonia.

Encourage your loved one to take deep breaths. This helps the lungs expand adequately, keeps the lung muscles firm and active, and helps to oxygenate the lungs. There are devices to help with this, such as "blow bottles" or incentive spirometers. Your patient should be instructed in their proper use. One simple technique that accomplishes the same purpose is to have your patient slowly blow up a balloon. Try this every four hours, or however often the doctor recommends.

Encourage your patient to cough and bring up lung secretions. The act of coughing will help to loosen secretions that may be clinging to the sides of the lungs. The aim is to keep the lungs free of excess fluids.

Note whether your patient's cough is productive. When she coughs, are secretions raised, or is it a non-productive, dry cough? Also note the amount, color, and consistency of the sputum. Is there any blood in it? If you see anything unusual, call your physician. Excess mucus may not indicate a problem, but blood, fever, or difficulty breathing can be cause for concern.

When your patient has pain from excess coughing, have her hold a pillow across her chest to serve as a splint, thereby cutting down on the pain caused by coughing. Patients with more serious respiratory difficulties may require more intense therapy.

Home care companies with staff respiratory specialists can come to your home to offer some of the more sophisticated services or oxygen therapies ordered by your physician.

Suctioning the Upper Respiratory Tract

Patients who are comatose, who have suffered strokes, or who are too sick to cough may have to be suctioned with a vacuum-like machine attached to a small catheter or tube. A doctor should prescribe this therapy, which can save the life of a patient who has excess mucus that she cannot remove on her own.

You will need a suctioning device, which is available either from the hospital, medical supply store, home care or respiratory service. The machine can be rented, and often is covered by medical insurance. You also will need a collection container (usually supplied with the suction machine), suction catheters, some sterile water, rubber gloves (not sterile), and lubricant, if you will be suctioning through the nose. Most of this equipment can be supplied along with the suction device.

Before you begin any procedure, tell your patient what you are about to do. Even if she is not alert, tell her; she may still hear you. *Do not attempt this procedure without training from a medical professional; practice it in his or her presence.* If your patient is contagious, get special instruction in how to protect yourself.

1. Wash your hands and prepare your equipment.
2. Position your patient. If she is alert, she should be on her back, with the head of the bed elevated. If your patient is comatose, she should be on her back with her head turned toward you and the bed slightly elevated. Cover her chin and chest with a towel.
3. If your patient can cough, have her cough just before you begin; this loosens secretions from the walls of the lungs and moves them up the respiratory tract.
4. Pour some sterile water into a container.
5. Open the catheter package and attach the connecting end to the tubing on the suction device. Leave the cover in place to keep the catheter tip clean.
6. Put on your gloves.
7. If you are suctioning through the mouth, have the patient turn her head toward you. If you are suctioning through the nose, have the patient lean her head and neck back to allow the suction tube to pass more easily.
8. Turn on the suction machine.
9. Take out the suction catheter, being careful not to have it touch the bed linens. Suction a small amount of the water, which will help the secretions to flow smoothly through the tube.

10. To see how far the tubing should go, take it and measure the distance from the tip of the patient's nose to her earlobe. This will tell you the amount of tubing that should be inserted into the patient.
11. Pass the suction catheter down the patient's nose or mouth, depending on where you were told to suction. Do not force it down the patient. If you meet any resistance, stop and seek help.
12. Remember to hold your finger over the opening on the catheter to exert suction pressure, and to take it off to stop suction.
13. Suction at 10- to 12-second intervals to prevent tissue damage and irritation. If you suction out a small amount of blood, it may mean you are suctioning too vigorously. Any large amounts of blood should be reported to the doctor.
14. If secretions seem to be accumulating in the tube, dip the catheter into the sterile water to help clean it out.
15. Continue until you are unable to obtain secretions and your patient sounds as if her lungs are clear—no more gurgling or wet sounds. Repeat as often as your patient needs it.

If the doctor wants you to obtain a sputum specimen (sample of the mucus your patient is coughing up), you can do so easily enough. Laboratory tests of the sputum sample will tell the doctor if bacteria are present; if so, he or she may decide to treat the patient with antibiotics.

Get a clean jar or plastic container. If a sterile container is recommended, get one from your doctor or hospital. Place it at the patient's bedside and have her cough mucus into the container; saliva only is not sufficient. You need a teaspoon of sputum for an adequate sample. If you are not delivering the sample right away, ask how you should store it.

Your doctor may allow you to take a fresh sample from the sputum container on the suctioning machine and place it in a clean container. To obtain a sputum sample by suctioning, you may need a special device that attaches onto the catheter to catch the sputum (called a sputum trap). You will have to be told how to use it before you can collect a sample from your patient.

Many respiratory ailments can be avoided, but even with the best of care, respiratory and lung problems may develop. Your observations and awareness of the symptoms will help to prevent some of the more serious complications.

Bed Rest and the Cardiovascular System

Bed rest causes sluggish blood flow and the pooling (stasis) of blood in some areas as the heart becomes accustomed to less work. Some symptoms of circulatory problems are shortness of breath; coughing; grayish or unhealthy skin color; leg pains; and redness, swelling, or warmth in the legs. Some patients with circulatory problems experience no symptoms at all.

To avoid these problems, especially if the patient is at an increased risk, the doctor may prescribe preventive anticoagulant therapy (heparin or Coumadin). A patient who takes anticoagulants should be careful not to cut herself because the drug affects the patient's ability to stop bleeding. If she does cut herself, apply direct pressure to the cut.

Movement also is one way to prevent circulatory problems from developing in the bedridden patient. If at all possible, get your loved one out of that bed! Encourage walking and exercise. If your patient cannot get out of bed, see that she is turned and repositioned often. If it's allowed, sit her up and dangle her feet over the side of the bed.

One of the biggest dangers to the circulatory system is a condition known as throm-bophlebitis. This occurs when the patient lies in one position and the blood pools or remains stagnant in one area. This can cause inflammation and clots within the veins, most often in the lower legs. These clots are called emboli, or if they are in the lungs, pulmonary emboli. The clots stick to the walls of the veins, but can become dislodged. If big enough to block a major passageway to the heart or lungs, such a clot could endanger your loved one's life—or even kill her.

To prevent this condition, have your patient wear loose clothes, no elastics in pajama legs, no tight stockings that stop at the knee, and keep the covers loose around the patient. When your patient is sitting up, do not let her sit all day with her legs down. Change her position and elevate her legs from time to time. Use anti-embolism stockings or elastic bandages on her legs to stimulate circulation and help to force the blood back up into the body. These must be individually fitted and applied in the following manner:

1. Elevate the leg for 20 to 30 minutes before applying stockings to enhance blood flow back to the heart.
2. Have the patient sit with her foot in your lap, or have her lie in bed.
3. Sprinkle some talcum powder on her foot to make the stocking slide. Grasp the foot and heel of the stocking and invert it over your hand, so that the stocking foot is inside the stocking leg.
4. Pull the foot portion over the patient's foot and pull the leg portion straight up the leg, getting rid of all wrinkles.

If the stockings are incorrectly fitted or applied, they can cause skin irritation or impair circulation. Do not massage your patient's legs because you might dislodge a clot from the wall of the vein. Thrombophlebitis is treatable, but can last for weeks or months.

Try simple bed exercises. Have your patient move her toes and feet up and down; then bend her legs at the knees and move them up and down. Tell her to do each exercise ten times every hour. If your patient is unable to do these exercises, do them for her.

Bed Rest and Skin Problems

The skin is the largest organ of the body! It protects us from bacteria or infections; keeps other body organs from drying out; helps control temperature; receives nerve stimuli that alert us to pain or temperatures; stores chemical compounds; excretes water and salts; and syn-thesizes important substances.

The outermost layer of the skin is called the epidermis, which consists of four or five layers of cells. The second layer, the dermis, is composed of connective tissue and encompasses blood vessels, nerves, glands, and hair follicles. Next comes the fascia, a broad band of fibrous connective tissue that surrounds muscles and other organs of the body. The thickness of the fascia layer varies depending on the organ that it covers. The fascia also contains arteries, veins, lymphatics, nerves, glands, and some superficial muscles. Underneath all of this is muscle, then bone. The skin is anchored to the muscles and bones by subcutaneous tissue composed of connective tissue and fat.

Anyone in bed for a long time is apt to develop skin irritation, abrasions, and, if extra care is not taken, bedsores. These problems may be caused by sluggish circulation; lying too long in one area; a patient's thinness; poor nutrition; paralysis that prevents movement; or bed linens that are coarse or not pulled tight. Your patient may have other medical problems, such as diabetes or an infection, that make her prone to skin problems. Poor nursing care and neglect are two major causes of bedsores.

The first sign of a pressure sore will be a small, reddened area on the skin. If allowed to progress, it will turn a bluish-gray, indicating superficial circulatory damage and skin weakening. There may be some blistering or broken skin. This condition can progress to deeper skin layers, then muscles, tendons, joints, and even bones. If your patient develops a fever, it may mean the bedsore is infected. Report this immediately to the doctor.

Ultimately, tissue death (necrosis) occurs, signaled by a black, blisterlike crust. The damage can be quite extensive and take months to heal. Treatment may even involve surgery (skin grafts and wound debridement) or hospitalization. There may or may not be a great deal of pain, depending on the amount of live tissue affected. All because of a little reddened area!

You should be especially concerned with pressure sores if you are caring for a comatose patient; one who is paralyzed, confined to bed with fractures, or in traction; a patient with progressive multiple sclerosis; an elderly, frail patient; some types of cancer patients; or anyone who will be in bed for a long time.

Concentrate on providing good skin care. Turn your patient frequently (ask the home care team how often), and watch the areas where bedsores are most likely to occur (figure 26). Give special attention to any reddened areas by massaging frequently with cream and keeping the patient off the sore. You can do this by positioning pillows around your patient to keep the area from touching the bedclothes. Keep bed linens soft and smooth. When you bathe your patient, be sure to dry her off well, leaving no wet, moist areas. Do not allow two skin surfaces or two bony areas to touch one another; it can cause pressure and, eventually, skin breakdown if left that way too long. Place a small pillow between the two areas. Keep your patient from lying on tubes or other objects.

Pay attention to your patient's diet because pressure sores develop more rapidly and are more resistant to treatment in patients in poor nutritional health. Offer a high-protein diet along with more vitamin C to promote tissue and cell regeneration and healing.

The best treatment for pressure sores is prevention. Sometimes, even the most conscientious nursing efforts will not be effective, so if your patient has a bedsore, you should not blame yourself. You cannot control some of the body processes that lead to bedsores.

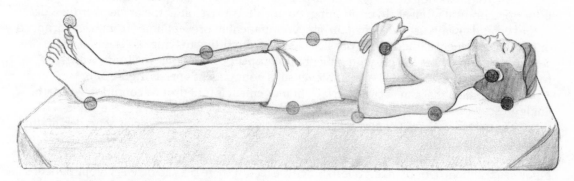

Fig. 26 Areas vulnerable to pressure sores

Pressure areas can develop quickly—within two to four hours in some patients. Continue with your preventive measures, but on a more vigorous level. Keep your loved one off the area; if you can, expose the area to air to dry it out. Turn the patient hourly, massage the area often, and get her on a high protein diet. Consult your doctor at once; you may be told to apply a dressing or bring your patient in for treatment. The nurses may be able to offer suggestions, such as sprinkling cornstarch on the sheets to make them smooth and less irritating. Ask your nurse about common household remedies; yogurt or egg whites can be used to treat bedsores. Your pharmacy probably stocks commercial remedies (Rest-On or Granulex) that are quite effective. *Follow whatever treatments your health care team recommends.*

Many devices can reduce the risk of bedsores. Adhesive-backed foam sponges can be cut into any size or shape, forming a doughnut effect so the sore does not touch the mattress. Special foam mattresses (egg crate mattresses) can be placed directly under the patient. Your loved one may have used one while in the hospital—she probably paid for it—so take it home and place it on top of her own mattress. Water mattresses and air pressure mattresses are available from medical supply stores. Use caution with these to avoid punctures. Machine-washable sheepskin blankets are soft and can be placed directly under the patient. Even when a patient is sitting up, be aware of increased pressure. Do not let her remain in one position too long. Place foam rubber "doughnuts" or water-filled cushions under your patient's buttocks. If she is in a wheelchair, make sure it has been properly fitted; a poor fit is one cause of pressure sores. Have your patient lift herself up periodically by doing a push-up from the wheelchair or chair. Remember to provide exercise to stimulate circulation.

Bed Rest and Muscles, Bones, and Joints

During prolonged bed rest, muscles can shrink from disuse, joints can become locked, and bones can lose valuable nutrients. Exercise and positioning are key here. Exercises must be done often and diligently; no exceptions! If your loved one is up and about, encourage walking or the use of a stationary bicycle, if your doctor approves. If your patient is unable to exercise her arms and legs, you will have to do the exercises for her. To exercise a joint, hold the extremity at the joint and gently move it through its full range of motion. Never force a joint beyond its own movement capabilities. If there is pain, stop and report it to your physician or physical therapist. Some patients may need pain medication before exercising.

Turn your patient frequently, as often as every two hours, and position her properly, using good body alignment. In positioning, do not allow extremities to dangle over the side of the bed and always use care when turning your patient to prevent limbs from being dropped or twisted. A patient should turn from side to side, from sitting to lying, and from back to stomach. Some devices can get your patient into proper position: pillows, foam wedges, footboards, backrests, blankets, or whatever suits your patient's needs (figure 27).

One problem that can occur from lack of movement is foot drop, a condition where the ankle muscles cannot hold the foot upright; the foot bends or drops down at the ankle. This may be corrected with proper and aggressive exercise; it can become a permanent, debilitating problem for the patient.

You can prevent foot drop by always keeping the feet in an upright position, either with pillows, a footboard, or blanket rolls to brace the feet. If there is a gap between your patient's feet and the footboard, place pillows in between to bridge the gap. Try these simple exercises: Flex and bend the feet at the ankle joint, or rotate the feet in a circular motion at the ankle.

These two exercises should be done ten times every few hours.

External rotation of the hip can occur when a patient spends too much time in bed. The hip joint tends to rotate outward, especially if your patient spends long periods on her back. This condition can be temporary or permanent, but almost certainly prevented. Roll up a small blanket or soft towel and place it tightly against the hips. This will help prevent the hip socket from rotating outward.

One of the most common threats to a patient confined to bed is a contracture. This is shortening of a muscle, and it happens when the muscle is not used or not put to its full range of use. A contracture can be prevented, but if left unattended can be quite difficult to correct. The best treatment is range of motion exercises on all extremities (figure 28).

Ankylosis is a stiffening or locking of any joint, causing immobility at the joint. This condition, too, is caused by lack of movement. Exercise and prevention are the best treatments. This can become serious and may require surgery to correct.

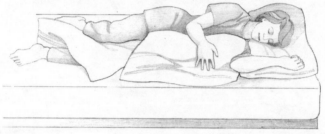

Fig. 27 Positioning with pillows

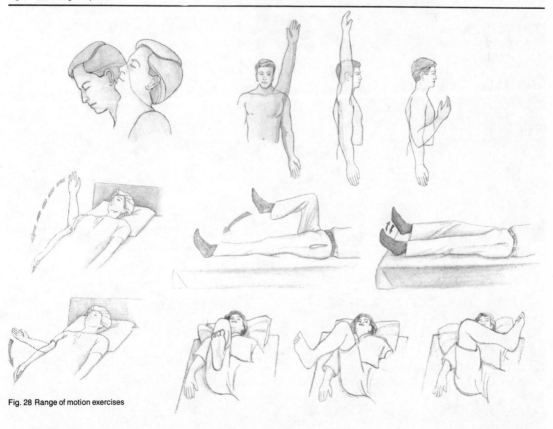

Fig. 28 Range of motion exercises

Care Giver's Checklist

1. Anyone confined to bed needs special care to prevent bedsores and crippling complications. Prevention is the key to avoiding hazards of bed rest.
2. Exercise is essential to keeping respiratory and circulatory systems healthy, and to keeping muscles, joints, and bones strong. Get your patient up and moving; if she can't get out of bed, provide exercises in bed.
3. Pressure sores can develop with frightening rapidity. Move your patient every two to four hours around the clock. Provide a nutritious diet high in protein and vitamin C.
4. Use special pressure mattresses, pillows, foam wedges, footboards, or other devices to position your patient and keep pressure off of sensitive skin.
5. Practice bedmaking for a smooth, wrinkle-free surface. Use fabric softeners on linens and give your patient loose, comfortable pajamas. Try sprinkling cornstarch on sheets to keep things smooth.

8   Medications

The twentieth century has seen many advances in drug therapy: a vaccine for polio; insulin to treat diabetes; penicillin, followed by a long line of antibiotics; and many anti-cancer drugs. The search for new and more powerful drugs continues in laboratories around the world.

Unfortunately, there is no drug to cure all ills. A drug, defined by the United States Food and Drug Act, is any substance other than food which, when taken into the body, affects living protoplasm. Drugs are categorized into broad groups: antibiotics, hormones, antiseptics and disinfectants, anti-cancer drugs, antihistamines, antidepressants, analgesics (pain relievers), anticoagulants, diuretics, and drugs to treat various anatomical disorders.

Drugs can be administered directly on the skin (topically), through the mouth (orally), under the tongue (sublingually), injected (intravenously, intramuscularly, or subcutaneously), by the use of sprays, or via catheters.

Whenever you are using a drug, know the following: What will it be used for? What is the proper dosage? What are the side effects and toxicities? What chemicals does the drug contain? How will this drug interact with other drugs? What is the route of administration? How long will it take for this drug to work? Under what circumstances or conditions should it not be used? What are symptoms of allergic reaction and how should they be treated?

All of this information should be available to you. Most drugs arrive at the pharmacist's with an insert containing these facts. Ask for the insert or make a copy. A number of drug books contain all of these facts; one such handy guide is the Physician's Desk Reference, or PDR (Medical Economics; Oradell, N.J.). It can be purchased in some book stores, especially in medical book stores (usually near major medical centers), or you can ask your pharmacist or doctor to give you the publisher's order form. A number of books about drugs have been written specifically for the general public (see the Appendix for suggested titles).

Whenever you are administering a drug, you should know exactly how much to give, how often, and for how long. Find out how the drug should be stored. By law, all drugs must be properly labeled, and you should refuse drugs that are not. The label will contain the following: the patient's name; the name of the drug; the proper dosage and how it should be administered; the drug expiration date; and any special instructions. Do not use old medications without checking first with your doctor.

Some drugs will require a doctor's prescription; others can be purchased over the counter at your pharmacy. Some labels will indicate if the prescription can be renewed without an order from the doctor, and how many times it can be renewed. Certain drugs, particularly narcotics, will require a special prescription form from your doctor commonly known as a "triplicate" prescription; your pharmacist will not supply these drugs without it. In most cases, these types of prescriptions cannot be renewed.

Some pharmacies will deliver to your home and take verbal orders from your doctor over the phone. Most pharmacists will not take verbal orders from anyone other than a doctor, unless you are calling to have a prescription renewed. Most pharmacies require you to pay them directly. You should check with your insurance company on coverage for out-of-hospital medications. Make sure your pharmacy is a participant in any prescription payment plan sponsored by your insurer. For tax purposes, save receipts for all medications; there should be one with the prescription number for each medication.

Order in advance to avoid running out of medications. If you need the doctor to call your pharmacy, try early in the day, and check to see what other supplies you'll need to administer the medications. Be sure you understand what is expected; if not, ask for help.

A drug may be marketed under many different brand names. Name-brand medications can be more expensive than generics, so ask your pharmacist whether there is another drug comparable to the drug that has been ordered. For example, the doctor may suggest that Tylenol be used to relieve your patient's aches. Tylenol is just one of many brand names for acetaminophen, and your pharmacist may be able to recommend a less expensive equivalent.

Medication Administration

Following the above guidelines for administering drugs, here is an example of what you may face: The doctor has ordered that your patient receive Digoxin (a heart rhythm drug). The dose is 0.25 mg (each tablet is equal to 0.25 mg). The doctor wants the drug to be given daily at 10 A.M., but only if the patient's apical pulse is over 60. (You can learn how to take an apical pulse in Chapter 6.) There are no special storage indications with this drug. One known side effect is that frequent use can slow the pulse below safe levels (which is why the doctor wants the apical pulse taken before each dose). Other side effects are loss of appetite, nausea, vomiting, diarrhea, weakness, headache, or dizziness. If any of these occur, you would report them to your doctor. For immediate treatment, you would have your patient lie flat in bed, keep her quiet, and await further orders from your doctor.

The doctor has told you to give the medication with any liquid the patient desires. Take out the medication and check the label on the container to be sure that you have the "three rights": the RIGHT drug, the RIGHT dose, and the RIGHT patient. If the patient appears fine, is without complaint, and her apical pulse is above 60, you can give the patient her medication with a glass of water or juice.

Prepare a list of all medications prescribed for your patient (chart 3). Find out which medications must be given without fail, and which ones may be skipped if there is a problem.

MEDICATION CHART

Drug, dose, time, route, date started, date ended, special instructions	Sunday 4/3/88	Monday 4/4/88	Tuesday 4/5/88	Wednesday 4/6/88	Thursday 4/7/88	Friday 4/8/88	Saturday 4/9/88	Side Effects/Problems
Colace one tab AM PM (bedtime) *Do not give if Diarrhea	10AM 11PM	10AM 11PM	10AM 11PM	(10AM) (11PM)	10AM 11PM	10AM 11PM	10AM 11PM	4/6 - held, due to diarrhea
Digoxin 0.25mg (one tab) Daily 10AM * Do not give if pulse is less than 60.	10AM (p.68)	10Am (p.64)	10AM (p=68)	10AM (p=70)	10AM (p.64)	10AM (p.62)	(10AM) (P.58)	4/9 - held, pulse =58 called doctor
Potassium one tsp. Daily - 10AM *Give with orange juice	10AM	10AM	10AM	10 AM	10 AM	10 AM	10AM	
Ampicillin 500mg four times a day 10-2-6-10 *Discontinue 4/12/88	10AM 2PM 6PM 10pm	10AM 2PM 6PM 10PM	10AM 2PM 6PM 10PM	10AM 2PM 6PM 10PM	10AM 2PM 6PM 10PM	10AM 2PM 6PM 10PM	10AM (2PM) (6PM) (10PM)	Complained of nausea. Doctor called. Medication discontinued 4/9/88
Tylenol 2 tablets for fever greater than 101° (orally) *Call doctor if no change								

Chart 3

If your patient misses a dose due to vomiting or some other problem, be sure to report it to the doctor. Never arbitrarily discontinue a drug without checking first with the doctor. Organize your medications chart according to the time schedule and keep all drugs in one area if possible, out of reach of children or a disoriented patient.

Bring the medications list with you whenever your patient sees the doctor or goes into the hospital, since it will certainly be of help. If your patient is being treated by several physicians, this chart will help one doctor avoid prescribing medications that may react unfavorably with drugs prescribed by another physician. Also record your patient's known allergies to any drug.

Oral Medications

Oral medications are anything that must pass through the mouth: pills, capsules, tablets, lozenges, syrups, and elixirs. Most oral medications are absorbed in the stomach or the intestines and are circulated through the bloodstream to the rest of the body. The outer coating of a pill will determine the amount of time before the drug goes into action. Some pills will act quickly, but have a short duration. Others are absorbed more slowly, thereby allowing for a longer action time. Generally, a pill will take effect in 15 to 30 minutes. Some factors that may affect this are the stomach contents (perhaps the patient has just eaten a large meal), or the amount of liquid given with the medication. Absorption time varies among individuals, and it is difficult to determine how long a pill will remain effective.

The oral route is the most popular, least expensive, safest, and the most convenient method of administering medications. When administering an oral medication, know what you are giving it for and some of the possible side effects; give the medication on schedule; supply the correct dose and follow special instructions; and be sure that your patient has taken it. Remember that some medications can discolor the urine or stool.

Some examples of special instructions are: Administer with orange juice; do not give milk products; take an apical pulse before administering; take the patient's blood pressure; give only when necessary; give extra fluids; take before, with, or after meals. These orders are important, and there are reasons that they should be followed. For example, a commonly used antibiotic, tetracycline, can cause discoloration of a child's teeth if the drug is taken during the mother's last trimester of pregnancy, or if it is given to children under eight.

Your patient may have problems swallowing pills. Some pills can be crushed and mixed with custard, ice cream, or applesauce. Your pharmacist may be able to supply the same medication in a powdered or liquid form. Some pills are scored with a line down the middle and can be broken in half for easier swallowing.

To administer medication to a patient in bed, be sure she is sitting upright. Never give a pill to a patient who is lying down, or to a patient who is unconscious or unable to swallow. (To give medications through feeding tubes, read Chapter 5 on nutrition. Pills may be crushed and mixed with liquid for administration through a feeding tube). Offer pills one at a time. If your patient is confused, stay with her until you are sure the pill has been swallowed; you may even have to check inside her mouth. If the pills cannot be taken orally, the doctor should be notified, and other routes considered.

Sublingual medications are given under the patient's tongue to avoid being absorbed in the stomach or the intestines. The pill must be placed directly under your patient's tongue and stay there until it dissolves. This usually takes a few minutes. During that time, your patient should not smoke, eat, or drink. This tablet should not be chewed. An example of this type of pill is nitroglycerine, prescribed for chest pain (angina).

Any *liquid medication* requires special attention to the dose. It may be in teaspoons, tablespoons, drops, drams, or a liquid unit of measure such as cubic centimeter (cc) or milliliter (ml). When you are pouring out a liquid medication such as cough syrup, be sure you have it at eye level to ensure a proper dose. Some pharmacists have medication spoons or cups with prescribed markings on them.

Most syrups and liquid medications have been flavored or sweetened to make them taste better. There is a tendency to wash down the drug with water or beverage, but with some medications, such as cough syrups, you should not do this. Check with your pharmacist to see if it is possible to mix the medications with orange juice or something tastier. Again, do not offer these medications to comatose or unconscious patients.

Inhalants

Hand-held inhalers deliver medication to the respiratory tract, where it is absorbed almost immediately. Some of these medications have serious side effects and should not be given if they occur. Check with your physician about this.

To administer an inhalant, your patient must be alert and able to assist you. Be sure the label on the inhaler is properly marked and the dose included. Your patient should exhale before you begin. Remove the mouthpiece cover; push the metal container into the plastic outer covering; invert the inhaler; and have the patient close the mouthpiece tightly over her mouth, so that there is a closed seal. She should inhale slowly as you or the patient push the bottom of the center container to release the medication. Repeat this procedure as often as specified, but remember that too much of the medication can decrease effectiveness. Rinse the mouthpiece after each use. The patient may gargle or have a drink to remove the taste.

Injectable Medications

When your patient is unable to take oral medications, needs a faster means of medication, or a particular drug requires it, the injectable route may be indicated. *Never administer injectable medications to your loved one without training from a qualified health care professional. Practice giving injections under the supervision of someone on the health care team.*

Before I discuss injectable medications, I want to stress safety in the use of needles and syringes. Always keep them out of reach of children or a confused patient; locking them up is preferred. Because of the worldwide health crisis posed by the AIDS virus, the disposal of needles and syringes has been revised in recent years. Used needles and syringes should be disposed of in an impenetrable needle container. Discuss proper disposal with someone on the health care team. It is generally felt most medical equipment should be incinerated and treated as contaminated waste.

If your patient is contagious, improper needle disposal could injure or contaminate a member of your family, your local trash collector, or a family pet. Also check to see how any excess medication should be destroyed.

If you stick yourself with a used syringe or with a syringe containing medication (this can be a problem on rare occasions), clean the area immediately with cold water and disinfectant (Betadine or Hebacleanse). Report this to the physician. In most cases, this will not be a problem, but in some instances, especially when the patient has an infectious disease, the risk exists that you may contract it.

Intramuscular Injections

An injection into the deep muscle tissue of the body is an intramuscular injection (IM). The medication given by intramuscular injection is rapidly absorbed due to the large blood supply there, thus allowing the medication to pass quickly into the bloodstream. The intramuscular route is used for injectable medications when large amounts need to be given. This route also may be used when a medication may irritate superficial tissues or the stomach and intestines.

Intramuscular injection is relatively painless if given correctly. Generally, pain is felt when the medication is particularly thick and irritates the tissues, or if a sensitive nerve has been touched. This discomfort usually is felt only as the medication is being injected. If the pain persists, it may indicate a problem and you should notify your physician.

The intramuscular injection is considered a sterile procedure. There are numerous sites for intramuscular injection (figure 29). Injections should never be given directly into a scar, birthmark, mole, burned area, or any other spot where there may be impaired absorption. If your patient has been receiving injections for a long time, it is often difficult to find unused areas. This can be a problem, possibly requiring alternate considerations by your doctor. As a general rule, no more than 5 cc/ml of medication should be given in one injection site.

You will need alcohol sponges, sterile syringes, sterile needles, and the medication. The syringe and needle size and length will be determined by the type of injection, location of the injection, and type and amount of medication (the larger the needle size number or gauge, the smaller the needle width). Be sure all injectable medication arrives unopened.

Here are some terms you may hear when you are being trained to give injections, and some of the reasons for these procedures:

Cleaning. Always wash your hands since you will be handling supplies and medications that will be injected into your patient. The medication preparation area should be as clean as possible.

Sterile. This means that the equipment, such as the needle, has been rendered free of organisms. Therefore, it is important that any part of the equipment coming in direct contact with the patient remain sterile.

Alcohol. In this case, it is used as an antiseptic to remove any organisms or bacteria that may be on equipment surfaces or the patient's skin.

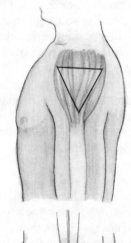
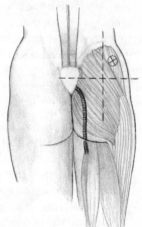

Fig. 29
Intramuscular injection sites

Injecting air into a vacuum vial. This is done to preserve the vacuum when medication is drawn out of the vial. Do this whenever withdrawing medication from a vacuum bottle. You should inject the same amount of air into the bottle as medication withdrawn from the bottle. (If you need 1 cc of medication, inject 1 cc of air.)

Single dose vial. Only one dose is provided in the vial. In some cases you will not use the entire amount, and you may or may not be allowed to save the excess for future use.

Multi-dose vial. When you have been supplied with multiple doses of medication in one vial, use it until it is finished or the expiration date arrives. Once you start to use a medication, always check the expiration date and how it should be stored.

Medication dose. Most medications are ordered in metric system units. (Consult the Appendix for a table of metric conversions.) An injectable medication is different from prescribing one pill or two capsules.

An example of how an injectable medication may be ordered is: Give 5 mg of Valium IM (intramuscularly) every four hours. You may have been supplied with a multi-dose vial labeled 1 cc = 5 mg. The vial contains a total of 20 cc, so there are 20 single doses of medication in this multi-dose vial. The patient would receive 1 cc of medication (5 mg) every four hours. Usually, your pharmacist would give you this information, and you would not be responsible for figuring it out alone. The medication probably would arrive from your pharmacist written as: Give 1 cc of Valium every four hours. Keep track of how much you are using so you do not run out.

Determining dose. The basics of this are done in the laboratory, long before the public sees the drug on the market. Researchers have determined how much medication is necessary to obtain a desired therapeutic effect. Your doctor, in turn, must determine your patient's dose based on age, height, weight, and present medical condition.

Preparing the solution. If you are lucky, your medication will arrive prepared and ready to use, but you usually have to prepare your own. Sometimes the medication comes premixed in the vial and you will have only to draw it into the syringe. Other times the injectable medication is powdered and must be mixed with a prescribed solution. There also will be times when you will have to combine two different types of medications in one syringe.

Do not give more than 5 cc/ml in one syringe to a patient. Even this amount will possibly be too much for a frail, underweight person without much fat tissue on her body. If the amount you must administer is too large for one syringe, you will have to give two separate injections in two separate syringes.

To prepare premixed solutions, take out the solution, prepare your clean work area, and gather all supplies (needles, syringes, alcohol sponges, and medication).

1. Check your medication label and be sure it is the right medication, the right dose, for the right patient. If the medication is being used for the first time, be sure it arrives sealed; if not, don't use it. Know how the medication should be stored; often it must be refrigerated after it has been opened.
2. Clean the top of the medication vial with an alcohol sponge.
3. Take the syringe, being careful not to contaminate the needle. Some syringes will come with the needle already attached, others will have the needle separate. Both the syringe and the needle should be in sealed, sterile packages. If the needle is not attached, take out the needle, being careful not to touch it where it will be connected to the syringe. Attach the needle cover securely to the needle base and keep it covered. Push the needle tightly into the top of the syringe and twist to lock it in place. Even if your syringe arrived prepared, make sure the needle is tightly in place.

4. Take the needle cover off in one swift motion. Draw back the same amount of air as of the drug you are using. For example, if you need 2 cc of medication, draw up 2 cc of air.
5. Take the syringe of air and inject it into the top of the vial.
6. Now invert the vial with the syringe still in the top, and keep holding the plunger part of the syringe.
7. Be sure you have the vial and syringe at eye level. Carefully draw out the required amount of medication. The tip of the needle must be immersed in solution, or you will not be able to obtain the medication. Withdraw the solution by pulling back on the plunger. Perhaps draw out a little bit more than the required amount, and slowly push the plunger back to the required dose (figure 30). This process also will eliminate air from the syringe.
8. Now turn the bottle back down and withdraw the syringe. Check to see that you have the exact amount of prescribed medication, and that you have removed excess air. To remove tiny air bubbles, gently flick the side of the syringe with your finger. As soon as you have withdrawn the syringe, replace the needle cap. Make sure you haven't contaminated anything. If you have, you must begin again using a new syringe or needle. Exchange any contaminated item for another sterile one.
9. You are now ready to prepare your patient.

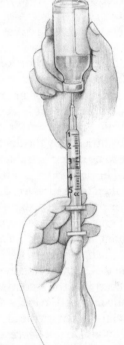

Fig. 30 Measuring medication

If you must mix injectable medications, they probably will come in a sealed vacuum vial containing the medication in powder form. Ask what you must mix this with; usually it will be a vial of sterile water or sterile salt water (labeled as normal saline or bacteriostatic sodium chloride). Find out how much to add and how to store the mixture. Know how long such a mixture will remain stable, both at room temperature and when it's refrigerated. Use a vial of mixed medication only as long as it remains stable; mark the vial so you don't forget and use a drug that has lost its effectiveness.

Draw up the mixing solution in the same manner that you used for premixed medication. Clean the top of the powdered vial with an alcohol sponge and inject the mixing solution into the vial. Turn the vial back and forth to create a pure liquid, with no particles unmixed. Using the same syringe, if it was not contaminated, draw up the medication in the same manner as for a premixed medication.

Ampules. Some medications come in glass ampules intended for single use only. All of these ampules are marked with the name of the medication and dose. They may read: 5 mg = 1 cc. The total in the ampule may be 3 cc. If your doctor has ordered that you give the patient a dose of 10 mg, you would give her 2 cc of medication (to equal 10 mg), and discard the rest.

To break the glass vial, the neck of the vial will have to be snapped off. You may be supplied with a metal file or special device that will help snap off the top of the vial. If not, you can snap off the vial by holding it upright and giving the vial a few gentle flicks on the side with your finger to be sure all of the medication has settled on the bottom. Take an alcohol sponge and wrap it around the neck of the vial to protect yourself from getting cut. Break the vial in a direction away from your body by exerting pressure on the top portion; it should easily snap.

Remove your needle cover and place the syringe directly into the broken ampule. (Ampules do not contain a vacuum, so you must not inject air first.) Pull on the plunger and draw up a little more medication than necessary. Hold the syringe at eye level and slowly push out the excess medication until you reach the exact dose on the side of the syringe. Be sure you have removed all air and that you have the exact amount. Recap the syringe and prepare the patient for the injection.

Combining Drugs. Sometimes you may have to mix two medications in one syringe. This must be ordered by the doctor; don't decide to do this on your own. Medications must be compatible to be mixed in the same syringe and to be injected into the patient's body at the same time. The procedure is similar to that of drawing up a premixed solution. Extra care should be taken to be sure you do not squirt any medication from the first medication into the container for the second drug.

To obtain a multi-dose from two vacuum bottles, clean the top of the first vial with an alcohol sponge. Draw back the amount of air required. Inject the air into the vial, *being careful that the tip of the needle does not touch the medication*. Withdraw the syringe and needle from the vial. Now, using the same syringe and needle, draw up the required amount of air needed to insert into the second vial and inject air into the second vial. Invert the vial and withdraw the medication in the usual manner. Remove excess air bubbles. Next, wipe the top of the first vial again with the alcohol sponge. Put the syringe that has part of the medication into the first vial. *Do not depress the plunger as you usually would.* Invert the vial and draw out the required amount of medication. You now have combined two medications in one syringe.

For two ampules, break open both as instructed. Draw up the desired amount of medication from the first ampule; remove air bubbles; then put the needle into the second one and draw up the second medication.

To combine drugs from one multi-dose vial and one ampule, clean the top of the vial with an alcohol sponge and break off the top of the ampule. Take your syringe with the needle attached and draw back the required amount of air to put into the vacuum vial. Put the air into the vial. Draw the required amount of medication out of the vial. Remove air bubbles. Now draw the second medication out of the already opened ampule.

Cartridge (Tubex) Syringes. This special syringe holds a prepared medication cartridge. All that is required is proper loading and preparation of the syringe. Most cartridge holders are made of plastic or metal. The metal holder will bend in half to load; most plastic holders are loaded from the side and will not bend. The medication cartridges will come from your pharmacist in a glass container holding the medication with the needle already attached. The name of the drug and the dose should be written on the side of the glass medication container.

To load a metal syringe holder, take the top portion of the syringe holder, pull it up, and the syringe should bend in half. Take your medication cartridge and place it down into the cartridge holder. It should screw into the bottom portion. Screw that section tightly in place (turn clockwise until you hear a click). You can now close the top portion over the medication cartridge by pulling up and out on the top plunger. Take the top and gently push it down so it touches the top of the medication cartridge. Gently turn the top so that you are screwing that portion into place (clockwise).

Take the syringe and hold it up to eye level. The needle should be pointed up, with the cover over the needle. If it has fallen off and the needle has been contaminated, you will have to begin again.

Now, take off the needle cover. Slowly push the top of the cartridge plunger up until you see one tiny drop of medication come out through the needle. Be careful to give the correct dose, since some of these cartridges will contain more medication than needed. If that is the case, before injecting your patient, push the excess medication out of the syringe until you reach the desired dose. Put the cap back on the needle.

To load a plastic cartridge holder, check the medication cartridge and be sure the medication and the dose are correct. Take the needle portion and slip it into the bottom part of the cartridge holder. You should be able to screw that bottom portion in place (clockwise motion). Then gently take the plunger portion and slowly push it down until it is touching the top of the medication cartridge. Gently screw that portion into place (turn clockwise). Take your loaded syringe and bring it up to eye level with the needle pointing up. Take off the needle cover and slowly push the plunger until one tiny drop of medication comes out through the needle tip. If you must, push out more medication to obtain the desired dose. Recap the needle.

To unload both syringes, reverse the process and turn counterclockwise. The injection is given using the same technique as with other syringes. Most medication cartridges can be stored at room temperature, but check to be sure.

Giving Injections

Ask a doctor or nurse for training before you administer any injection. A good way to practice giving an injection, before you try the real thing, is to use an orange or a grapefruit. Use sterile water in vacuum bottles to practice drawing out medications and injecting them. Properly dispose of practice syringes. Always wash your hands before giving an injection.

1. Gather your equipment in a clean, uncluttered, well-lit area.
2. Check your medication label and dose. Be sure it has been stored as directed. Find out whether you should wear gloves when handling the medication and injecting your patient.
3. Prepare your injection and bring it to your patient. Let the patient know you are about to inject her so she doesn't jump or move away.
4. Select the injection site. It's a good idea to rotate injection sites. You can keep a record on your medication chart as to where you placed each injection. For example, if you gave the last injection in the right buttock (RB), give the next one in the left buttock (LB). Rotate through all recommended injection sites (both buttocks, upper arms, and top of the upper thighs); ask someone on the health care team to review appropriate sites for your patient. Some medications can be given only in specific areas. Another way to remember the last injection site is to apply a small Band-Aid, even though your patient may not need one.

5. Have the patient expose the injection site and clean it thoroughly with your alcohol sponge, using a circular motion. Do not throw it away; save it for after the injection. Allow the area to air dry. Be careful not to touch the area you have just cleaned.

6. Remove the needle cap, using caution not to contaminate the needle. Take your thumb and forefinger and spread the skin at the injection site. Hold the syringe in your dominant hand for the injection. The tip of the needle should be no more than four to five inches from the patient.

7. With the syringe at a 90 degree angle, stick the needle into the patient. The motion should be a quick, firm thrust. (You are not throwing darts!) Once the needle is inserted (it should be in at least three-quarters of the needle length), remove the hand that was spreading the skin. Your other hand should still be holding the syringe.

8. Take the top of the plunger with your dominant hand and gently draw back, just enough to check for blood. There may be tiny blood vessels in the area; if you are in one of them, you will see blood. If so, stop the injection, remove the syringe, and massage the injection site with an alcohol sponge. You will have to start over with a new syringe; do not re-inject medication that has blood in it. If you pull back the plunger and there is no blood, slowly inject the medication by pushing down on top of the plunger.

9. After all the medication has been injected, gently withdraw the syringe and massage the injection site with an alcohol sponge. If your patient is on anti-clotting drugs, anti-cancer drugs, or any other medications that interfere with clotting, apply added pressure until the bleeding stops. You may wish to apply ice to help stop the bleeding and cut down on bruising.

For the patient receiving frequent injections, you can apply a warm, wrung out washcloth to enhance absorption and repair tissue damage. Hot baths, if allowed, also will help. In patients who have had frequent injections, you may find any of the following situations: the medication takes longer than usual to be absorbed; the medication tends to leak back out of the tissues; there is decreased effectiveness; and there is an increased possibility for abscess formation. If you feel your patient may be experiencing any of these problems, consult your physician.

Your patient may need a special form of deep, intramuscular injection called a Z track injection, although it is not commonly used. This method prevents leakage of certain medications, such as iron, into the subcutaneous tissues. When done correctly, the medication will be sealed into deep muscle. Ask someone on the health care team for specific instructions if you are told to give this type of injection.

Sterile Abscess

Sterile abscess is a possible complication of intramuscular injections that appears when pus accumulates or an infection occurs in an injection site. This can be caused by any of the following circumstances: too much medication injected into an area at one time; contaminated equipment; failure to rotate sites; extremely irritating drugs; or when your patient has been receiving injections for a long time.

Some symptoms of sterile abscess are swelling or pain in the area; warm to touch; redness; skin breakdown with pus formation; and fever. If you note any of these symptoms, notify your doctor right away. Do not continue to inject in that area. You may be told to apply warm, moist packs to the abscess and refrain from using that area for injections. The doctor may prescribe antibiotics or possibly even surgery to drain the abscess.

Subcutaneous Injections

The same procedures for intramuscular injection should be used for subcutaneous injections (page 97). The only difference is that a subcutaneous injection (Sub-Q) should be administered into the subcutaneous tissues, as opposed to deep muscle layers. This method of injecting medication is still faster than the oral route, but will provide a slower, more sustained action than that of an intramuscular injection. It also will cause less damage to the surrounding tissues, blood vessels, and nerves because it is not as deep. The medication is absorbed mainly through tiny blood capillaries. Because this injection is given at a superficial tissue level, smaller amounts of medication should be given, generally no more than 2 cc at one time.

The sites chosen for subcutaneous injection can be the same as those for intramuscular injection (figure 31). However the technique is different and the needle and syringe sizes usually will be smaller.

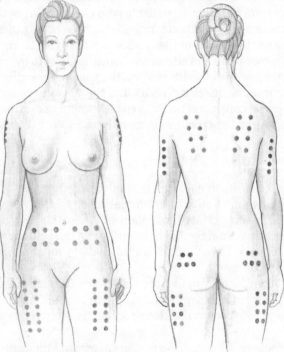

Fig. 31 Subcutaneous injection sites

Prepare your medication, equipment, and the patient using the same methods as for intramuscular injection. Select your injection site. Tell the patient you are about to give the injection.

Cleanse the skin with an alcohol sponge and allow the area to air dry for a moment. Remove the needle cover, taking care not to contaminate the needle. Using your non-dominant hand, gently pinch a one-inch area on your patient's skin. The needle point should be close to the patient's skin and should enter the patient's body at a 45 degree angle. (Depending on the medication and the patient, you may sometimes give this injection at a 90 degree angle.)

Insert the needle quickly with one motion, holding the patient's skin until the needle has entered. Now release the hold on your patient's skin. Before injecting the medication, pull back on the plunger to check for blood (this rarely occurs with a subcutaneous injection). If there is blood in the syringe, withdraw the needle. Prepare a new syringe and needle, a new injection area, and repeat the process. If there is no blood, slowly inject the patient's medication. Remove the syringe and gently massage the area with your alcohol sponge. If your patient is taking certain medications, her clotting mechanism may be impaired. If necessary, exert a little pressure to stop the bleeding. Dispose of your material appropriately.

If your loved one is diabetic, she may need insulin injections if the disease cannot be controlled through diet or oral medications. Refer to Chapter 14 on care of the diabetic patient for information about insulin injections.

Intravenous Medications

(Most information on intravenous therapy is contained in Chapter 5 on nutrition.)

Intravenous medications are given to patients who cannot take medications orally; when the intramuscular or subcutaneous method is not adequate; when a faster absorption rate is needed; or when the required amounts of medication are too great to inject. Because of rapid rate of absorption, all the more care and attention should be given to the procedure. Intravenous medications enter directly into the bloodstream via the vein and the effects can be felt immediately. Because a catheter must be inserted directly into the vein and remain there during the course of the therapy, special consideration is given to keeping that catheter in place and to preventing infection. If your patient requires intravenous delivery of fluids or medications, see Chapter 5.

Pain Control

Pain is defined as a sensation that causes discomfort, distress, or suffering. The physiologic process of pain is initiated by the stimulation of specific groups of nerve fibers or nerve endings. The nerve fibers feed into the thalamus, where the body first becomes aware of pain. These impulses are transferred by the thalamus to the cerebral cortex in the brain, where they are acknowledged as pain. Here the pain is analyzed, the location identified, and the intensity evaluated. Then you say "OUCH!"

In some instances, it will be easy to identify the source and stop the pain; in others, it will not be so easy. Pain can be intense and unrelenting; it can be sharp and jabbing; or it may be sporadic discomfort. How pain is described is important, and often represents something specific to the doctor.

First determine the source. Often, this is not an easy task. Pain cannot be seen or felt by another person, although certain conditions and illnesses are known to cause pain. The cancer patient may have pain as the cancer spreads to other body organs. The tumor or parts of the tumor may be sitting on an organ and compressing nerves in the body, thereby rendering pain.

Pain may serve as an early warning sign of a health problem. If the patient is having abdominal pain, perhaps her appendix is inflamed and needs attention. If she is experiencing chest pain, her body may be signaling heart problems, or that a heart attack is taking place. In all cases, pain is to be considered a symptom that something is wrong, and proper attention should be sought.

The types of pain treatment may be non-medical (hypnosis, biofeedback, guided imagery); medical (surgery, medications); or acupuncture. Electrical stimulation devices may counteract the impulse that carries the pain message to the brain.

People respond differently to pain. A pain threshold is the point at which an individual will begin to feel pain, and it is reached in varying degrees in different people. It is much easier if your patient is able to speak and tell you where the pain is and what it is like. Other times, there may be no verbal response. This can depend on the patient's age, ethnic background, upbringing, and the way she was taught to respond to pain. Perhaps your patient was raised in a family where it was considered a weakness to complain or cry. Your patient may fear that if she admits to having pain, she may have to return to the hospital, or that it is a prelude to death.

Some non-verbal responses to pain may be facial grimacing, tensed muscles or clenched teeth. Your patient may lie curled up in her bed in a fetal position. Body responses to pain may be an elevated pulse, perspiration, or loss of appetite. Report all verbal and non-verbal communications of pain to your physician.

Make sure your patient understands the cause or source of her pain, if possible. This could decrease anxiety which may aggravate her condition. You may want to discuss with your doctor the possibility of using placebos in place of addictive pain-killers. Sometimes placebos, which contain inactive substances, satisfy a patient's psychological need for medication. Your patient must not know that placebos are being used; they can be helpful in determining the need for pain drugs. The following factors should be considered in pain management. Is it acute or chronic? How viable is your patient? Will she be up and about, carrying on daily activities such as driving a car or going to work? Have other methods been tried and were they effective? Does your patient have a life expectancy of less than one month? All such variables must be considered.

Since most medications given for severe pain are narcotics (strong drugs associated with addiction), emphasis is given to alternate methods of pain control, unless it is acute and short-term. Some other means of pain control are distraction; talking to your patient; promoting relaxation; being with your patient and reassuring her; and even helping to prevent pain from occurring. The care giver can offer all these techniques.

Depending on the nature, intensity, and duration of the pain, some of these techniques will work. Some patients may use pain as a means of getting extra attention, and if that is the case, examine the reasons for this need. Is the patient afraid? Does the pain occur only at night when she is alone? Does the pain seem to be relieved when she receives attention? The care giver must be tuned in to the patient to recognize some of these subtleties.

Never offer pain medication because you are too busy to take time to talk to your patient. Try to help her relax. Offer quiet music; tell the rest of the household to be quiet; suggest a massage or a cup of hot herb tea (avoid caffeine, which only serves to stimulate the patient); avoid bright lights or darken the room, if you think it might help. Try to make the patient as comfortable as possible.

Distraction is not easy to accomplish with a person in pain. Talk to her to get her mind off the problem. Play a game or have her do some prescribed care such as her foot exercises or deep breathing. Put on her favorite TV program. Try anything you might be able to think of that will take her mind away from the pain.

Other pain relief measures that your patient can be taught are guided imagery and self-hypnosis. Guided imagery is using one's imagination to obtain a desired effect. In this case, the desired effect is relaxation and pain relief. To learn guided imagery, your patient must be able to concentrate, follow directions, and use her imagination. This is difficult for the heavily sedated patient, or the patient with severe pain, because these patients have trouble concentrating.

Here is an example of guided imagery: The patient is told to close her eyes, try to relax, and focus her mind on tiny, fluffy, floating clouds. She must convince herself that each time she breathes, using slow breaths in and out, she is slowly allowing these fluffy clouds to carry her pain out with them. She must practice this exercise at least several times a day, using whatever image works best for her. Whenever the pain starts to occur, before it is allowed to progress, she should use this form of imagery.

Hypnosis and self-hypnosis also are ways to alleviate pain. There are many respected professionals who practice hypnosis for medical purposes. Ask your doctor to recommend someone who does this form of therapy, since it can be quite effective. Initially, the patient will work with the hypnotist and then will be given a tape to play at home. She can use this whenever pain approaches.

The Oriental practice of acupuncture has been investigated and is increasingly accepted as a useful weapon in the fight against pain. Acumassage, acupressure, and acupuncture (which uses fine needles) are three methods sometimes used to relieve pain. Ask your health care team about this practice and whether such therapy might help your patient.

A number of centers throughout the country specialize in pain control. Ask your doctor about them. A number of large teaching hospitals also have pain control departments. For a pain clinic directory, write to:

Committee on Pain Therapy and Acupuncture
American Society of Anesthesiologists
1515 Busse Highway
Park Ridge, IL 60068

Medications used for pain control are categorized as analgesics. There are opiates and their derivatives (morphine, codeine, laudanum and paregoric, Hydromorphone, Pantopan, and Methodone); synthetic analgesics (Demerol, methadone, Levo-Dromoran, and Talwin); and analgesics used for minor pain (aspirin, Tylenol, and Darvon).

Analgesics are given orally, injected intramuscularly or subcutaneously, or sometimes given intravenously. Analgesics interfere with the conduction of nerve impulses, or by altering the perception and response to pain in the brain. Some of these drugs are extremely powerful and their use should be limited. Most are considered narcotics and are closely controlled; they should be locked away even when using them in the home.

Pain medication for your patient will be ordered by a specific dose, but the frequency may be determined by the patient's need and the established interval between each dose. A doctor may prescribe "Demerol 50 mg IM every four hours, as needed." The amount the patient receives must remain at 50 mg. If you find the dose is ineffective, call your physician and report it. The doctor may either increase the dose or decrease the time interval. *Do not make adjustments on your own.*

Many pain medications have common side effects. They can induce sleep or fatigue; depress the respiratory system; cause dizziness; produce nausea and vomiting; cause constipation; cause depression or mental confusion; and be habit-forming.

A patient requiring pain medication should know that these drugs are available if she needs them. Sometimes, the doctor may prescribe various types of pain medications for varying degrees of pain. There may be oral and injectable doses available. This should be the patient's choice, based on severity of the pain.

It may be appropriate to offer pain medication just before your patient will be moved or undergo a particular activity or procedure. Provide adequate time for the medication to work (about 20 to 30 minutes for oral medications; 10 minutes for injectable ones).

One common mistake patients make is that they wait too long before taking pain medication. They should request pain medication at the onset of pain; if they wait until it has peaked, the pain will be more difficult to control. However, sometimes out of fear and anticipation that the pain will reoccur, patients take pain medications every four hours, whether they have pain or not. This is not recommended.

The judgment made by the care giver is difficult, since pain is subjective. It is somewhat like the dilemma of a parent with a crying baby. How long can the parent let the baby cry before going into the room and picking up the baby? If the baby is picked up, will she cry every night? There will be times when you will feel torn, in much the same way as the parent who tends to a crying baby. You can only abide by the doctor's orders and report problems with pain management to the physician.

In spite of all your efforts, some patients will continue to have pain and may require medication either by an intravenous route or through an implantable disk. These drugs are delivered on a slow, continuous basis.

The issue of drug dependence is very delicate and difficult. Sometimes, after prolonged use of some pain medications, your patient will require more of the medication, perhaps more frequently. This may be because the patient builds up a tolerance to the medication; other times it is because the patient has become physically or psychologically dependent. Some patients can take the same amounts over a long period of time, and when the pain is resolved, discontinue the medication without any problem. Others may not be able to stop so easily. It is unclear why this occurs. Some researchers feel it is due to the body's chemical composition; others believe it is related to a patient's mental strength. No one knows for sure.

If your patient has a problem with drug dependence (which neither the patient nor care giver should feel responsible for), it is a consequence of these types of medications. Withdrawal attempts must be made. With some medications, it is dangerous to abruptly stop the drugs if the patient has been taking them for a long time. Withdrawal probably will require hospitalization under close supervision by the doctor and hospital staff.

Sleeping Medications

Sleep is important, especially for someone who is ill. A patient should not be allowed to suffer more than two nights without sleep. Report any problems to your doctor and try to ascertain if there are underlying problems interfering with your patient's inability to sleep.

Sleeping medications are classified as sedatives, barbiturates, and hypnotics. Drugs such as chloral hydrate, Dalmane, Seconal, Nembutal, phenobarbital, or Amytal are used to induce sleep or promote a sedated state. Most of these drugs require a prescription. They usually are given orally in a tablet, capsule, or pill, and come in different strengths. In rare instances, they are injected when the patient cannot take the drug orally.

Most sleeping medications have the same common side effects: dizziness, mental confusion, dependency, respiratory depression, mental depression, hangover effect, emotional disturbances, and nightmares. Sometimes, when these drugs are combined with other drugs, they have the opposite effect and make a patient extremely agitated, restless, and unable to sleep.

When medicating your patient with a sedative, be sure she does not get out of bed on her own at night. Ask her to let you know if she needs to get up; keep a bell at the bedside. Leave a bedpan or urinal within reach. If the patient has a bed with bed rails, put them up. Avoid falls by keeping obstacles out of the patient's path. Keep a night-light on. Take extra caution with elderly people; they tend to really feel the effects of sleeping medication and may become confused or disoriented.

Most doctors will order sleeping medication for the hour of sleep, and perhaps a repeat dose if needed. Do not wake your sleeping patient to give her a sleeping pill. If your patient asks for a sleeping pill after 4 A.M., it is usually not a good idea to offer it, since she will still feel the effects during the day. Use common sense here. If you have a patient without a prescribed sleeping medication, and she is having trouble sleeping, ask your doctor to prescribe one.

Other methods you can use to help your patient sleep are much the same as those for pain control: promote relaxation; create a restful environment; play soft music; avoid distractions; offer a cup of tea or hot milk at bedtime; avoid beverages with caffeine; or have the patient use a form of guided imagery. If these methods fail, then the patient may need to resort to sleeping medications. Some of them will promote dependence, making it more difficult for the patient to sleep without them.

Tranquilizers/Depressants

Depressants or tranquilizers act by blocking stimulation of areas in the central nervous system. There are various categories of these drugs: phenothiazine derivatives (Thorazine, Sparine, Stelazine, Valium, Librium, Serax, Haldol; rauwolfia derivatives (Serpasil, Moderil, Rauval); and muscle relaxants (Soma, Robaxin, Atarax, Vistaril).

Some of these drugs have multiple uses; all of them have similar side effects: drowsiness, constipation, dizziness, mental confusion, headaches, hallucinations, double vision, tremors, slurred speech and dry mouth. Some or most of these side effects may be eliminated by adjusting the patient's dose.

These drugs usually are given orally, but they also can be given by injection (intramuscular or subcutaneous) or intravenously (either by direct injection or by continuous drip infusion). The route will be based on the patient's need. If any of these medications are given via the injectable or intravenous route, the patient should continue to lie down for a few hours so her reactions can be observed.

A level of tolerance may be reached with some of these drugs. This can mean that it will take greater amounts of the same drug, or more frequent intervals, to obtain the desired effect. Patients taking these types of drugs for a long time may build up a physical or psychological dependence. The use of these types of drugs should not be taken casually, but in some patients, there will be no other choice. The physician will have to ultimately make this determination.

Whenever a patient is taking tranquilizers or depressants, she should be watched closely. If she appears to need help walking, guide her so she does not lose her balance and fall. The patient's usual sense of good judgment may be impaired, which is why she should not drive or operate machinery. Sometimes the dose may be too strong. If your patient is sleeping a great deal, is confused, or appears not to be herself, consult with the physician.

Suppositories

Suppositories are medications in the form of a small solid mass given either rectally or vaginally. This route is used to relieve constipation, pain, infection, vomiting, nausea, fever, or to treat a specific problem.

The medication is absorbed in the rectum or vagina through the mucous membranes, and then into the bloodstream. Drugs are given this way for a number of reasons: the patient cannot take the drug orally; the patient is vomiting; the drugs will not work if they come in contact with the digestive enzymes of the stomach; or the taste is offensive. This route provides another effective alternative to the traditional oral route.

Suppositories melt from increased body temperature in the rectum or vagina. As they melt, they are absorbed slowly into the body. For this reason, all suppositories should be refrigerated; otherwise they will melt and you will be unable to insert them, or their effectiveness may decrease.

Rectal Suppositories.   Two of the most common uses of rectal suppositories are to treat constipation or fever. To insert, you will need the suppository, a rubber glove (unsterile) or finger cot (slips over one finger only), and a lubricating jelly. Wash your hands before you begin.

1. Have the patient roll over on her left side, with her knees pulled up, if possible.
2. Put the glove or the finger cot on your dominant hand.
3. Unwrap the suppository, take your lubricant, and apply a small amount on the tip of the suppository.
4. Spread the patient's buttocks with your ungloved hand to expose the anus.
5. Gently insert the suppository (the tapered end first), using your index finger. (The patient can take slow, deep breaths to help relax rectal muscles.) The suppository should be inserted about 1 to 1½ inches (past the rectal sphincter).
6. The patient should try to retain the suppository. She can make herself comfortable, or continue to lie on her left side.
7. Remove glove and discard appropriately. Wash your hands.

If the suppository is to relieve constipation, the patient must try to retain it for at least 20 minutes, for it to be effective. Keep the bedpan nearby if she cannot go to the toilet. The suppository should be given 30 minutes before meals. You and the patient should know that some suppositories discolor the stool.

Vaginal Suppositories.   The most common reason for this type of treatment is to treat infections or vaginal irritation. Some vaginal medications come with an applicator to make insertion easier. The insertion will vary depending on whether the patient will be inserting it herself. Most vaginal medications will contain directions on insertion, as well as important information on the medication. You will need the medication, gloves, medication applicator, and a sanitary pad.

If you are inserting the medication for the patient:

1. Wash your hands.
2. Have the patient urinate first.
3. Ask her to lie down, flat on her back.

4. Have the patient pull up her knees.
5. Gently spread her knees apart.
6. Place a glove on your dominant hand.
7. Remove the wrapper from the suppository or place the medication into the applicator as directed.
8. Spread the labia (lips of the vagina) and insert the suppository about two inches into the vagina, using your forefinger. (If you are using an applicator, insert it into the vagina until you reach the end of the vaginal canal. Push the plunger in, release the medication, and remove the applicator.)
9. After insertion, have the patient continue to lie flat for ten minutes. Apply a sanitary pad for drainage and discharge.
10. Discard your used equipment, wash the applicator with soap and warm water, and save for reuse. Wash your hands.

For self-insertion, tell your patient:

1. Wash your hands.
2. Prepare the suppository, or vaginal applicator.
3. Find a position that is easiest for you. Perhaps use the method you would use to insert a tampon.
4. Using your forefinger or the vaginal applicator, insert the medication as far into your vagina as you can reach (as when a tampon is inserted).
5. Apply a sanitary napkin, since the medication will melt in your vagina and some will leak out.
6. Wash your hands and the applicator with warm water and soap.

Patients should not wear tampons for this type of treatment. Tampons will only serve to absorb the medication.

Drops: Eye, Nose, Ear

Drops may be prescribed for your patient. Be sure to follow safety guidelines that apply to all medicines.

Eye drops, or any other types of eye medications (ointments, creams), can be used to treat infection, dilate or constrict the pupils, and lubricate. Before applying any type of eye medication, be sure of the following: What is it being used for? How should it be applied? Which eye should it go into? Should it be used in both eyes? What are some of the side effects?

Wash your hands before you begin. To apply eye ointments or drops:

1. Remove your patient's contact lenses, if she wears them.
2. Check the medication. Read the labels. Are you sure which eye to treat?
3. Have the patient lie flat on her back, with the head of the bed slightly elevated. Have proper lighting.
4. Use a cotton ball moistened in warm water and wrung out to remove eye discharge or crust. Have the patient close her eye for this. Start from the inner part of the eye outward, using a fresh cotton ball each time. Never use the same cotton ball for both eyes.
5. When the eye has been cleansed, have her tilt her head back slightly.
6. Prepare your medication.

7. Tell the patient to direct her eyes away from you.
8. Pull the patient's lower eyelid down with your non-dominant hand.
9. For drops: Using your dominant hand, drop the prescribed number of drops into the lower eyelid sac. (Pinch the dropper gently and release; for each pinch you should have one drop of medication.) Do not let the eye dropper touch the patient's eye. Now have the patient blink once.
10. For ointments: Squeeze the ointment tube with your dominant hand, while holding the lower lid down with your other hand. Squeeze the medication in a thin line by starting from the inner area of the eye, outward across the inner, lower eyelid. When you have finished, have the patient squeeze her eye shut for a moment, and then open and roll her eyes in a circular motion to allow the medication to be absorbed.

Wash your hands after the procedure. If you are doing both eyes, wash your hands between administrations of medication. Do not place medication directly into the tear ducts (on the lower lid in the inner area).

Ear drops are used to treat an ear infection, to help soften excess wax, or to alleviate pain. Check to see how your medication should be stored. If it is refrigerated, never administer it cold; allow it to warm to room temperature. Be sure you have the correct medication, know the prescribed dose, and are treating the correct ear.

Wash your hands before you begin. To administer ear drops:

1. Prepare your medication.
2. Have the patient lie flat with the ear you wish to treat up.
3. Gently take hold of your patient's ear at the side, pull it up and back.
4. Clean any drainage with a cotton swab. Do not enter the patient's ear canal with the swab.
5. Place ear drops directly into the ear canal. Do not let the dropper touch the ear canal; hold it just above it. Have the patient lie on her side for ten minutes.
6. If the other ear requires medication also, do the other one at this time. Wash your hands between each treatment. Some doctors recommend a cotton ball be placed into the patient's ear to prevent the medication from leaking out.

Always wash your hands when you are finished. Your patient can be taught to do this, although it is awkward. It is easier to have someone administer the medication to the patient.

Nose drops are given to loosen nasal secretions and nasal congestion, relieve inflammation, and for allergy symptoms. Wash your hands before you begin.

1. Check your medication.
2. Have your patient lie flat on her back, with her head tilted back. You can use a pillow rolled under her neck and shoulders to accomplish this.
3. Push up the tip of the patient's nose and hold it there.
4. With your dominant hand, place your medication dropper just inside the patient's nostril (center) and release the prescribed amount of medication. (You can then do the other nostril.)
5. Have the patient remain in that position for five minutes.

The procedure is the same for nasal inhalers, except that the bottle must be inverted and is placed in the patient's nostril. The bottle is then squeezed while the patient sniffs up the medication.

Some nasal medications contain antihistamines that may cause restlessness, anxiety, increased pulse, and palpitations. If your patient experiences any of these side effects, report them to your doctor.

Topical Medications

Topical medications are placed on the skin or a specific outer organ of the body (ear, nose). Most of these medications come as creams or ointments. Topical medications are used to treat itching or local skin irritations; fight infection; treat burns; and for skin disorders.

Check the label on the medication to be sure you have the correct medication and strength. Strength is important to note because sometimes there are slight differences; 1 percent or 2 percent are two different strengths, and you should use only the strength that has been ordered.

In some cases, the patient may be allergic to the creams or ointments. The doctor may ask you to try an application to a small area first, before proceeding to a larger surface. Find out if the doctor wants a protective dressing applied; if the area should be exposed to the air; how long the cream should remain on the patient; how often it should be applied; and to what areas.

Some creams or ointments may irritate an untreated area. Ask whether gloves should be worn to apply the medication. Some creams and ointments will stain, as many contain an oil base, so don't use your best bed linens. Always remove the previous application before giving another. The doctor may or may not want the patient to bathe in between applications.

Find out how much ointment to apply. In most cases, just a bit will provide a smooth covering of the surface being treated. Either wear gloves or use a tongue depressor to spread the ointment or cream. Wash your hands before and after treating the patient.

When applying the ointment or cream, use long smooth strokes, going in the direction of the hair growth. If a dressing is required, find out what type—one with a non-stick plastic coating is best. If you are wrapping an area with gauze or an elastic bandage, be sure it is not wrapped too tightly. Report any adverse reactions to the physician. Do not give another treatment until you have spoken with the doctor about the problem.

To remove ointment or cream, take a gauze sponge and gently wipe away the excess, using the same long, smooth strokes in the direction of hair growth. Always keep an extra tube or jar of medication on hand. Store it appropriately, and pay attention to expiration dates.

Care Giver's Checklist

1. Whenever a drug is prescribed for your patient— whether it is a simple analgesic or a complex medication for a serious disorder—you should know the following:

   • What is the drug prescribed for?
   • What is the proper dosage?
   • What are the side effects and toxicities and how should they be treated?
   • How will it react with other drugs?
   • Under what conditions should it not be used?
   • What is the administration route (oral, intravenous, injection)?
   • When will it take effect, and how long will the effect last?

   Your pharmacist or doctor can supply all of this information. Be persistent about answers to these questions for each prescribed medication.

2. Draw up a medications chart indicating each drug, dose, times given, route, dates started and ended, special instructions, and patient reactions. Keep the chart current and take it to the hospital or doctor whenever your patient has an appointment.

3. Remember the "three rights" of medication administration. Always be sure you have the right patient, the right drug, and the right dose before giving the drug.

4. Read drug labels carefully. Check the expiration date and for special instructions about administration or storage. If an injectable or intravenous drug must be refrigerated, take it out 30 minutes before using to allow it to warm to room temperature. Some injectable medications must be mixed before administration and will lose their effectiveness within 24 hours.

5. Treat all drugs with respect. Your patient may develop a dependency on pain-killers or tranquilizers. This is not your fault, nor your patient's, but withdrawal must be accomplished under a doctor's care.

9 Elimination of Body Waste

Body elimination is a highly personal routine that can be quite distressing for anyone confined to bed. If your patient must use a bedpan or urinal, offer privacy; be sure other family members or visitors do not intrude. Keep your patient covered, if possible. You may leave your patient alone, but stand outside the door in case you are needed. Supply toilet tissue at the bedside, and a little air freshener. Empty bedpans and urinals quickly; do not leave them for any length of time at the patient's bedside. Use a small towel to cover the bedpan or urinal after your patient has finished.

Always allow the patient to wash his hands after using the urinal or bedpan. Be sure to wash your own hands before and after handling urinals and bedpans.

Offer the bedpan or urinal to the patient before meals, but be sure to remove it before the food arrives. Provide a bell so your patient can ring if he needs your help.

For the care taker, this chore may not be easy. Even nurses never quite get used to emptying dirty bedpans. Try not to show offense when you remove the bedpan or urinal. Empty the contents into the toilet after measuring output, if your doctor requires it. Be sure to thoroughly clean bedpans and urinals with heavy duty cleansers or disinfectants. Bedpans and urinals do not need to be sterilized.

Bedpans and urinals are plastic or metal, reusable, and can be found in most pharmacies or medical supply stores. Urinals for men are easy to insert and to use in a sitting position, although some men have difficulty urinating while sitting. Urinals usually have an attachment making it easy to hang them at the bedside. If the patient is able, he may be allowed to stand by the side of the bed to urinate. If he is unsteady on his feet, you may have to stand next to him for support.

Urinals for women are shaped to fit into the perineal/vaginal area, but if not placed correctly, they can leak and soil the bed. They can be used while sitting or standing.

Bedside commodes, which are like portable toilets, can be kept in your patient's room if a bathroom is not close by or the patient is unable to walk a great distance. A bedside commode can be rented from most medical equipment suppliers. Care should be taken if your patient needs help using the commode. Clean the commode bucket as often as necessary, just as you would bedpans and urinals. Some patients may ultimately use all three devices at different times. Ask your health care team what equipment will be best for your patient. If you want to protect the bed, place a disposable pad or piece of plastic underneath the bedpan. Disposable pads, which absorb wetness just like a disposable diaper, can be obtained from your pharmacy or medical supplier. Order these supplies before your patient's discharge; many will be covered by insurance.

Bedpan Placement

The technique for putting your patient on a bedpan will vary depending on how much help he needs. The way your patient is placed is key. It can make the difference between a wet or dry bed! Patient comfort is important, too. Don't leave your patient on the bedpan too long. If your loved one is confused or apt to fall out of bed, do not leave him alone. If there are safety rails on the bed, leave them up. When using a hospital electric bed, raise it to an easy working height for you, but if you must leave your patient alone, be sure to lower the bed level first. Sprinkling talcum powder or cornstarch on the top of the bedpan will make sliding easier.

The patient who is able to help should be sitting up. He can do a push-up type movement with both arms to raise his buttocks, or turn slightly to one side while you gently push the bedpan underneath. If your patient can bend his knees, it will be easier for him to lift himself up onto the bedpan. An overbed trapeze may be useful; your patient could lift himself up just enough so the bedpan slides under. Once the bedpan is positioned, you may have to support the patient with pillows to make sitting easier. To remove, have your patient lift up as you pull out the pan.

The patient who needs help should be flat in bed. Have your patient turn as far as he can on his side. Place the top of the bedpan (rounded seat portion) up against the top of the buttocks, just below the tailbone (coccyx). Steady the bedpan in place with one hand. Have the patient gently roll back toward you onto the bedpan. Once he is on top of the bedpan, slight repositioning may be necessary. The bedpan should be placed in such a way that urine will flow into the pan (there should be a four- to five-inch gap in the front of the bedpan, if you have done it right).

Once you are sure of position, raise your patient to a sitting level. If you are not using an electric bed, you will either have to stay with the patient to provide back support or prop him up with pillows. Remove the bedpan by lowering your patient flat in bed again, rolling him over on his side and off the bedpan. Be sure that the patient is wiped, cleaned, and dried throughly. For women, be sure to wipe the perineal area from front to back, using a different tissue each time. Some patients will need additional cleansing with a warm, wet cloth.

The technique is the same for the patient who cannot help you. Depending on how large or heavy the patient is, you may need another person. In most instances, one strong body should suffice. However, if you are alone, *do not try this without safety rails on the bed.*

Go to the opposite side of the bed, take the patient gently by the shoulder and buttocks, and roll the patient toward you. If the bed level is low, bend at your knees, spread your legs a short distance apart, and with a smooth, pulling motion, roll the patient toward you. Always be careful to not strain your back or other muscles.

Now go to the opposite side of the bed. Take the bedpan, positioning the top rounded surface just below the patient's tailbone (coccyx), hold it in place, and in a gentle motion, pull the patient back toward you. Place the hand not supporting the bedpan on the patient's hips and guide him onto the bedpan. This is not an easy procedure; you may find the patient isn't centered on the bedpan and you will have to start over again. With practice, you will develop a coordinated method that will work for you. The procedure is reversed to remove the patient. Carefully clean and dry your patient afterward.

There is a smaller type of bedpan, called a fracture bedpan, for patients in bed with fractures. If your patient is not too large, you may find this type of bedpan easier to use since it is more shallow. However, it cannot hold much urine and spills more easily. Placement and positioning are the same. The handle on the back of this bedpan goes under the tailbone. Most fracture patients are encouraged to use this type of bedpan because of limited movement.

Intake and Output

Even if your doctor has not ordered intake and output monitoring for your patient, you should at least be alert to indications of any problems. Intake is anything placed into the patient's body: fluids, food, intravenous solutions, tube feedings, blood or blood products, nutritional supplements, or liquid medications. Output is anything passed out of the patient's body: urine, stools, diarrhea, vomited food, blood, wound drainage, or excessive sweat. Report any unusual observations to your physician.

Watch for things that may influence intake and output. Is your patient taking in less food and fluid than usual? Is he having diarrhea? Is he vomiting frequently? Is he losing large amounts of fluid from a drainage tube? Is he urinating less than usual, or not at all? Is he losing large amounts of blood? All of these things can influence intake and output.

If your patient is placed on intake and output monitoring, *everything* that goes into his body and *everything* that goes out of his body must be recorded (charts 1 and 4). The metric unit of measurement is used, and I have provided some common household measurements on the charts along with their metric equivalents. To measure output, get a graduated measuring device from a medical supply store or pharmacy. Everything must be accurately recorded, otherwise the doctor may prescribe treatment based on incorrect information. Keeping accurate records will help your doctor make a diagnosis, or verify that a problem exists. If you are unclear about how to measure, have someone on the health care team explain it to you.

It is easiest if you tabulate measurements for each eight-hour period, although the doctor may request that this be done hourly. Then total the intake and output for each 24-hour period. If your patient will be on strict intake and output, he and all family members should know it. This will ensure that no urine is flushed away without measuring, or not a single glass of water is taken by the patient without first recording it. Tape a reminder message over the toilet. If your patient is alert, he will be able to help you with this. Give him pen and paper at his bedside to keep track of his intake.

To measure output, put a urinal or bedpan at the patient's bedside or by the toilet. All urine should be placed in this urinal or container and measured before discarding. If the patient has to move his bowels, it is better if the bowel movement and the urine are kept separate. This may be easier to accomplish with the male patient. Have him use the urinal first; then have him move his bowels in the bedpan or the toilet. In most cases, the bowel movement will not have to be measured, but only recorded as occurring and the approximate amount (small, medium, or large). If your patient is experiencing large amounts of diarrhea or liquid stools, the doctor may want this output to be measured as well.

If your female patient must urinate and move her bowels at the same time, have her urinate first into a container or bedpan, then move her bowels into the toilet. If the patient is bedridden, or cannot do two movements separately, use a bedpan. After the patient has finished, empty the urine into the measuring container and record. Then place the stool into the toilet.

If the patient has liquid stools and urine combined in the bedpan, it will not be possible to separate the two. In this case, measure the entire contents and record the amount as stool and urine.

It will be difficult to measure exact amounts of urine and stool loss in an incontinent patient (one who has no bowel or bladder control). In most cases, you will only be able to record the fact that it occurred and the approximate amount.

Other forms of output are measured in much the same manner. Place an emesis (vomiting) basin at the patient's bedside. Pour the vomitus into the measuring container and record the amount. If you are not able to measure it, record the occurrence and approximate

FLUID OUTPUT SHEET

Date 4/8/88	Urine	Stool	Emesis	Drainage / Other	Bladder Irrigation Through Foley Catheter				Total
					Type (Solution)	Amount In (Rate)	Amount Out	*Balance	
7 AM to 3 PM									
7 AM					Normal Saline	500 cc/8°			
8 AM									
9 AM									
10 AM									
11 AM			50 cc						
12 N									
1 PM									
2 PM						500	1800	1300	
Total			50					1300	1350 cc
3 PM to 11 PM									
3 PM					Normal Saline	500 cc/8°			
4 PM									
5 PM		ɫ loose stool							
6 PM									
7 PM									
8 PM			75 cc						
9 PM									
10 PM						500	1500	1000	
Total			75 cc					1000	1075 cc
11 PM to 7 AM									
11 PM					Normal Saline	500 cc/8°			
12									
1 AM									
2 AM			50 cc						
3 AM									
4 AM									
5 AM									
6 AM						500	1200	700	
Total			50					700	750 cc

*Subtract the amount of irrigant infused from the total urinary output to determine actual urinary output from a patient who has a urinary catheter and requires bladder irrigation.

24° Hour Combined Total	3,175

Chart 4

amount. To measure drainage from a drainage tube or urine catheter, disconnect the retrieval container and empty the contents into the measuring container and record. If you have a dressing or sheet that shows drainage, note the approximate amount and source (such as blood or pus). Record excessive perspiration, although you will not be able to measure the amount.

The Urinary Tract

The kidneys, ureters, urethra, and bladder are the organs that make up the urinary system. Basically, these organs work in a synchronized fashion to filter, reabsorb, and eliminate fluids and waste products from the body. The kidneys provide a filtering system. Blood is circulated through them and wastes are reduced to urine, which is passed through the ureters and on to the bladder. Urine is stored in the bladder until nerve impulses signal that the individual must empty his bladder. The bladder is emptied by muscles that contract and relax, pushing the urine through the urethra and out of the body.

If there is a problem in any one of these areas, complications can occur. Some of these may be: the kidneys are unable to filter waste products; the system is blocked; the bladder's muscles are inefficient; or there is a problem transmitting nerve impulses to and from the brain.

Your patient may be having urinary tract problems if inadequate or excess amounts of urine are passed. If some urine remains in the bladder (urinary retention), it can cause infection, fever, pain, high blood pressure, mental confusion, skin irritation, nausea, vomiting, and possibly convulsions. Other danger signals are blood in the urine; a strong odor to the urine; changes in the color or consistency of the urine; or edema (fluid retention).

Your patient may experience weakness, abdominal pain, fullness or bloating, and gastrointestinal problems. There can be loss of appetite, excessive thirst, or even hemorrhage. Urinary incontinence also is a sign of urinary tract problems. If you observe any of these symptoms, report them to your doctor immediately. Some may represent other medical problems.

Generally, your patient will have multiple complaints, not just a single symptom. A patient confined to bed is at an increased risk for urinary tract problems and his urine output should be observed. The average person puts out 1,500 to 2,400 cc/ml a day (about 2 to 4 pints). This varies, depending upon how much fluid the patient takes in; his blood pressure and blood concentration; whether he is taking medication that makes him urinate more frequently; his diet; his body temperature; and general health. The amount of fluid the patient takes in daily should be somewhat consistent with the amount of fluid passed out of the body over 24 hours. If not, there could be a problem.

Fluid Control

The doctor may put your patient on a restricted fluid diet or a diet requiring increased amounts of fluid. Either way, it is important to follow the guidelines. If something prevents you from doing this, you should report it to the doctor.

The average person takes in six to eight glasses of water or fluid a day. Increased fluid intake may be prescribed to keep the urine clear and dilute; improve blood volume and circulation; enhance elimination of body wastes; decrease fever; raise blood pressure; provide adequate hydration and nutrition; replace lost fluids and electrolytes; increase urine output; or as part of a combined regime to treat certain medical problems. Do not make fluid adjustments on your own; some patients require very careful monitoring. Even if extra fluids are prescribed for your patient, too much fluid over a short period of time can cause fluid overload. A very delicate fluid balance must be maintained. In deciding whether to increase or restrict fluids, the doctor will consider your patient's height, weight, age, kidney function, amount of fluid needed, and overall physical condition.

Fluid Increase. Generally, if fluid increase is taken orally, give one-quarter of the total at night and the rest throughout the day. When fluids are increased, the amounts can be as much as 3,000 to 4,000 cc/ml a day. Offer the fluids in small, more frequent servings, rather than in large quantities all at once. If he is able, the patient should take some responsibility in this aspect of his care. Keep a container of fresh water, juice, or other liquid at his bedside. Encourage him to drink; offer things he likes, but pay attention to dietary restrictions. Offer juices, soda, milk, water, tea, coffee, ice, custard, gelatin, oatmeal, or ice cream. As a general rule, anything liquid at room temperature is considered a liquid. Be sure to keep a bedpan or urinal nearby since increased fluids will increase urine output.

Fluid Restriction. Fluid restrictions will vary from one individual to another. Again, the patient's height, weight, and age will influence the amounts. Patients may be placed on fluid restrictions for high blood pressure, cardiac problems, fluid retention problems, urine retention problems, and other urinary problems.

The amounts allowed can vary from 600 to 800 cc/ml a day; even as low as 400 cc/ml a day in severe cases. Restricting fluids may prove to be harder than encouraging the patient to take increased fluids. Your loved one may be thirsty, and you won't be allowed to let him drink. Try to spread fluid intake equally throughout the day and evening. In between, give your patient ice chips to suck on, although these count as fluids and should be measured. The doctor may allow the patient to suck on hard candies.

Your patient's mouth will be quite dry. Offer more frequent mouth care; let him swish mouthwash around in his mouth several times a day. Be sure your patient's intake and output are monitored closely, and that you adhere to the restricted amounts.

Urinary Tract Infections

Infections of the urinary tract can result from a problem within the system, or as a secondary response to infection in other areas of the body. Some common causes may be improper catheter technique; contaminated equipment; prolonged use of a catheter; stasis or limited flow of urine out of the bladder; kidney stones; contaminated irrigating solution; or inadequate amounts of fluid intake. In most cases, prevention or prompt medical attention can decrease the incidence of urinary tract infections.

Some signs of a urinary tract infection are fever; cloudy urine; increased odor; pus or mucus in the urine; altered blood values (indicating infection); change in urine output; increased pulse; chills; and gastrointestinal complaints. Treatment will be made based on the results of urine, and possibly blood, analysis. If the urine specimen has been contaminated or left sitting at room temperature for a long time, results may be altered. The most common treatment is antibiotic therapy, and increased fluid intake is important. Fluids should be increased so that there is a urine output of at least 1,500 to 2,000 cc/ml a day, unless otherwise indicated by your doctor.

A variety of medications are used to treat the urinary tract and kidneys . Many drugs are excreted through the kidneys. Drugs that may have a direct effect on the urinary tract are diuretics; anti-cancer drugs; some antibiotics; drugs that alter pH of the urine; and drugs that anesthetize the urinary tract. Kidney disorders may interfere or even prevent the elimination of these drugs. This can cause severe damage to the kidneys or produce toxic levels of these drugs throughout the body. With some extremely toxic drugs, such as chemotherapeutic agents, it is necessary to establish adequate kidney functions before these drugs are given.

Some drugs, when eliminated through the kidneys, will change the color of the urine. Don't be surprised when your patient's urine is blue, or orange, or even red after he takes these drugs. When urine is meant to be red, you have to be careful that it is not blood as well; the red color may mask actual bleeding. In this case, look for the formation of blood clots or any strands of red in the urine. Bleeding may be an important indicator of kidney irritation from drugs. Be sure you know your medication and what to expect from it. If you already are aware of side effects, you will not be surprised or unnecessarily worried.

Obtaining Urine Specimens

When obtaining any type of urine specimen for analysis, you should know: What type of specimen is needed? How much urine is necessary? What equipment is needed? How should the specimen be stored? How soon must it be sent to the lab or doctor's office? Label the specimen with the following: the patient's name, the contents, date and time the specimen was obtained, and type (sterile or unsterile).

Urine specimens are obtained to determine a number of patient conditions and will help to rule out other problems. A urine specimen may be needed to check for microorganisms when evaluating for infection. The specimen is checked for color, volume, composition, odor, pH, specific gravity, and abnormalities (blood, pus, mucus). A "normal" urine sample should be a clear yellow and have a faint aroma. Normal volume is 1,200 to 1,500 cc/ml a day; the pH is 4.6 to 7.5 (acid); and the specific gravity is 1.005 to 1.025. Urine should show no abnormal amounts of protein, blood, sugar, pus, bacteria, or crystals. Observe your patient's urine daily for any abnormalities and report them to your doctor.

There are two types of urine specimens; sterile and unsterile. The unsterile urine specimen can be collected by having the patient urinate into a bedpan, urinal, or other container while at the toilet. If possible, it's better to have the patient urinate a small amount and then obtain the remaining urine for the specimen. About half a cup is necessary for evaluation.

To obtain a sterile or "clean catch" midstream urine specimen, the technique is somewhat different. This type of specimen must be uncontaminated. The patient's genitals should be cleaned with soap and water. The sterile container for the specimen usually comes with cleansing towelettes. Cleansing must be done three times, using a different towelette each time. For men: If your patient is uncircumsized, the foreskin of the penis should be lifted back. Begin at the center of the penis (urinary meatus) and, in a circular clockwise motion, clean to the outer surface. Do this three times, discarding the towelette each time. For women: Spread the labial folds (vaginal lips) open. Take the towelette and wipe down from front to back. Do one side, discard; the other side, discard; and then the center and discard. Continue holding the labia apart. Ask your patient to urinate a small amount to wash away any remaining bacteria. Then fill the container half way with urine and empty the rest of the bladder into the toilet. If your patient lacks this kind of control, it is sufficient only to clean the area as directed and collect the urine in the sterile container. Neither you, nor the patient, should touch the inside of the sterile container.

You also can obtain a sterile urine specimen from a catheter. There are two techniques for this: one involves opening the drainage system, which presents an added infection risk; the other involves collecting the urine with a needle and syringe inserted into a special adapter on the catheter. *Ask someone on the health care team for instructions in how to obtain these specimens and avoid exposing your patient to infection.* Don't just empty urine out of the patient's drainage bag for a sample because the urine may have been in the bag for some time, or the bag may have some microorganisms inside. In some cases, your doctor may allow you to take a specimen directly from the bag. To obtain a specimen from a catheter that has irrigating solution infusing, shut off the irrigating solution and allow the urine to drain for 30 minutes. Clamp the section of the brown catheter above the "Y" site for 30 minutes. Collect the specimen using whatever technique is recommended by your health care team.

Incontinent Patients

Patients who are unable to control bladder and bowel movements are termed incontinent. The causes of incontinence are many. Your patient may have neurological damage, making the relay of these messages to the brain impossible or delayed. The patient may be elderly, confused, or forgetful. Perhaps your patient lacks the necessary muscle control.

This type of patient will be difficult to manage, both from a practical sense and because of medical complications of incontinence. You may be able to deal with the problem by placing your patient on the toilet or bedpan at frequent intervals. This can be an effective way to keep the patient's bed dry, but it puts a tremendous burden on you. Some patients have problems only with urgency, and this can be solved with a bedside commode or bedpan placed close by.

Two major concerns with the incontinent patient are keeping the patient—and the bed— dry and clean, and looking after the patient's skin. Frequent episodes of incontinence cause skin to become irritated, just like that of a baby in diapers. Urine contains toxic substances that irritate and break down the skin surface if proper care is not given. The incontinent patient should be checked every two hours. With a man, you can try leaving a urinal between his legs, with his penis placed inside the urinal opening. Wrap a towel or absorbent pad around the urinal. It will not be easy to do this with a woman.

Disposable, absorbent pads can be bought in bulk from a medical supplier or pharmacy. Put them on the bed, covered with a folded sheet or soft under pad; the patient should not lie directly on these. Roll your patient to one side; roll the under pad materials halfway (in the way you change an occupied bed); and place beside the patient. They should touch the patient's lower back to the middle of the thigh for proper absorption. Now have the patient roll over the materials and pull them through. Be sure the bed is free of wrinkles. Removal is done in the same fashion: Prepare your fresh materials; turn the patient on his side; roll all the soiled materials in against the patient; place your clean ones in at the same time. Roll the patient over the materials, remove the soiled ones, and pull through the clean ones.

With the incontinent patient, not only should the linens be changed, but the patient should be cleaned throughly. Use a wash basin of warm water and soap. Clean the entire area; buttocks, lower thighs, in between the legs, and genitals. Remember, when cleaning a female patient, always cleanse by going from front to back, and by using a different section of the towel each time. Rinse with a second basin of water. Be sure to dry the patient well, giving special attention to areas where two skin surfaces overlap. You may put some talcum powder on your patient—but not too much.

Check with your pharmacy, medical supplier, or supermarket for absorbent disposable briefs sized for adults (Depend is one widely sold type). These are useful for fully incontinent patients, or those with less severe problems with bladder control.

In some patients, even frequent attention will not be an effective or efficient way of managing incontinence. Special devices, such as catheters, may be recommended by the health care team. If your patient is male, a condom catheter can be applied directly on the penis. This external device is connected to a drainage tube and bag for urine collection. There is no risk of internal complications with this type of device, but it is often difficult to hold in place and can fall off.

Proper and secure placement is important. Clean your patient's penis carefully with soap and water. Rinse it thoroughly and dry. Roll the condom over the penis. You will have either a Velcro™ or rubber tape-like piece to secure the condom in place. Wrap it tightly, but not so tightly that you cut off the circulation.

Some condom catheters come with an adhesive strip that is wrapped around the penis first, about one inch from the scrotum. After the adhesive strip is secure, remove the adhesive covering from the other side; this will stick to the condom sheathe. Now roll the condom over the penis. Connect the condom to the drainage tubing and bag.

The condom catheter should be removed daily, in order to clean and air out the penis. Check the skin for irritation. If there is irritation, perhaps you have applied the condom incorrectly or your patient's skin is extremely sensitive, possibly limiting the use of this type of catheter. Inspect the catheter for twists or kinks in the tubing. Empty the drainage bag at least every eight hours.

Urinary Catheters

Special rubber or plastic sterile catheters may have to be used on some patients with urinary tract problems. A catheter may be recommended if blockage prevents passage out of the patient's bladder or if excessive amounts of urine are retained in the bladder. Frequent incontinence, obtaining sterile urine specimens, or infusing special solutions are other reasons to place a catheter.

This small, sterile catheter is passed up through the patient's urethra and into the bladder. It is known as a Foley catheter, retention catheter, or indwelling catheter. Catheter placement usually is done by a nurse, doctor, or orderly, at home or in the hospital. It is a relatively simple procedure, and the insertion will cause little or no discomfort. There may be some circumstances when the care giver, or even the patient, will be instructed in catheter insertion.

The most important consideration in catheter placement is that it must be done under sterile conditions. If not, infection can result. After placement of the catheter is ascertained, usually by the appearance of urine flowing through the catheter, a small balloon at the end of the catheter is inflated with air or a sterile water solution. This is done to be sure that the catheter remains in the patient's bladder.

If it is to be left in place, the catheter is connected to a closed drainage system. The urine will drain out of the bladder, through the catheter, into the connecting tube, and into a sealed drainage bag. This is done by gravity, so the bag must always be at a lower level than the patient. If it remains at the same level as the patient, or higher, the urine will not drain out of the bladder. If your patient is in bed, the drainage bag should be placed below the bed. These bags are made to hook onto the bed. The same technique should be used if the patient is in a chair, although the bag should be off the floor. You may need to be creative; if you have nothing to hang the bag from, perhaps a coat hanger, some string, or a safety pin can be used to help hang the bag beside the bed or chair.

The catheter can be held in place with tape; in women, tape it to the inner thigh, for men, to the thigh or abdomen. This will help to avoid direct tension or pulling at the catheter insertion site. This sturdy tubing should pass over the patient's thigh and out to the side of the bed. It can be fastened to the side of the bed by using a rubber band attached to the drainage tube and secured to the bed with tape.

The tube should not be kinked or obstructed. Some common signs that the catheter is not draining properly may be: the catheter has slipped out of the patient; there is wetness under the patient; urine is leaking around the catheter insertion site; the tubing is kinked or closed off; the drainage bag is not lower than the patient; the patient's abdomen is enlarged; or the patient complains of pain. If you see any of these signs, check the drainage system. Make sure it is positioned properly, the catheter is in the patient, and there are no leaks, holes, or punctures. Be extremely careful if using scissors or sharp devices near the catheter or tubing. Is the bag hanging below the patient? Are all connection sites in place and tightly secured? If you check all these areas and don't find the source of the problem, contact the home health team.

If you or your patient are taught to do catheter insertion at home, be sure to note the amount of urine removed from the bladder following insertion; this may be significant to your physician. Some doctors do not want more than 800 cc/ml of urine removed at one time. Ask your physician about this. If the patient has urine in his bladder beyond that amount, your doctor may recommend that the catheter be clamped for a short time before allowing additional drainage.

If your patient is turning or will be getting up to walk, don't forget the catheter tubing and bag—it always goes with the patient and must be kept low. Both men and women can wear catheter leg bags, which make movement with a catheter less confining. Leg bags come in various sizes to meet individual needs and can be used by patients with indwelling catheters or by men with external condom catheters.

The top of the bag should be just below the knee and the bottom portion should be attached to the calf, on the outside of the leg. It should be tight enough to secure the bag, but not so tight that circulation is impaired. Be sure the plug is in the bottom of the leg bag. Clean all connection sites with an alcohol sponge before disconnecting and connecting the catheter to the leg bag drainage tubes. Be sure the tubes are not bent or kinked. The leg bag can be emptied by raising the patient's pant leg, taking out the plug, and draining the urine into a measuring container. Empty the bag regularly; if it gets too full, urine can back up into the bladder and cause infection. Be sure to record output, if required, before disposing of urine.

After removing the leg bag, it should be cleaned throughly with soap and water and left to air dry. Have two extra bags available.

If your loved one is restless or confused, he may accidently pull out this catheter, inflated balloon and all. Such a patient may need to be restrained (see page 21). If your patient pulls out the catheter, it may cause trauma to the urinary tract, such as slight bleeding or irritation. Report this to your physician. Catheters sometimes fall out on their own. The balloon may not be inflated properly or it may have a leak. If the catheter has been left in place for a long time, the balloon can slowly become deflated. If your patient's catheter does fall out, your doctor will determine whether it must be reinserted. Even if you have been trained in catheter insertion, *do not make this decision on your own and never use the same catheter.*

Whenever your patient has a catheter in place, you should be supplied with a catheter clamp. Use only this special clamp and no other unless you have permission from a health care professional. Catheters are clamped for a number of reasons: to temporarily stop the flow of urine from the bladder; to provide bladder muscle exercises; to obtain urine specimens; to connect new tubing; or whenever disconnecting the catheter.

The clamp must be placed on the tubing you wish to block off. If you want irrigating solution to go into the patient, but do not want urine flowing out, clamp the clear portion of the connecting tubing. To block flow out of the bladder, clamp the brown portion of tubing above the "Y." Be sure you vary the area you clamp each time, so that one section does not become worn. Don't forget to unclamp the catheter as ordered. If you forget, the patient's bladder will fill up with urine and he may complain of pain, an urgency to urinate, or a bloated abdomen. Check immediately to see whether you forgot to unclamp the catheter. The clamp should be clean, not sterile, and can be washed with soap and water.

Daily Catheter Care

Instructions for daily care of catheter patients vary from hospital to hospital. Here are some standard procedures for daily urinary catheter care; if they differ from your instructions, be sure to follow guidelines set by your home health team.

Observe your patient regularly for catheter placement and urine output. Make sure drainage tubes are clear, not kinked, and that urine flows freely. Care for the catheter when your patient has his daily bed bath. (A patient with an indwelling urinary catheter cannot take a tub bath or shower.) Always wash your hands before you begin.

1. Clean the genital area with soap and water, leaving the actual catheter area until last.
2. Inspect the entire catheter system for problems. It is common for mucus or crust to accumulate around the area where the catheter is inserted. Note any irritation or discharge.
3. Organize your catheter care equipment (kits are available) and put on sterile gloves. You will need sterile cotton balls, cleansing solution, a solution container, a wastebasket, and proper lighting.
4. Take a sterile cotton ball and dip it into some cleansing solution. For women, hold the labia apart as you cleanse; for uncircumsized men, push back the foreskin. Remove any crust or drainage by starting close to where the catheter is inserted and wiping away. Do this three times, using a new cotton ball each time, or until all of the drainage is removed. Some doctors recommend an antibacterial cream or ointment applied at this time.
5. Untape the catheter from the leg, check the skin for irritation, remove any excess adhesive, and wash the area. Reapply the tape on another section of the inner thigh, or use the opposite thigh. You can place a rubber band on the drainage tube (use a slip knot), and attach a safety pin to the rubber band. The excess tubing can now be pinned or taped to the edge of the bed so it isn't left hanging.

The catheter drainage bag should be emptied at least every eight hours. Use a large measuring cup, big enough to hold large amounts of urine without overflowing. The bottom of the catheter bag should have a nozzle with a clamp attached. Put the nozzle inside the container, unclamp the nozzle, and allow the urine to flow out of the bag into the container. When the bag is empty, reclamp the nozzle and insert it into its special bracket. Place the bag in proper position. Measure and record your patient's output.

Opinions vary as to how long the catheter should remain in place. A common recommendation is that the catheter should be changed every 30 days. If it becomes blocked, if there is increased sediment, or if you note leakage, the catheter and tubing may need to be changed. Check with your doctor to find out how often your patient's catheter should be changed. You may want to remind someone on the health care team when a catheter change is due.

Irrigating the Catheter

Catheter irrigation is recommended to help keep the drainage system open and free of sediment, to flush a catheter plugged by sediment, or to instill antiseptic or medicated solutions into the bladder. Open or closed drainage techniques are used; ask someone on the health care team for training in closed drainage catheter irrigation, which requires a needle and syringe.

Open drainage catheter irrigation is more common. *This procedure requires sterile technique.* You will need irrigating solution, a special irrigating syringe and receptacle, sterile gloves, bedpan or basin, a plastic absorbent pad, and an alcohol sponge. Sterile irrigating kits are available. If the irrigating solution has been refrigerated, warm it to room temperature first. Always wash your hands before you begin.

1. Place the absorbent pad partially under the patient's buttocks; the other portion should be under the catheter connection site.
2. Place your equipment next to the patient's bed on a clean, flat surface. The patient should be lying flat in bed. Clamp the catheter.
3. Place all supplies on the sterile field. If you are using a kit, the inside wrapper provides a sterile surface.
4. Pour the irrigating solution into your sterile receptacle (do not instill cold solution).
5. Fill your irrigating syringe with 50 cc/ml (or a specified amount) of irrigating solution. Leave in the receptacle until ready to use.
6. Open your alcohol sponges and place on the sterile field. Put on your sterile gloves.
7. Clean the catheter connection site with the alcohol sponge. Disconnect the catheter. If the patient is able to help, he can hold the drainage system portion of the catheter while you hold the patient's catheter with your non-dominant hand.
8. Take your irrigating syringe and connect it to the catheter. Unclamp the catheter.
9. Slowly push the prescribed amount into the patient's catheter. If you need to refill the syringe to meet the prescribed amount, do so. Do not force the solution into the catheter. If it does not flow smoothly, stop the irrigation and report the incident to the doctor. There probably is something blocking the catheter.
10. Now hold the catheter over the bedpan or container to catch the excess drainage from the irrigation. The catheter tip should not touch anything or it will be contaminated.
11. Wipe the catheter tip and the drainage tube connection with the alcohol sponge, allow them to dry, and reconnect the two pieces.
12. Discard all used equipment. Wash your hands, and the patient's, if he helped.

Bladder Irrigation

Your patient may need to receive solutions directly into his bladder. This process, known as bladder irrigation, is a relatively easy procedure. Be extra careful about giving the proper solution and medication dose, and establishing the correct flow rate (usually 30 to 60 drops per minute). Bladder irrigation requires a three-way catheter; one portion for the infusing solution, another for the urine to flow out, and a third piece to inflate the balloon inside the bladder.

Continuous bladder irrigation means that solutions will be infused on a continuous basis into the patient's bladder. The solution usually is sterile water, sterile salt water, or a solution containing antibiotics. This process can be used to break up blood clots; break up or dilute particles in the urine; or to treat or prevent infections. Check to see how these solutions should be stored, that they are labeled correctly, and that the expiration date is on the label. They may or may not be pre-mixed. The mixing procedure is much like that of adding a medication to an IV solution (see Chapter 8 on medications). The bottle should arrive sealed, unless it has been premixed. In that case, the seal may be broken.

If you will be adding the medication yourself, be sure you have the exact dose. Once the medication has been added, most solutions require refrigeration. Warm the solution to room temperature (about 30 minutes). Do not infuse cold; it will cause muscle spasms and cramps. Find out how fast to run the infusion, how much to give the patient, and over what period of time. Your doctor or nurse will provide you with the rate.

If your doctor has asked you to record urine output, be sure to subtract the amount of irrigating solution infused. Calculate this every eight hours. For example, if your patient's total urine output over eight hours is 1,000 cc/ml and the amount of irrigating solution was 500 cc/ml, then the total urine output is 500 cc/ml. The total urine flow should be equal or slightly more than the amount of solution infused.

Before beginning bladder irrigation, wash your hands and gather your equipment.

1. Prepare your solution, check the label and medication dose.
2. Place the solution and container on a flat surface. Insert the administration tubing into the top of the container; most of these are inserted by a spike adapter or by screwing a cap in place.
3. Close the flow clamp, invert the container, and place on the pole provided to hang the solution. The pole should be at the foot of the patient's bed.
4. Slowly open the flow clamp and allow the solution to run down the tubing until it runs out through the connecting tip (just a few drops). Reclamp.
5. Wash the "in" outlet on the catheter with an alcohol sponge. Connect the bottom tubing to the outlet. Be careful not to contaminate any connection sites with your hands.
6. Slowly open the flow clamp and adjust your drip rate. (See page 55 for calculating drip rates.) Mark your bottle for easy observation of flow rate. To keep the flow rate clamp from moving, place a piece of tape over the clamp after you have adjusted the flow rate.
7. Be sure you have your next bottle or container of solution ready before the one in place runs out. Check to see that the solution and urine flow are not impaired in any way. Watch the drainage bag; it may need frequent emptying.

8. On your intake and output sheet, record the type and amount of solution and time of infusion. Your patient's urine should be clear and free of sediment at this time. Report any unusual observations or problems to your doctor.

Intermittent bladder irrigation is the same procedure, but done only at specific intervals. The doctor's order may read: bladder irrigation of normal saline, every four hours, infuse 100 cc/ml over 30 minutes. The flow rate probably will be calculated for you; if not, see page 55. Between irrigations, the entire irrigation tubing may be disconnected, or you will clamp only the irrigation portion. Record the amount of solution for each infusion, and remember to subtract that amount from the total urine output at eight-hour intervals. Find out how long the solution can be used before it will have to be discarded and how frequently you should change the connection tubing.

Removing a Catheter

The catheter can be removed by deflating the balloon within the bladder. *Never remove the catheter without specific instructions from your physician.* Wash your hands before you begin.

1. Clean the portion where the catheter was inflated with an alcohol sponge.
2. Attach the syringe.
3. Pull back on the plunger and withdraw the exact amount of air or fluid that had been injected into the balloon when the catheter was inserted.
4. Grasp the catheter and gently remove it. If you feel any resistance, it may indicate the balloon is not completely deflated. Try again. If you still feel resistance, *do not attempt to remove the catheter.* Call your doctor.
5. Dispose of the used catheter.

Be sure to record the final amount of urine in the catheter bag. Your patient may feel the need to urinate, so offer a bedpan. However, the bladder probably will be empty and your patient will not actually have to urinate for a few hours. Watch for the first urination (probably within four to six hours). By this time, if your patient is not urinating, or passing only very small amounts of urine, report this to the doctor. Encourage fluids after the catheter is removed. If the catheter has been in place for a long time, the muscle tone of the bladder may be weak. Your doctor may order bladder toning exercises before removal of the catheter.

Other Types of Catheters

Other types of catheters are inserted into the bladder, but not through the urinary meatus. Some catheters are surgically inserted directly into the bladder or a kidney. The catheter may be clamped off and used intermittently, only when the patient needs to empty his bladder. The basic care of the catheter is the same, although sterile technique may not be required. In the case of a surgical incision, a tube is left in place until healing occurs around the catheter. You will be given specific instructions in care of the incision. The doctor will determine when it is appropriate for the patient to begin removing the catheter.

Some of these tubes require irrigation, cleansing of the catheter, fluid monitoring, and dressing changes. They can become plugged, requiring prompt attention. These tubes usually are placed when the patient has long-term chronic needs, or when the lower portion of the urinary tract is not functioning due to surgery, disease, or obstruction. Care of these patients is highly individualized; consult your health care team for guidance.

Urinary Stomas

A urinary stoma is created when surgery diverts the passage of urine into a portion of the patient's intestine. This loop of the intestines is then led out through the wall of the abdomen and a temporary, or permanent, opening is left in the abdomen. (When ureters are looped out through the abdomen, it is called a ureterostomy.) Care of the stoma will depend on how much time has elapsed since surgery. Usually, a bag is attached over the stoma to collect urine.

Immediately following surgery, the skin around the area is quite sensitive and special care must be given to this area. Your patient will be hospitalized about two weeks. Since urine is constantly being drained out of the stoma, a tight seal is necessary between the stoma, the urine collection bag, and the skin. Leaks can cause skin problems.

Pay attention to urine odor. If it is foul-smelling, it may indicate medical problems. Fluids usually should be increased to flush the system and decrease sediment or thick, foul-smelling urine.

The urinary appliance and its accompanying pieces of equipment may be disposable or reusable. The equipment will depend on the placement and size of the stoma, the patient's activity, and economic resources. As healing occurs, the stoma will shrink, requiring frequent measurements for appliance fittings. Eventually, the stoma will shrink to a permanent size and shape.

Daily Stoma Care

The frequency with which the collecting appliance should be changed will vary based on the patient's needs and the doctor's recommendations. It usually is changed weekly. The bag is emptied as often as necessary and should not be allowed to become so full that it pulls on the appliance holder, loosening the seal. Most bags have a valve that can be opened to drain off urine. A special drainage system may be used at night, so that urine flows freely without interrupting the sleeping patient. Leg bags are available for urine collection; some patients prefer these because they bulge less.

A deodorizer can be used in the bag or a few drops of vinegar can be placed in the bottom of the bag to prevent odor. The patient also can control odor through diet. Increasing fluid intake, cranberry juice, and foods or juices containing ascorbic acid will help cut down on odor. Your doctor may prescribe an oral preparation that will help with odor control.

When changing an appliance, provide privacy. A good time to do this is early in the morning, before the patient has had anything to drink. Always wash your hands before beginning.

1. Gather your equipment.
2. Moisten the adhesive covering with soap and water, or use a special adhesive solvent. (Some patients use only plastic skin barriers.)
3. Before removing the appliance, the patient should bend over quickly to allow optimum emptying of urine. Remove the appliance. If the stoma continues to seep urine, the patient can place a clean piece of gauze or a tampon in it.
4. Wash the skin with soap and water. (Don't use oily soaps.) Gently pat dry with a towel. Check the skin for irritation.
5. Make every effort to keep the skin dry and free of urine. Apply adhesive or skin barrier as directed by your home care team. Allow it to air dry before applying the bag.

6. Center the appliance over the stoma, making it adhere tightly to the adhesive surface.
7. Put on the appliance holder belt, if your patient wears one, making sure it is not too tight.

Urine crystals on the stoma are more common if your patient wears reusable appliances. These are white, gritty particles that may cause irritation or stoma bleeding. To prevent this, make sure the pouch is properly cleaned, keep urine acidic, and make sure the appliance fits well. To clean a reusable appliance, rinse it in warm water and soak it in vinegar, soap, and water for 30 minutes. Rinse and allow to air dry. Sprinkle with cornstarch to prevent brittleness when storing. Your patient should have a minimum of two appliances so a clean one is always available.

Your patient may be trained to do his own care, and if able, should be encouraged to do so. Your loved one may have a problem accepting this condition at first. Contact your nurse, doctor, or social worker about local ostomy associations to provide support. Read the end of this chapter for more information about the psychology of the ostomy patient.

Bowel Function

Food digestion and absorption occur in the small and large intestines. The stomach empties into the small intestines, which are about ten inches long, where nutrients are absorbed. In the large intestines, certain vitamins are manufactured, absorption of nutrients is completed, and feces (stool) are formed. The expulsion of feces takes place in the lower segment of the large intestine, which is about five feet long (extending from the ileum to the anus).

Digested food and food by-products are moved along the intestines by means of a churning, wave-like movement. When one area of the intestines becomes full, the walls contract and squeeze the digested food along into the next section. By the time food arrives at the large intestines, digestion and absorption are almost complete. These contents may remain in the large intestines for three to ten hours. During this time, the contents become solid or semisolid as a result of fluid absorption.

The same motions push the fecal material into the rectum. Distension of the wall of the rectum stimulates nerves in the area, indicating a reflex for the patient to move his bowels. The feces are then pushed out of the body through the anus. A number of problems can occur in this process. If the churning motion speeds up, diarrhea may result. If this motion slows down, there may be constipation or an intestinal obstruction. If there are abnormal amounts of gas released in the process of food breakdown, the patient will have gas trapped or escaping out of the intestines (flatus). If there is a problem with the transfer of nerve impulses that indicate the need to defecate, there may be bowel incontinence. Some of these problems can be easily corrected; others will require diagnostic testing or even surgery.

External factors that may affect bowel function are diet, bed rest, decreased activity, and some drugs. Internal problems may be caused by prolonged retention of fecal matter, blockage caused by a tumor or structural defect, infection or irritation to the intestinal wall, or lack of food and fluid intake.

Some common symptoms of intestinal problems are fullness or bloating; loss of appetite; indigestion; excess gas; no bowel movement for more than two days; excess bowel movements; change in bowel habits; anemia; changes in stool color and consistency; excess odor; or blood or mucus in the stool. One or more of these symptoms may indicate a problem that needs medical attention.

Diarrhea

Diarrhea is defined as loose, watery stools occurring frequently. The patient with diarrhea has increased movement or irritation to the intestines, causing most substances to be moved out of the intestines at a much faster rate than usual. The stool does not stay in the intestines long enough to become formed. Diarrhea can cause irritation of the rectum and surrounding skin; loss of fluid, nutrients, vitamins, and minerals; and electrolyte loss resulting in muscle weakness, tremors, or convulsions.

To treat diarrhea, stop putting food into the intestines; let them rest. Medications that will relax intestinal spasms may be taken if the doctor recommends them. Some of these are sold over the counter; others require a prescription. Some drugs used to treat diarrhea are Lomotil, Kaopectate (kaolin and pectin), bismuth, and paregoric. Antispasmodics, sedatives, or tranquilizers are sometimes prescribed for diarrhea.

If fluid loss has been excessive, it must be replaced. This may not be possible via the oral route, as the intestines are irritated. Some patients may require intravenous replacement of fluids. A patient with frequent episodes of severe diarrhea will become dehydrated and need prompt fluid replacement.

For the bedridden patient with diarrhea, keep the bedpan or bedside commode nearby. Put an absorbent pad beneath your patient. Allow your patient to wash his buttocks often with soap and warm water. If you are washing the patient, be gentle; the anal area will be extremely sore and irritated.

After your patient's colon has rested, foods should be introduced slowly. Start with clear liquids: broths, tea, ginger ale, water. Then advance to full liquids: soups, ice cream, Cream of Wheat. If the patient tolerates these, try semisolid foods and then return to a regular diet.

Hemorrhoids

Hemorrhoids are varicose veins in the rectum and anal area. They can occur inside or outside the anal sphincter. External hemorrhoids appear as small, reddish-blue lumps, and can be quite painful. Certain conditions can predispose a patient to hemorrhoids, such as pregnancy, constipation, diarrhea, tumors, and hereditary factors. Look for the following symptoms indicating hemorrhoids: swollen, painful lumps outside the anal area; pain during bowel movements; or slight bleeding in the anal area. These symptoms will vary depending on the size and location of the hemorrhoids.

Over-the-counter hemorrhoid creams and ointments contain local anesthetics. Most of these creams will not require a doctor's prescription (Nupercaine, Anusol, Preparation H). The cream is applied to the external hemorrhoid as needed. The care taker can use a piece of gauze, tissue paper, or a cotton swab to apply the cream. This does not require sterile technique. The patient should be encouraged to take warm baths, which may help relieve pain. Try to avoid constipation, which increases hemorrhoid pain. Changes in diet or medications to soften the stools will help.

When the condition is serious, surgical removal may be necessary. This is one of the most common surgical procedures done on adults. It is relatively routine, sometimes even done on an outpatient basis. General care of the post-operative hemorrhoidectomy patient (one who has had a hemorrhoid removed) consists of caring for the dressing site (if there is one) and providing pain medication. There usually is a great deal of pain after the surgery. Help your patient get comfortable. Sometimes patients are given a rubber doughnut ring to sit on so there is no pressure to the surgical area. However, some doctors feel that this ring may add pressure.

Consult your physician about this. Provide stool softeners so your patient will not have to strain when moving his bowels.

Sitz baths often are recommended to improve circulation and promote healing. The pelvic region is immersed in warm water (110 to 115° F or 43.3 to 46.1° C) for 15 to 30 minutes. You may have to add more warm water during the bath to maintain the temperature. A portable sitz bath basin or bathtub can be used. Help your patient into the bath, if necessary. If your patient cannot tolerate this, remove him from the bath and report it to the doctor. When your patient has finished the bath, pat the area dry with a clean towel. If a dressing needs to be reapplied, it should be done at this time. Have your patient lie on his side while you apply the dressing, which usually is a clean gauze pad. After a sitz bath, your patient should lie in bed for 30 minutes to allow circulation to return to normal. Sitz baths are not recommended for a patient who has a cardiac condition, is bedridden, or confused.

Constipation

Most people establish a "normal" bowel routine, but circumstances may alter it from day to day. Sometimes changes bring on constipation, which is an abnormal infrequency of stools (feces). When a patient is constipated, the color and consistency of the stools can change (they will be abnormally dry).

Illness may affect a patient's bowel routine. A tumor or mass may be positioned so that the intestines are partially or completely blocked. Prolonged bed rest, certain medications, or diet may affect intestinal movement so that passage of stool is slowed down, or even stopped.

Whenever a change in the patient's bowel pattern is noted, it should be reported and the causes investigated. The doctor can establish a diagnosis based on a number of observations. Any information you or the patient can provide will be helpful. The doctor may feel the patient's abdomen for fullness, bloating, or tenderness. Diagnostic X-rays may be ordered. Radiographic dye may be passed through the gastrointestinal tract and photographed so the doctor can observe the medication's passage. Some devices allow the physician to look into the gastrointestinal tract for problems.

In some patients, constipation is caused by bed rest, diet changes, pain medication, or poor eating habits. These problems may be corrected with stool softeners, diet changes, laxatives, or enemas. If your patient still has no relief, the doctor or nurse may have to manually check the rectum for impacted stool. This should be done only by a qualified medical professional.

Prevention is the most effective treatment for constipation. If your patient is allowed, offer foods high in roughage and fiber (fruits with skins, prunes, whole grain cereals and breads, vegetables). Provide plenty of fluids. Encourage exercise. A patient on medications that may cause constipation (narcotics, sedatives, some antibiotics) should prevent this condition through diet, stool softeners, or laxatives. This is one important reason for knowing as much as possible about the medications your patient takes and their possible side effects.

Get your doctor's permission before administering oral laxatives or cathartics. Be sure you are using the correct preparation and proper dose, know when to give it, whether it should be mixed with anything, and when it will work. Make sure your patient will have easy access to the bathroom or a bedpan. You may have to help a patient who will be using a bedpan; try to place him in a high sitting position.

Avoid excessive use of laxatives; they can diminish normal bowel activity if used too often. If there are no results, the doctor may order that the medication dose be repeated, or that alternatives, such as enemas, be used.

Constipation can be treated with any of the following:

Stool Softeners.　　　These medications act as wetting-agents, permitting water and fatty material to penetrate and mix with fecal material, resulting in a softer stool. These usually are taken daily and their use should be discontinued if the reverse effect occurs (diarrhea or loose, runny stools).

Contact Laxatives.　　　These drugs act by stimulating the nerve endings in the lining of the intestines. This causes movement inside the intestines, helping to move the stool along and out of the intestines. If taken orally, results are seen in six hours; if taken by rectal suppository, results can occur in 20 to 60 minutes. A contact laxative is one of the gentlest forms of laxatives.

Bulk Cathartics.　　　These medications help to increase bulk in the intestines. They must be mixed well in water, fruit juice, or milk. Bulk cathartics contain salt, so a patient on a salt-restricted diet should not use them. Follow the medication with an additional glass of water for best results. Bulk foods can be used in place of this medication (raw vegetables, fruits, bread, cereals, other grain products).

Lubricants.　　　These medications lubricate and soften fecal contents, making movement along the intestines easier. A common lubricant is mineral oil. It should not be given with meals; it doesn't taste very good. Mixing it with fruit juice may help to conceal the taste. Give your patient a slice of orange or lemon to suck afterward to cut the oil taste. Results usually occur in six hours. The best time to take this preparation is before bedtime.

Irritant Laxatives.　　　These laxatives increase movement in the intestines by irritating the intestinal lining and muscles. Castor oil is a well-known irritant laxative. It does not taste very good; try mixing it with fruit juice. This is a very powerful laxative that usually works within six hours. Don't use this to relieve mild constipation; it is generally used to provide full bowel cleanout for X-rays.

Saline Laxatives.　　　These laxatives act by binding water in the stool and providing liquid bulk in the intestines, helping to promote evacuation of stool. Milk of magnesia is a saline laxative used for mild constipation. Expect results within six hours.

Suppositories.　　　Rectal suppositories irritate the lining of the intestinal mucosa, stimulating movement in the intestines and the urge to move one's bowels. They usually are small, solid, cone-shaped masses composed of a glycerin base. (See page 105 for insertion techniques.) The suppository should be retained as long as possible, at least 20 minutes for optimum results. Keep a bedpan or commode close by. Most suppositories should be kept refrigerated until ready to use.

Enemas

An enema is the instillation of a solution into the rectum. There are two basic types of enemas; the retention enema and the irrigating enema. The retention enema is held in the rectum for at least 20 minutes, often longer. Most of the oil-based commercial products are used as retention enemas (Fleets). A retention enema acts by mechanical irritation on the walls of the lining of the rectum, eventually stimulating bowel evacuation.

With an irrigating enema, solutions are run into the patient's rectum. The patient will feel cramping and, usually within 15 minutes, the enema will be expelled. Irrigating enemas come commercially prepared or must be mixed at home. They contain a large amount of water mixed with soap or other bowel irritants. An irrigating enema acts by stimulating movement along the lower intestines, causing distention or swelling that will trigger the message to the patient that he must move his bowels.

Enemas can be used to clean out the bowel for diagnostic tests; to relieve constipation; or to relieve gas or other intestinal disorders. Medicines also can be instilled through an enema to sooth irritated tissues, counteract bacterial conditions of the intestines, or change the pH within the intestines.

An enema should not be used on someone who has had recent colon or rectal surgery, a recent heart attack, or any acute abdominal pain.

Do not force entry of the enema tubing and do not infuse the solution too quickly. Be very careful if your patient has hemorrhoids. Have your patient gently bear down when the tube is inserted. Make sure the enema solution is not too hot or cold. Enemas can cause dizziness, weakness, or make a patient faint. Discontinue the enema if any of these symptoms occur and report to your doctor. No more than three enemas should be given in a 24-hour period, and additional enemas should not be given unless ordered by a doctor.

Chronic use of enemas or laxatives can cause irritation to the lining of the intestines, create problems with muscle tone, and cause anal sphincter problems. Eventually the patient must rely on laxatives or enemas as the only means of bowel evacuation.

If your patient's output is being measured, be sure to record the amount of stool obtained. If your patient had poor results, report this to the doctor. Some patients need oral laxatives as well as an enema for effective evacuation.

To administer an enema, have the proper amount and type of solution, an enema administration kit, lubricant, absorbent pads, rubber gloves, and something to hang the solution from (IV pole or hook). If the enema is to be warm, it should be no hotter than 100 to 105° F (37.8 to 40.6° C). If the enema is too hot, it can burn the patient. The amount of solution will vary. The normal volume for an irrigating enema is 750 to 1,000 cc/ml. A retention enema is a lot less voluminous, usually 100 to 350 cc/ml.

Have your patient urinate first, if necessary. The patient should be positioned on his left side, with his knees pulled up. A sitting position will not allow for the solution to extend far enough into the rectum, and will serve only to trigger rapid explusion. Place absorbent pads under the patient to prevent the bed from becoming wet and soiled. Have a bedpan or bedside commode nearby, or have close access to the toilet. Provide patient privacy for this procedure and always wash your hands before you begin.

1. Prepare the enema. Check for the right solution, the amount, and any substance to be added. Be sure that the tubing has been clamped before you start to fill the bag with solution. If you are using water as a base, fill the bag with water first, then add the soap. Gently mix the solution around, being careful not to create a bag full of bubbles. Hang the bag on the pole and open the clamp so that the solution is allowed to run through the full length of the tube. Re-clamp.
2. Lubricate the tip of the enema tube (the portion that will be inserted into the patient's rectum). Put on your rubber gloves.
3. Tell your patient to relax; slow, deep breaths may relax the muscle around the rectum (anal sphincter).
4. Spread the buttocks so that you are able to see the rectum.
5. Gently advance the tubing into the patient's rectum Ask your doctor how far to introduce the tubing; generally the tubing should be placed about four inches inside the rectum. Never force the tubing. You may feel some resistance, especially if the patient has a large amount of stool in the lower rectum. Try to release a small amount of the enema solution to loosen up the stool so that the tubing may be advanced. If there is excess stool in the rectum, the tip of the tube

may become plugged with feces. If so, take out the tubing, clean out the tube, and begin the procedure again. If you still meet resistance, remove the tube and consult your doctor or nurse.

6. After insertion (the solution bag should be slightly above the bed level), open the clamp on the tubing and begin the flow of the solution into your patient. If this is a retention enema, the flow will be much slower than an irrigating enema in order to promote retention of the enema. You can adjust the flow rate by using the clamp or lowering or raising the enema bag. (Raising it increases the flow rate.) If the solution runs too fast, it can cause severe cramping, rapid dilation of the intestines, and possibly intestinal injury.

7. Keep a close watch on your patient's tolerance. If he complains of severe cramping, pain, or the need to move his bowels, stop the infusion. This may only be caused by increased muscle tension. Tell your patient to relax and continue with his deep breathing. Gentle massage to his abdomen may relieve the cramping. You do not want the patient to expell the enema at this time, if at all possible. You can try to press the buttocks together to retain the enema. Now try to continue with the enema. Whenever the patient complains, stop the flow, wait a few minutes for the cramps to subside, and continue. The aim is to give as much of the prescribed solution as possible.

8. Stop the flow of solution while there is a small amount left in the bag, so that you do not introduce air into the intestines. Gently remove the tubing from the patient.

9. Your patient should try to retain the enema as long as directed. For an irrigating enema, 15 minutes; for a retention enema, 30 minutes. The patient can continue with his breathing techniques in an effort to provide muscle relaxation and distraction.

10. When the patient is ready to expell the enema, he can be helped onto the bedpan or bedside commode. If your patient will be walking to the bathroom, hold his arm; he may feel weak or faint.

11. Remove and dispose of all soiled equipment and materials. Most enema equipment can be cleaned with soap and water and reused.

12. Results of the enema should be observed and reported. Look for amount, consistency, color, and the presence of any abnormalities (blood or mucus). Your patient should be encourged to rest in bed for 30 minutes following an enema.

Commercial, small-volume retention enemas can be administered by the patient or the care giver. It's best to give this type of enema before a meal. Use the following procedure:

1. Follow preliminary steps listed above for all enemas.
2. Take the plastic covering off the top of the container.
3. Most commercial preparations are pre-lubricated; you may wish to apply an additional amount. Insert the container's nozzle into the rectum.
4. Squeeze the container, emptying the contents into the rectum. The patient should try to retain this as long as possible, at least 30 minutes for a good result.
5. Discard the used container.

Sometimes barium is given in a liquid form, which the patient either drinks or receives through an enema. Barium contains a special material that enables it to be seen on an X-ray.

This substance can become hardened in the intestines and cause bowel obstruction if it is not removed. Your patient may need an oral laxative or enema to remove this from the intestines. Following a procedure using barium, your patient's stool will appear a chalky white for 24 to 72 hours after the test.

Stool Specimens

Stool samples are collected for a number of reasons. The doctor may want to evaluate the amount, odor, color and consistency of stool, and check for bacteria or abnormal substances. If you must obtain a stool sample, find out the following: How much do you need to collect? When should it be collected? What should you put it in? How should you store it? What does the doctor want you to do with it?

The patient will have to move his bowels in a bedpan for you to collect a stool sample. When he has finished, he must not contaminate the specimen with toilet paper or urine. If he also needs to urinate, have the patient do that first in a separate container. To collect stool, you will need a container and something to remove the stool with. Put on rubber gloves, remove the stool from the bedpan with a tongue depressor, and place it in the container. Seal the container and label it with the patient's name, contents, and date and time of specimen collection. Be sure you know whether the specimen should be refrigerated; this can be very important.

Your doctor may ask you to check your patient's stool for the presence of blood. You may be able to easily see it, or it may go unnoticed (occult blood). The color of the stool (black, tarry) may indicate bleeding, but remember that some medications, such as iron, will give the stool that same appearance.

If you will be checking for blood at home, use a test kit available from your pharmacy. Ask your doctor to recommend a brand. Each kit will have specific instructions; some use tablets, others use filter paper slides. Find out if you should save any positive samples. If you are to save positive slides, be sure to label them. Do not test any stool samples mixed with urine because it affects the accuracy of the test. If you are using tablets, check the expiration date on the label. If your patient is taking medications that would affect accuracy, stop them 48 hours before the test. Iron, steroids, aspirin and vitamin C can affect the results, as can red meats, poultry, fish, and some vegetables. Check with your doctor about this.

Colostomy

A colostomy is a surgically formed opening of the colon. Part of the colon is brought through the patient's abdomen and an opening (stoma) is formed for the passage of fecal matter, creating a sort of artificial rectum. The procedure is done for various medical purposes and can be temporary or permanent.

An external bag may be worn on the abdomen to collect fecal matter. In some patients, bowel training can be done so that it is not necessary to wear the bag at all times; the patient may need only gauze over the stoma. It will take six to 12 weeks for bowel function to become regular after a colostomy. Your patient may still feel the need to move his bowels after the surgery; this is normal and will subside.

Pay attention to potential management problems: odor; care and protection of the skin; collection of fecal material; and psychological concerns of the colostomy patient. Remember that the same things that affect "normal" bowel routine will affect the colostomy patient. Illness, certain foods, infections, changes in diet or fluid intake, or prolonged bed rest can disrupt the colostomy patient's bowel routine.

Although it is no longer routine, your patient may be trained to perform colostomy irrigation so he won't have to wear a colostomy bag. This method is not suitable for all patients; check with the health care team.

Colostomy Care

Care of the ostomy patient may appear cumbersome and time consuming at first, but it will soon become an easy process. Perhaps you and the patient should do the procedure together until your patient feels comfortable enough to take it on alone. Provide ample privacy and time for care. Do not rush; choose a period when you will both be relaxed and free of interruptions.

The care giver should participate in any hospital teaching and do the procedure under supervision at first. However, your patient may feel strongly about doing his own care, and wish to be left alone to perform it. Allow him to do so. Be sure you have a complete list of equipment and where you can find it. Get the names of health care professionals you can call with questions or problems. Your hospital may have an enterostomal therapist on staff.

Drainage from the colostomy is usually liquid for the first few weeks following surgery. Once the patient is back on solid foods, the stools begin to form. Most of the care done in the hospital probably will be somewhat different once the patient returns home. A good deal of teaching will be done with the patient and his family before discharge. Most hospitals have nurses on staff that specialize in this type of care. By the time the patient is discharged, he should feel confident managing most of his own care and he should be encouraged to do so. Even the bedridden patient can be taught to do his own care. You may want a visiting nurse or home care nurse to make regular home visits to check on patient progress and to assist with management.

There are many different types of colostomy pouches and ways of adhering them to the body. Your patient and the ostomy specialist will have to decide what best meets his needs. Most colostomy equipment can be purchased from pharmacies or medical supply stores. If you are using special supplies or equipment, find out the names of manufacturers, sizes, lot or order number, and what the equipment is called before your patient is discharged. Make a list of these supplies and the quantity you will need. In most circumstances, clean (not sterile) supplies are used.

Colostomy care should become a routine part of the patient's daily hygiene. Empty the bag or pouch when it is one-third full, or in the morning (before breakfast) and at bedtime. Spray the bathroom and the pouch with deodorizer before emptying (Greer Guard Pouch Deodorant is one type often used). Drop a wad of toilet tissue into the toilet before beginning; this will prevent splashing when you empty the bag. Wash your hands before you begin.

1. Remove the pouch clamp, or the entire pouch if you are planning to change equipment or do stoma care.
2. While sitting on the toilet, empty the pouch into the toilet; remove as much of the fecal matter as possible.
3. Flush the toilet. Clean the tip (where the clamp goes) with toilet paper. Use a syringe of water to flush extra matter from the pouch.
4. Close the pouch. Wash your hands.

Stoma Care

During this care, the skin should be inspected closely for irritation. Report any irritation; perhaps improper technique has been used in bag application or the equipment does not fit. Observe the stoma; it should be a pinkish-red color. Changes in color may indicate problems. Bleeding during stoma care may be normal, but it is *not* normal for the stoma to bleed when the patient is wearing the colostomy pouch.

Many colostomy patients undergo cancer treatments and they should know that chemotherapeutic agents (5-fluorouracil, bleomycin) will make the stoma deep red or purple. Other drugs (methotrexate, adrenocorticoids) can cause skin breakdown. It is difficult to get the skin to heal while the patient is undergoing chemotherapy or radiation treatments. Radiation may make the stoma purple and cause blistering, inflammation, ulceration, bleeding, or other complications.

When caring for the stoma, remove the bag or any dressings covering it. Put disposable soiled supplies in a plastic bag and throw them away. Wash your hands and collect equipment.

1. Wash the stoma area carefully with a solution of mild soap and water. If there is any skin irritation, use only water. Cleaning can be done with gauze sponges. A piece of gauze can be placed over the stoma to catch any seepage.
2. Be sure the skin is dry and free of fecal material before you apply any skin preparations.
3. Skin preparations can be used to prevent irritation and skin breakdown (Vaseline gauze, aluminum powder, Karaya powder, Amphogel). Apply as instructed around the stoma. These substances should be removed occasionally for cleaning and air exposure. This also will allow you to check the skin condition under these preparations.
4. Apply skin adhesive or protective barrier.
5. Put on the plastic collection bag, centering it over the stoma. Press the adhesive to the skin for 30 seconds, allowing the warmth of your hand to seal it. Press out excess air and close at the bottom.
6. Attach belt, if used.

Your patient may have skin problems, usually from fecal leakage out of the bag or stoma. To prevent this, be sure the bag has been attached properly, that it is the right size for your patient, that the lower portion of the pouch or bag has been sealed, and that good cleansing and skin care are given. Substances in the stool can irritate the skin and every effort should be made to assure that the stool and the patient's skin do not touch one another.

Ask how often the adhesive surface must be removed and the area cleaned; a special solvent is available to remove the adhesive. Solvents should not be used for regular cleansing. As the stoma heals, it will tend to shrink and the patient may find the bags do not fit properly. Usually six months is needed until the stoma reaches it permanent size.

Some doctors tell the patient or care giver to gently stick a gloved finger into the stoma each time care is given to help prevent the stoma from becoming too narrow. Ask your doctor about this. Most patients will be allowed to take a tub bath or shower; whether the bag must be worn will depend on if there is drainage from the stoma. A shower during a pouch change will help remove any residue. Some doctors recommend putting gauze or a tampon into the stoma to plug stool drainage during skin care.

Keep extra bags or pouches on hand. They can be cleaned in a mild solution of soap and water, or soaked in a weak white vinegar solution to remove odor. Let them air dry. Most colostomy bags are odor proof, and there should be little concern about odors. The most effective means of control is to make sure the bag is properly sealed so odors do not escape. If this is a problem, commercial deodorizers can be placed in the bag; a few drops of white vinegar or an aspirin will do the same.

Diet is another way to control odor. Avoid foods that create gas (fish, eggs, onions, and vegetables such as asparagus, cauliflower, or cabbage). Oranges, parsley, yogurt, and buttermilk will help control odor. Diet control also can help control stool consistency. Your doctor may prescribe oral medications to control odor.

Belts are no longer routinely worn, but your patient may want one for added support. Most belts are machine washable.

Ileostomy

An ileostomy is a surgical procedure like a colostomy, but involving the ileum portion of the intestine rather than the colon. An ileostomy can be temporary or permanent. Because the ileum is used, stools will be loose or watery, so your patient will need to wear a collection bag at all times. This can cause collection and skin care problems.

The ileostomy patient needs added skin protection and special skin barriers because of caustic enzymes in the stool. The pouch or bag must fit properly and stick to the patient's skin so there is no leakage. The collection bag can be changed as often as necessary, or stay on the patient for as long as a week. The bag should be emptied as often as needed, usually every four to six hours. The bag can be rinsed out by using a syringe filled with tap water that is squirted around the inside of the bag to remove fecal matter. Some bags can be snapped off for emptying and rinsing. Most of these pouches are odor proof. Commercial deodorizers can be placed in the pouch to offer added protection against odors.

Proper pouch fit is important. One way of making sure is with a measuring guide that has several hole sizes. Find the hole that fits over the stoma; there should be about 1/8 inch excess around the stoma. Once you have found the proper size, trace that onto your skin barrier and cut out the hole. When changing the bag, use the steps described above for colostomy patients.

Psychology of the Ostomy Patient

Whether the ostomy will be temporary or permanent, your loved one may have a number of problems adjusting to this external means of emptying the bowels. One major factor will be how the family responds to the procedure. If the response is one of revulsion or discomfort, the patient may adopt the same attitude. One of the key adjustment periods occurs in the hospital. If the postoperative period is plagued with problems, your loved one may take longer to adapt. For example, was there excess leakage? Were there odor problems? Was the patient allowed to sit in fecal contents while waiting for the nurse to come? All of these experiences can affect how the patient will adjust.

Another major factor will be the reason for the colostomy or ileostomy, and whether it will be permanent or temporary. Often, a colostomy is performed for cancer of the bowel, which undoubtedly presents other concerns for the patient. If the ostomy is temporary, it may be easier to accept. However, sometimes the doctor may find it impossible to reverse the condition and the ostomy will become permanent.

Most of us consider feces as a necessary, messy component of body waste. For the ostomy patient, the process is now in full view. Seeing feces exit from the patient's abdomen, often in uncontrolled quantities, can be devastating. Show your loved one that he will still be accepted and able to carry on with a minor adaptation in his daily care. The care giver must understand and accept this, too. If you will be performing some or all of his care, it is important that the patient feels accepted. If you walk into his room dressed as though you are about to drain the septic tank, your patient may be demoralized. It is not necessary to wear gloves during any part of the procedure, except when placing a finger into the stoma.

Talk openly with your patient. Let him know he is loved. Sexual dysfunction can be a problem for ostomy patients. Consult with a specialist or seek counseling if this complication occurs. Encourage visitors, if he will allow them. Acceptance may be slow, but it will come. Seek out local ostomy support groups. These include ostomy specialists, other ostomy patients, and their families. They can be very supportive and offer first-hand tips on home care. The American Cancer Society keeps a list of ostomy patients who will meet with your loved one before and after the operation to lend emotional support. For information about support groups, or a national publication, "Ostomy Quarterly," contact:

United Ostomy Association
2001 West Beverly Boulevard
Los Angeles, CA 90057

For a directory of outpatient resources, write to:

International Association for Enterostomal Therapy
5000 Birch Street
Newport Beach, CA 92660

Care Giver's Checklist

1. Waste elimination can be one of the most difficult aspects of home care. Your attitude is important; if you show distaste or resentment when emptying a bedpan or helping with colostomy care, your loved one may adopt—or even magnify—these negative feelings. Seek out home care specialists or local support groups to help you maintain a positive outlook.
2. Urine and stool specimens can be valuable in evaluating illness. Know how to collect the specimen, label and store it, and how long it can be kept before evaluation.
3. Urinary incontinence can be managed with catheters. These need special care; do not attempt this at home until you have performed the procedures in the presence of a health professional.
4. Bed rest, illness, and diet can affect bowel function. Stool softeners, laxatives, or enemas may be prescribed to treat constipation or promote regular bowel function. Remember that chronic use of these can result in dependence; eventually, the patient may require laxatives or enemas as the only means of bowel evacuation.
5. A urinary stoma, colostomy, or ileostomy can pose physical and psychological challenges to your loved one. Participate in hospital teaching so you will understand the dynamics of daily care, even if your patient will be caring for himself. Don't hesitate to call on local support groups or the health care team for assurance and encouragement.

10 The Circulatory System

Blood vessels form a complex network to transport blood from the heart to various regions of the body. Blood-filled arteries divide and branch off to form arterioles, which divide into tiny vessels known as capillaries. Within the capillaries, an exchange of substances takes place between the blood and body tissues. Capillaries reunite to form minute veins called venules, which merge and branch off to form larger vessels known as veins. Veins carry blood back to the heart. In short, arteries carry blood away from the heart; veins return it to the heart.

Blood transports oxygen from the lungs to red blood cells, and it carries carbon dioxide from the cells to the lungs and kidneys. Blood also carries nutrients from the digestive system to the cells; transports waste products from the cells to the kidneys, lungs, and sweat glands; takes hormones and enzymes to the cells; regulates body pH and body temperature; prevents fluid loss through clotting; and protects the body against infection. It's almost easier to describe what blood doesn't do!

The heart pumps blood throughout this vast network of arteries, arterioles, capillaries, venules, and veins. The heart is set into action by stimulation of the nervous system. A large muscle surrounding the heart (myocardium) provides continuous pumping action, with rest periods only while the heart chambers fill with blood. The right side of the heart receives blood via the veins; the left side receives oxygenated blood from the lungs and pumps it out to the arteries.

Problems can occur in any part of this complex system. The heart muscle can weaken, causing heart and circulatory problems. Blockage in a major artery or vein makes passage of blood to or from the heart difficult. Heart conduction problems affect the normal, steady rhythm of the heart. These problems can originate within the system itself, or as complications of other medical conditions.

Circulatory Problems

Thrombophlebitis is inflammation of a vein due to clot formation, usually caused by prolonged bed rest or inactivity. It is most common in the large veins in the lower extremities. Symptoms of this condition are pain; leg cramps; tenderness over a vein; swelling; warm to touch; redness or other changes in the leg's color; and sometimes fever.

The best treatment is prevention. Provide regular exercise for the bedridden patient or patient with limited movement. Change your patient's position frequently and get him moving! He should be encouraged to walk as much as possible, if allowed. Avoid prolonged sitting; elevate his feet periodically. Avoid tight clothing that restricts circulation. Anti-emboli stockings or support hose may help. (See Chapter 3 for tips on avoiding bed rest complications.)

The treatment will vary depending on the severity of the condition. Although bed rest may have contributed to the problem, sometimes the prescribed treatment is strict bed rest with periodic elevation of the leg to prevent the clot from becoming dislodged and going elsewhere in the body. Never rub or massage an affected area for this reason.

Warm, wet towels may be recommended to decrease swelling. The best type of heat for the patient with thrombophlebitis is moist heat. Heat dilates the blood vessels and promotes circulation. Take a small hand towel, run it under warm tap water (not too hot or you'll burn your patient), wring it out and apply it to the affected limb. Put an absorbent pad or some plastic wrap around the towel to retain the heat. Your doctor must prescribe this type of therapy; ask how long to leave the warm pack in place and how often to provide the treatment. It's usually done for 20 to 30 minutes every four to six hours. There can be much pain with this condition and pain-killers may be necessary.

If the condition is serious, the patient may be placed on anticoagulant therapy to keep the blood thinned out. (Sometimes the clots are surgically removed.) Anticoagulants may prevent extension of an existing blood clot or stop more clots from forming. Anticoagulants can be given orally, by injection, or intravenously. The two most common types of medication for this are heparin and coumadin. When a patient is on anticoagulant therapy, it's sometimes necessary to do blood tests to monitor anti-clotting effects and to determine daily doses. If the patient is at home on anticoagulant therapy, outside lab services may perform these blood studies. If none is available, the patient will have to go to the doctor's office or hospital for blood tests.

Anticoagulants have serious side effects, such as hemorrhage. Watch for signs of internal or external bleeding. Some indicators are nosebleeds; blood in the urine or stool (stools will be black or tarry); bleeding from the gums; bruising; or hemorrhage. If you note any of these, do not administer the anticoagulant, try to control excessive bleeding, and call the doctor at once. If your patient is receiving injections, apply pressure to any post-injection site until bleeding stops. Do not bump or bruise your patient. Your patient should not use a straight or safety razor; an electric razor is recommended. Don't administer aspirin or substances containing aspirin; acetaminophen is OK.

Anti-clotting effects will continue for several days after the therapy is discontinued. Serious bleeding problems can be corrected by administering drugs to enhance clotting (vitamin K), although blood transfusions may be necessary.

Edema (increased swelling) occurs when body tissues contain an excessive amount of fluid. It can be generalized or local and is caused by decreased blood circulation; inflammation; obstruction; or organic problems within the heart, kidneys, or lungs.

Again, the best treatment is prevention. Sluggish circulation, bed rest, or inactivity can predispose a patient to edema. Encourage movement and exercise. Don't leave your patient's legs in one position too long. Use varying levels of elevation and movement, if prescribed. Avoid clothing or shoes that impair circulation.

There may be diet restrictions for the patient with edema. Salt, which is known to retain fluids, should be avoided, as should any foods with high salt content such as bacon, seafood, some cheeses, and pork products. Check food labels for salt content. Don't use salt as a seasoning, although the doctor may allow a salt substitute. Diets should be adequate in protein, high in calories, and rich in vitamins. Fluids may be restricted to as little as 600 cc/ml in a 24-hour period. If fluids are restricted, provide frequent mouth care for your patient. Offer mouthwash or hard candies, if allowed. Lemon and glycerine swabs are refreshing and increase saliva production. Ration fluids throughout the 24 hours, giving the largest amount during the day.

The doctor may prescribe medications that increase fluid output via urine (diuretics).

Patients must have adequate kidney and cardiac function to take these drugs. Some commonly used diuretics are Lasix, Hydrodiuril, Edecrin, Aldactone. These have some common side effects associated with the loss of large amounts of body fluids: dehydration; electrolyte imbalance; muscle weakness; tremors; confusion; and clotting disorders.

Shortly after the medication is taken, increased episodes of urination should occur. Provide a bedpan, urinal, or easy access to a bathroom. Accurate intake and output should be recorded for all patients on diuretic therapy. Know what your patient's urine output should be and report any discrepencies to your doctor. Some physicians will want the patient weighed daily for an indication of fluid loss. Check the legs for swelling; you may be asked to take daily measurements.

Since potassium is lost when a patient is on diuretics, a supplement may be needed. You can provide natural potassium through diet with foods such as bananas, fresh vegetables, peas, nuts, molasses, fresh fish and fresh poultry.

Edema can cause shortness of breath and your patient may require oxygen therapy.

Stroke

Strokes occur when there is a sudden loss of the arteries' ability to carry blood to the brain. Brain cells are extremely sensitive to a lack of oxygen, and if the condition exists too long (sometimes just a few minutes), brain damage will occur. Since brain cells do not regenerate, much of the damage is irreversible; the extent depends on the severity of stroke and its location in the brain. For example, if it occurs in the part of the brain involving speech, then speech will be impaired. Stroke, also called cerebral vascular accident (CVA), ranks third as a cause of death for people over 45, and is the leading cause of disability in the elderly.

Conditions that predispose a person to strokes may be diet; high blood pressure; blood clots; heart disease; stress; or other disease processes. Patients can experience a gradual onset of symptoms (transient ischemic attack, or TIA) or sudden onset of symptoms that may or may not eventually lead to a major stroke. There may be no no symptoms at all prior to a massive cerebral hemorrhage.

Immediately after the stroke, the patient may be unconscious and it will be difficult to determine the extent of damage. The patient's face may be bright red and he may have difficulty breathing or swallowing. His pulse will be slow, but the impulse felt will be strong. His blood pressure may be elevated. The patient may remain comatose for several weeks and then recover, or he may never regain consciousness. The longer the coma, the poorer the prognosis. A series of neurologic studies will have to be done to evaluate the damage.

The post-stroke patient may experience impaired concentration and attention span; impaired memory, especially of recent events; scattered thoughts (talking about unrelated topics); inappropriate responses to social situations (crying when he should be laughing); an inability to understand requests or commands; paralysis or partial paralysis; and speech disorders (aphasia). Along with these problems there may be long-term complications. The level of your loved one's care will depend on the extent of damage.

Stroke patients often are placed on anticoagulant therapy to keep the blood free of clots or to prevent existing clots from developing further. The major emphasis in the treatment of the stroke patient is to prevent further complications (pneumonia, bedsores, loss of muscle tone) and to provide aggressive therapy to restore as much function as possible. This begins as soon as the patient is able and the doctor has decided there is hope for rehabilitation. Generally, the patient will remain in the hospital during the acute stroke phase and may continue to be hospitalized for some of the initial rehabilitation. Beyond that point, the patient may be transferred home or to a rehabilitation unit for further therapy.

As soon as the patient's condition stabilizes and he begins to show improvement, he's on the long road back to recovery. In some patients, this will involve re-teaching almost all aspects of daily living; learning to feed himself, clothe and bathe himself, and even how to speak and walk. Realistic goals must be set. What can be expected in rehabilitation? How long will it take? What will the results be? Many of these questions cannot be answered now, or even several months from now. Some indicators are the amount of residual brain damage; patient commitment and ability to concentrate; and commitment from the rehabilitation team and family.

Progress most likely won't be seen in leaps and bounds. It will be measured not in days, but rather in weeks and months. Little things that we take for granted, like being able to lift a fork, will take on new meaning. Your loved one will need patience, reassurance, great effort on your part, and lots of tender loving care.

Your patient will be encouraged to get out of bed as soon as he is able. Inactive muscles will atrophy, shorten, or shrink from disuse. Regular exercise is important. If the patient is able, he should participate fully; if not, he will have to have exercises done for him. Joints also may become fixed or limited without exercise. Your patient can do strengthening exercises while in bed or sitting in a chair. Have the patient squeeze a tennis ball, knit or crochet, flex, and extend and rotate muscles and joints. If a physical therapy program has been set up, the care giver should participate. Help your loved one do exercises as often as required.

Bowel and bladder control must be considered. Take your patient to the toilet often; he may forget or not realize he has to go to the bathroom. Limit fluids after 9 P.M. If he wets or soils himself, do not scold him. Ask at your pharmacy about fitted absorbent disposable briefs for adults. The post-stroke patient should not strain when he moves his bowels. This could increase internal pressure and loosen another blood clot. To avoid constipation, your patient may need laxatives or stool softeners. You can help to prevent this by providing high fiber foods in the patient's diet (raw vegetables and fruits, wheat, and whole grain products).

Hemiplegia is paralysis or loss of movement on one side of the body. When a stroke occurs, the clot or hemorrhage usually takes place in one side of the brain (often the right side). There is a crossover of nerves as they lead down the spinal cord, so when a stroke occurs in the right side of the brain, the left side of the body is affected. The centers for speech, movement, and other bodily functions are in the right side of the brain. Often, a stroke patient's mouth may droop to one side, or his leg or arm on one side of the body is weakened or paralyzed. You may see the stroke patient leaning or drooping. If the stroke has affected his dominant side, he will have to be trained to use his non-dominant hand.

Help the hemiplegic patient sit up on his own by tucking pillows around his affected side. There is some disagreement about which side to stand on when helping a stroke patient walk. Some feel it is safer to support his unaffected side; others feel you should stand at the affected side. Ask your doctor or therapist for guidance. It is sometimes helpful if the stroke patient wears a sling on his affected arm to provide support and balance. Most stroke patients will be encouraged to use a walker or a three-pronged cane held in the unaffected hand.

While eating, a stroke patient may drool out of the paralyzed side of the mouth. This is due to lack of swallowing control and the inability to keep his lips closed because of paralysis. To help to prevent this, try to turn him toward his unaffected side. If you are feeding the patient, place small portions of food in the unaffected side of his mouth. Feed your patient slowly and give him time to chew. He may need to have his food put in a blender or food processor. Even if your patient is able to feed himself, he may need some help. Place his food near the unaffected side and offer to cut it up. Drinking straws are helpful, as are plates with sides or silverware with thick handles (figure 17).

Anticipate your patient's needs before he must struggle with asking; his speech may have been affected by the stroke. He most likely began speech therapy while in the hospital and is continuing therapy at home. Be patient. Do not cut off your loved one in mid-sentence; give him time to finish what he is saying. When we feel people do not understand us, we often tend to shout at them. This is a mistake with a stroke patient since hearing usually is not affected. Stand in front of your patient and speak slowly and clearly.

The speech disorder in stroke patients is called *aphasia*, which is a loss of the ability to understand spoken and written language. There are many forms of aphasia. Some are not associated with intellectual impairment, but often there is a degree of intellectual impairment when aphasia is caused by a stroke. *Expressive aphasia* is when the patient may know what he wishes to say, but is unable to express it. *Auditory aphasia* is when the patient has difficulty understanding the spoken word. Such a patient's speech will be garbled or appear to make no sense. Some patients may indeed understand, but their words will make no sense. Sometimes your loved one will realize this and be frustrated; other times he may not be aware of his errors. Your patient also may have problems with reading and writing.

In the beginning, basic, simple sentences are best. Talk to him, tell him what is going on around him, orient him to the time, day, and date. Tell him what you are going to do. For example, tell the patient "Here is the bed" while pointing to the bed, and then say, "Now I am going to put you in bed."

Stroke victims usually have short attention spans. Even so, never be tempted to treat your patient like a child; he is not a child and does not feel like a child. Try to temper your own frustrations, at least when you are with your patient. Just because he does not appear to understand you or respond appropriately doesn't mean he has lost the sensitivity and feelings we all have. You would be surprised how much he is taking in and how aware he is of his surroundings.

If you participate in his speech therapy, provide a quiet environment free of distractions. Picture flash cards are a good means of associating the written word with a picture of the object. Say the word, point to the object, and have the patient repeat after you. Praise him when he is right and encourage his efforts. Never lose your temper or scold him when he is incorrect. Tell him the correct word gently, leave the card alone, and go on to the next. You can come back to that one later. Crayons and a drawing pad can be helpful, too. Work on the alphabet.

Early on, the keys to success are basic, repetitive exercises. When your patient appears tired or frustrated, it's best to stop. Early in the day seems to be a good time for therapy since your patient should be rested and ready to go to work. Subtle mental exercises can continue all day. For example, at the dinner table, point to his daughter and ask, "Who is that?" If he appears puzzled, tell him, "This is Julie, your daughter." Give him time to answer and do not cut him off until he finishes, even if he is wrong.

The Comatose Patient

The comatose patient may be transferred home because the doctor feels there is little hope of rehabilitation. The patient's condition has stabilized, there is no further need for hospitalization, and the patient goes home, if the family is equipped and willing to meet his needs. Such a patient will be totally dependent.

This type of care is commonly called custodial care. You will have to see that the patient receives adequate nourishment, that bodily functions are looked after, that complications of bed rest are avoided, that movement is provided, and that the patient is comfortable and free of pain. The psychological needs of the comatose patient vary; it is difficult to determine his level of awareness since you receive no feedback. Some health professionals believe the comatose patient never loses his sense of hearing, vision, or touch and that the patient should continue to receive these important stimulants.

If you and your family want to take on this care at home, check your medical insurance policy first to see what kind of coverage is available. Will it cover costs for professional nurses or unskilled nursing care (nurses' aides or sitters)? What about physical or respiratory therapists? Will it cover medical equipment? Is there a cap on reimbursement for any of these services? Try to remove yourself emotionally when making this decision. Decide what will be best for your patient, your family, and your budget. If home care is not appropriate, research other avenues such as nursing homes or rehabilitation centers.

The comatose patient should be repositioned as often as every two hours. Perform range of motion exercises on all extremities. Prevent bedsores with frequent skin care. A comatose patient is a good candidate for an air mattress, water bed, or other pressure relief device. A hospital-type bed will make caring for him easier. You will be providing full hygiene: bathing; mouth care; eye, ear, and hair care. Refer to Chapters 3 and 7 for information about caring for bedridden patients.

A comatose patient is unable to swallow; if food or liquid is given, the patient will choke and the food or fluid may be taken into the lungs. This can be a life-threatening complication. Feeding tubes or intravenous tubes may be placed in this type of patient. For information about alternative nutrition, refer to Chapter 5.

The comatose patient will be incontinent, with no control over the passage of urine and feces. In most of these patients, an indwelling urinary catheter will be put in place. The bed will need to be protected with absorbent pads. Additional cleansing and skin care will be required. Because of bed rest and diet, your patient may have problems with constipation, diarrhea, or frequent bladder infections. Observe your patient for these types of problems and report them to your doctor (see Chapter 9 for more information).

With the comatose patient, you will need to be sure the airway is open. Since this patient will have a diminished swallowing reflex and won't know when to cough, he is prone to choking and respiratory problems. Some of these can be prevented by positioning the patient on his side, rather than flat on his back. When he is on his back, the bed should be slightly elevated. Your patient may require suctioning to remove excess mucous secretions (see page 82); oxygen therapy may be prescribed. One of the most common causes of complications, or even death, in the comatose patient is aspiration. This occurs when mucous secretions or fluids have been drawn into the lungs, usually resulting in pneumonia.

Protect your patient from accidents or falls. Safety rails should be on the bed; never leave your patient unattended when the rails are down. Keep your loved one warm and out of drafts. Protect him from injury. Watch your loved one closely; some of his needs will be obvious, others will be far more subtle. For example, he won't be able to tell you he is lying on a misplaced object. You'll know only when you turn your patient and see a reddened area. Look at facial expressions: Does he appear comfortable? Is he grimacing, restless, or clenching his teeth? Observe his skin: Is it dry or moist? Warm or cold? What is the temperature? Your patient's response to pain will depend on the depth of his coma. He may not know when something is too hot or too cold. You must bear that responsibility and safeguard your patient.

Remember that your patient may have a level of awareness, even if he is unable to respond. Never say anything in his presence that you do not wish him to hear. Keep his environment quiet and restful, but allow for some stimulation. Play soft music, hang bright colors around the room, and bring in family members and visitors.

Caring for a comatose loved one is emotionally and physically draining. Taking on this care means that someone must always be at home. This can pose a tremendous financial and social burden on your family. Consider your decision carefully before committing yourself to such a demanding task.

Peripheral Vascular Disorders

Peripheral vascular disorders are mostly diseases of the blood vessels that supply the extremities, usually the lower extremities. Vascular disease can be caused by diabetes; changes in the vascular system in the elderly; progressive heart disease; blockage in the veins or arteries; varicose veins; or Raynaud's disease.

Common symptoms of vascular and circulatory problems are cold extremities; absence of pulse in an extremity; skin discoloration; leg pain, which can be severe; swelling; and skin ulcers. The symptoms signal a diminished blood supply to the area, causing inadequate oxygenation of the cells and tissues (ischemia). The extent and severity of these symptoms will vary depending on the area and degree of obstruction.

Peripheral vascular disorders may be acute or chronic. In the acute condition, the problem may be corrected and the patient can go on with his normal routine, although he may be at risk for future circulatory problems. A chronic condition could involve daily care for the rest of his life, or just preventive measures to avoid future problems.

Diagnostic procedures can determine the location and severity of any blockage. Treatments may include anticoagulant therapy, which will help dissolve the blood clots; vasodilators to dilate the blood vessels; or positioning to make it easier for the blood to flow. Sometimes surgery will remove the obstruction.

Pain associated with this circulatory condition varies with each patient. It can be unrelenting for some; for others, it can be relieved by changing position or stopping an activity and resting, thus improving circulation. It is often described as an achy, cramping pain. There is medication available that may help; sometimes aspirin alone is sufficient. Narcotics usually are not prescribed because of the long-term nature of the problem. If pain medication has been ordered, offer it when the first symptoms of pain occur. This may help the medication take effect before the pain peaks. Never offer medication in anticipation of pain; offer only when necessary.

Sometimes, even the weight of the bed covers can cause discomfort. You can use a bed cradle or footboard to lift the sheets off the patient. Check with your doctor before offering to massage the legs.

Avoid things that cause blood vessel constriction (vasoconstriction): smoking or other tobacco products; cold temperatures; and restrictive body positions (crossing the legs, kneeling, sitting, or standing for long periods). Keep the extremity warm with extra layers of clothing or warm socks. A diet high in protein and vitamins B and C is recommended. Warm baths may help, but use caution with heat when your patient has impaired circulation. These patients often have diminished nerve sensation and cannot tell if something is too hot. These methods may help to relieve the symptoms, but will not correct or reverse any organic disorder.

Ask your health care team about the dynamics of positioning a patient with circulatory problems. Elevating the legs will promote circulation, but only venous circulation (veins carrying blood back to the heart). You also want to promote arterial circulation (blood carried away from the heart and into the extremities). When your patient is in bed, keep him flat; do not elevate his legs unless ordered by the doctor. Don't let your patient remain in one position too long; alternate between sitting and standing. If he is sitting in the chair, he should keep his feet on the floor.

Exercise may help to develop alternate circulation to the area, known as collateral circulation. Have your patient lie flat in bed and lift his legs straight up (one at a time) for two minutes; you may help him if he needs it. Then have him sit on the edge of the bed with his legs dangling while exercising his feet for three or four minutes. Now have him lie flat in bed for five minutes. He should try to do this series of exercises three times a day to promote full circulation. If your loved one cannot tolerate this, the best overall exercise is walking. Pain indicates your patient has overdone it and should rest.

Foot Care

The feet are last in the body to receive blood during the circulatory process, so special attention must be paid to your patient's feet if he has circulation problems. Keep them warm, even if it means wearing socks to bed (cotton socks are best). Apply a fresh pair daily. Do not use hot water bottles, heating pads, or other heating devices to provide warmth; you may burn your patient. Do not allow him to walk in bare feet. Always protect his feet to avoid bumping or bruising. Don't let him wear socks, stockings, or clothing that constrict circulation. Socks or stockings should not bag at the ankles.

Bathe his feet daily with warm water and mild soap. Dry them thoroughly and in between each toe. Apply cream or lanolin to prevent dryness. Do not cut toenails; use a nail file and file nails straight across. Do not cut calluses, corns, or anything on the feet. If his feet need attention, call in a professional foot doctor (podiatrist or chiropodist). Report any unusual looking sores, blisters or infections.

Leg ulcers or open sores are a common problem with diminished circulation of the lower extremities. Sores, cuts, or bruises can take weeks, even months, to heal since there is a decreased blood supply nourishing the cells and tissues. These areas are easily infected. Open sores that don't need surgery will require sterile dressings to protect against further damage or infection. Your patient may have to stay in bed during this period.

If you are changing your patient's dressing, use sterile technique (see Chapters 3 and 12). Nothing unsterile should touch the wound. Wash your hands before and after treating the patient.

Ask your doctor how often the dressing should be changed. These dressings usually are applied wet, soaked in medication or petroleum jelly. Never apply lotions or creams with bare fingers; wear gloves or use a sterile applicator or tongue depressor. If you are wrapping bandages around the leg, don't wrap too tightly (see page 173). Report any changes in the condition of the wound, such as excess drainage or bleeding. Fever may be a sign of infection.

Bypass Surgery

Surgery may be required to bypass an obstructed blood vessel. In some cases, it will be possible to remove the obstructed or deteriorated area and reconnect the vessel. More often, grafts are used to circumvent the blood flow around the blocked area. The advantage here is that there is less surgical trauma; the area is left alone and a piece of blood vessel, or an artificial substitute, is used to bypass the occlusion (blockage). The type of surgery is determined by the vessel, the amount of deterioration, the patient's physical condition, and what is needed to restore the vessel.

Postoperatively, it is important to ascertain that the graft or resection has been effective. This is determined by your doctor, but you can help by checking for signs of success: Is the leg warm to the touch? Is your patient free of pain? Can you feel a pulse in the area? Is the skin color healthy?

Know how to care for the surgical incision. Will dressings need to be changed? How often? What activities are best for your patient? Can he be out of bed? If so, he should avoid prolonged periods of sitting or standing in one position. Find out if leg exercises are prescribed; if so, be sure your patient does them. Smoking should be avoided along with anything else that causes vessel constriction. The full effect of the surgery may not be seen for a few months, although the doctor can ascertain circulation and functioning soon after the surgery. Your patient will be the true indicator; what's most important is how he feels as a result of the bypass surgery.

Blood Disorders

Blood cells are formed in the liver, spleen, thymus gland, lymph nodes, and the bone marrow. These organs all participate at various phases of cell development. Problems with the blood may occur during early development of blood cells, creating abnormal or nonfunctioning cells. Some of these problems may be inherited; others develop from injury to an organ (liver, spleen) or from an organic disorder in the body.

Treatment will depend on the cause of the problem, if it can be established. Some common types of blood disorders are anemia; leukemia; clotting problems; bleeding disorders; some forms of cancer; or hemophilia. Diagnosis may be made by laboratory examination of the blood or bone marrow. Common treatments for blood disorders may be whole blood transfusions; replacing individual blood components (platelets, white blood cells); removing the patient's spleen; phlebotomy (removing excess blood); or transplanting bone marrow. There are ways to remove suspected impurities or abnormal cells by pumping blood through an elaborate filtering system and returning it to the patient without impurities or abnormal cells.

Anemia is an abnormal condition in which your patient has a low number of red blood cells demonstrated by low hemoglobin or hematocrit levels. Anemia can mean that the patient simply is missing important nutritional elements, but it also can be an indicator that other processes are taking place within the body.

Some common symptoms of anemia are weakness or fatigue; shortness of breath; the patient feels cold; bone and joint pain; excessive blood loss; loss of appetite; feeling faint; a rapid pulse; and possibly heart palpitations. Generally, the more rapidly the condition occurs, the more severe the symptoms will be. If your patient is experiencing any of these, report them to your doctor. Anemia can be diagnosed through a blood sample to determine the type of anemia and course of treatment.

In iron deficiency anemia, a common blood disorder, the patient is unable to meet an increased need for iron. Iron is needed for production of hemoglobin (red blood cells). In some cases, iron can be replaced through diet with iron-rich fruits, eggs, meat (liver), fish, green leafy vegetables, and whole grain breads and cereal.

An iron supplement may be prescribed until the problem is corrected. Iron therapy should not be taken for long periods of time. The drug usually is discontinued when the patient's hemoglobin reaches the desired level. Iron preparations are best absorbed when taken on an empty stomach, or just before meals. They should not be taken with milk, or chewed, since iron can stain the teeth. If an injection is recommended, you'll need instructions in a special injection technique so the iron does not leak into subcutaneous tissues.

Your patient's stools will be black while taking iron supplements. Some other side effects may be nausea and stomach disturbances; insomnia; diarrhea; or constipation. Iron is a relatively safe drug, but it is possible to give a patient too much iron. Some signs of this are a feeling of fullness in the head; fast pulse rate; insomnia; and skin eruptions. If you note any of these symptoms, report them to your doctor.

Excessive bruising, black and blue marks, or small hemorrhage areas on the skin may indicate a *bleeding disorder.* These problems can result from lack of platelets (the clotting element in the blood) or from an abnormality in the blood vessels. Look for indications of bleeding taking place elsewhere in the body: black stools; blood in the urine; nosebleeds; a wound that will not stop bleeding; blood on toilet tissue after a bowel movement; vaginal bleeding; bleeding gums; or skin pallor. You may see tiny purplish-red dots on the patient's body (petechiae), most frequently on the abdomen or legs. These may indicate an acute problem, or may result as a side effect of an existing condition or treatment. If they appear, report this to the health care team. In many cases, the disorder can be treated with an infusion of platelets.

Emphasize safety so your patient doesn't accidentally cut himself; bleeding will be difficult to control. Your patient should use only an electric razor, not one with a blade. If you give him an injection, be sure to apply added pressure afterward. Treat any bleeding by applying pressure to the area and elevate, if possible. Call the doctor; you may be told to bring your loved one in immediately for treatment. Your patient should not take aspirin products because they alter the blood's clotting mechanism.

Leukemia is a white blood cell disorder that can affect the lymphocytes, the granulocytes, and monocytes—all components of the white blood cell. Leukemia usually is signaled by a marked increase in the number of white blood cells, which may prevent other healthy cells from functioning. The disease can be acute or chronic; acute forms are more common in people under 25, chronic forms in people over 40.

Early symptoms of leukemia are chronic infections, bleeding problems, fatigue, bruising, fever, anemia, or nosebleeds. Sometimes, these early symptoms go unnoticed and are passed off as a cold or sore throat until they refuse to go away.

Diagnosis may be made through blood studies and bone marrow examination. The treatment for leukemia is vigorous and may include anti-cancer drugs; radiation; treatment of the symptoms and accompanying infections; blood transfusions; or bone marrow transplants.

Both the disease and the treatment may cause problems. Leukemia patients often have bouts of infections requiring prompt medical attention and usually some form of intravenous antibiotic therapy. Your patient may be hospitalized during the acute phase and then discharged home on antibiotic therapy. If so, you will need to know how to manage antibiotic intravenous therapy and what equipment will be needed. (Read Chapters 5 and 8 for more information about home care of the IV patient.)

Watch your loved one for any indication of infections. A fever, chills, a wound that will not heal, pus or drainage from an area, mouth sores, or urinary tract problems are all signs that may indicate infection. Report them to the health care team.

Nosebleeds are common among leukemia patients, and may be difficult to control. To stop the bleeding, pinch both nostrils. Have the patient sit with his head slightly tilted forward with a basin beneath; tell him to spit out any blood. Never place the patient flat on his back. If he is unable to sit up, put him on his side.

A cold ice pack can be applied to the bridge of the nose to try to constrict the blood vessels and stop bleeding. Notify your doctor if the bleeding does not subside after a few minutes. Your patient may need to be taken to the emergency room where doctors will pack the nose to stop the bleeding. The amount of blood loss should be considered; a serious nosebleed may have lowered it to dangerous levels.

Consult with the health care team until you are familiar with all of the anti-cancer drugs prescribed for your patient. Most of them have serious side effects such as nausea and vomiting; mouth sores; hair loss; or alterations in the patient's blood count (bone marrow suppression). To treat the disease, toxic levels of anti-cancer drugs must be given.

If your patient has mouth sores, avoid solutions that may cause further irritation (salt, mouthwash). Oral medications may treat the problem; check with your doctor. Offer frequent mouth care; use soft toothbrushes or a Water Pik.

Diet also is important. Because of the disease, the treatment, or both, your patient may have no appetite. Cancer drugs may alter his sense of taste or your patient may complain of a metallic taste in his mouth. If your patient has nausea and vomiting, anti-nausea medications may be prescribed. Medicate your patient at the first sign of nausea; don't wait until he's vomiting. If your patient vomits shortly after receiving medications, call the doctor.

After episodes of vomiting, offer your patient clear liquids (broths also help to replace the loss of salt). Slowly progress to bland and solid foods. If your patient has mouth sores, he may be able to tolerate only bland foods with no spices. Offer small, frequent feedings; liquids are especially important. To maintain your patient's nutritional health and body weight, provide high calorie, high carbohydrate, and protein nourishment. Ask your doctor about commercial diet supplements. Your nutritionist may be able to recommend a recipe book written especially for the cancer patient. If your patient has severe problems taking food orally, alternate methods (intravenous, total parenteral nutrition) may be prescribed.

Caring for the leukemia patient can be a constant battle. There will be periods of remission when the patient is considered disease free, and relapses when the disease is active. The length of remission varies, although some people never attain it. Emotionally, this burden of disease and treatment can take its toll. It helps to know as much as possible about the disease. (See the Appendix for recommended reading.) Your doctor and the entire health care team will be supportive and provide solutions to some of your patient's problems. Ask for help; it is there for you! Seek out hospital or community support groups. For more information, write to:

The American Cancer Society
777 Third Avenue
New York, NY 10017

High Blood Pressure

High blood pressure (hypertension) is a major cause of death in adults and has been called the "silent killer" because the victim may be unaware he has the disease. Normal blood pressure in a relaxed adult is 110 to 145 mm of mercury for the systolic (top number) and 60 to 90 mm of mercury for the diastolic (bottom number). Hypertension can be described as a persistent elevation above 140/90. An increase in the lower number (diastolic) is the most significant because it shows elevated pressure even during the resting phase of the heart cycle.

High blood pressure may be caused by obesity; diet; kidney disease; age; stress or tension; and other organic diseases. Hypertension is placed into two categories: primary refers to the condition when it is not related to other organic causes; secondary means the hypertension is a result of other physiologic conditions (tumors, kidney disease).

Patients with high blood pressure may complain of headache, blurred vision, dizziness, insomnia, and nervousness. Uncontrolled hypertension can cause vision, heart, kidney, and brain problems.

High blood pressure can be treated with medications, diet, weight control, avoiding salt, and by altering life-style to limit stress. Management through drugs is achieved by reducing the amount of sodium in the body with diuretics, thus lessening the cardiac output by the heart and reducing pressure in the vessels. Some of these drugs have a tranquilizing effect; all of them have possible serious side effects. Look for excessive fluid loss; drowsiness; headaches; dry mouth, gastrointestinal problems (stomach upset, vomiting, constipation, diarrhea); nightmares; and mental depression. Sexual problems or impotence may be a side effect of some medications. Never discontinue these drugs unless your doctor approves.

A patient with high blood pressure should rise slowly when going from a lying to a sitting position. If you are monitoring your patient's blood pressure, keep an accurate record. Ask the doctor when, and how often, to take it. Establish what the desired blood pressure range should be and let your doctor know when it is not within that range. Use good judgment about whether to tell your patient what his blood pressure is; for some, this knowledge creates additional anxiety. (See Chapter 6 for information about taking blood pressure.)

Your loved one may have a hard time adjusting psychologically to his condition and the requirements of altered life-style. Consult books on stress and behavior modification. The habits of a lifetime are not easy to change, but your patient should be encouraged to try. Some form of psychotherapy may be helpful as a way of understanding self-inflicted stress. Help your patient plan a much-needed vacation and give up the 14-hour work days; there is always tomorrow, if he watches his health.

If he is overweight, your patient may be put on a calorie restricted diet. Help him follow it by making meals appetizing and appealing; emphasize quality rather than quantity. Salt probably will be restricted; ask if salt substitutes are allowed. Read labels for sodium content. Cholesterol and fats may be restricted, too. Caffeine and alcohol should be taken in moderation; tobacco use should be discouraged.

Congestive Heart Failure

Congestive heart failure does not mean the heart has stopped working. It is a condition in which the heart is unable to keep up with the job of pumping blood throughout the body, resulting in inefficient circulation. It can be caused by heart problems, by other organic problems, or by factors causing the heart to work harder.

One of the first signs of congestive heart failure may be that the patient tires easily after exertion. Simple tasks such as walking or climbing stairs may make your patient short of breath and tired. He may have trouble breathing when lying flat, or he may develop a cough (usually associated with the production of sputum or mucus). His feet or ankles may become swollen. As the problem progresses, these symptoms may become more severe. The patient may experience increased difficulty breathing. Gasping for air or rapid, noisy, gurgling breathing are signs that would indicate an emergency and rapid action should be taken.

In treatment, your patient may be placed on oxygen. Bed rest is necessary so that the heart is allowed to rest. A heart medication may be given to slow down the heart and strengthen its beat. In most cases, heart disorders are treated medically and surgery is reserved as an alternative when these measures fail, or when there is extensive heart damage.

Diuretics may be prescribed to rid the body of excess fluid. Be sure that the medication is given as prescribed (often with orange juice) and taken on time. Some of these drugs cause potassium loss; check with your doctor to see if potassium replacement is a concern. Foods that provide potassium are bananas, fresh vegetables, orange juice, peas, nuts, molasses, fresh fish, and poultry.

Fluids may be restricted and careful attention should be paid to urine output. Your doctor may want you to measure and record all output to evaluate the effectiveness of the medication. Check the extremities for signs that swelling is decreasing. Watch for signs of dehydration (decreased urine output, dry mouth, shaking and muscle tremors, dry skin) since too much fluid can be lost. Other side effects may be nausea, vomiting, headaches, palpitations, dizziness, drowsiness, and tingling of the extremities. Report these to your doctor.

Your patient may return home on a salt-restricted diet. No table salt may be used, although the doctor may allow a salt substitute. Read *all* labels for sodium content; some medicines contain salt. Avoid foods high in sodium (fish, ham, bacon, nuts, potato chips, ketchup, peanut butter, bread, butter, and milk). Use pepper, lemon juice, or other herbs and spices to flavor foods. Watch your patient for excessive losses of sodium through increased sweating or urine loss. Ask your doctor if replacement is necessary.

Heart Attacks

During a heart attack, the blood supply to the the muscle surrounding the heart (myocardium) is impaired, usually as a result of blockage of a major vessel by an excess of fatty plaques, increased exercise or work, blood clots, or from direct trauma.

The symptoms that precede it may be severe pain in the chest radiating to the shoulder and arm (usually the left); increased perspiration; a feeling of fullness; indigestion; fever; decrease in blood pressure; a fast, weak pulse; or feeling faint or weak. Some of these symptoms will be more subtle and the patient may not even realize what happened. The amount of damage that occurs can vary from mild to severe. Fever alone may be an indication that heart damage has occurred, signaling tissue death (necrosis) in the area.

Emergency handling of the situation can mean the difference between life and death. If the patient has heart problems and is taking nitroglycerine, offer this medication first. Ask your doctor about whether you should provide multiple doses of nitroglycerine in an emergency. Call the paramedics. Make the heart attack victim lie down; keep him comfortable and warm; and loosen any clothing. If he is having trouble breathing, place a few pillows under his head. If possible, have someone with him constantly. If he must vomit, turn him on his side; don't let him vomit while lying on his back. Contact your physician's office and tell the doctor you are on your way to the hospital. Try to stay calm; don't create excess anxiety.

An electrocardiogram and blood tests will help to establish the diagnosis and extent of damage. The patient's vital signs (temperature, pulse, respiration, blood pressure) will be taken frequently. The most critical period occurs in the first 48 hours. Your loved one may require pain medications, oxygen, a heart monitor, and special drugs. Rest is imperative. Your patient's hospital stay will vary depending on the extent of damage and the amount of progress toward recovery. The prognosis will depend on the extent of myocardial damage and the severity of the vessel occlusion.

Upon discharge, the patient will be required to rest at home before returning to work or other activities. Your patient may be confined to bed or allowed short periods up in a chair. If he appears weak, don't let him walk alone; have him hold on to you. Just because your patient has been discharged from the hospital does not mean he is well enough to pick up where he left off. The damaged heart must be allowed to heal; recuperation may last several months.

You may have to adapt your home while your loved one recovers. If his bedroom is on the second floor, perhaps put a bed downstairs. If you live in a five-story walk-up, climbing the stairs probably would be unhealthy at this time. Your patient should not be allowed to exert himself and stairs may be too taxing.

After your loved one comes home, watch for these symptoms: shortness of breath or difficulty in breathing; chest pain; swelling of the feet or ankles; changes in pulse rate or blood pressure; and complaints of weakness or fainting. Notify the health care team if any of these occur.

Your patient may go home on a number of medications. Know what they are; what they are taken for; how frequently they should be taken; and what side effects to expect. If you are monitoring vital signs, make sure you understand how to take them and keep accurate records (see Chapter 6). Find out if special exercises are prescribed and carry out the doctor's orders.

Your patient should not strain his heart in any way. Hard bowel movements and constipation can cause straining. Doctors often recommend stool softeners for these patients. Enemas may be prescribed. Tell the doctor if your patient has to strain to move his bowels.

A special cardiac diet probably will be prescribed. Salt, cholesterol, and caffeine may be restricted. The patient should avoid foods that make his digestive tract and heart work too hard. Soft foods are best at first. Avoid large, heavy meals. If your patient is overweight, he may be put on a calorie-restricted diet. Don't "cheat" in this important area; the patient's diet before the heart attack may have contributed to the cause. For free publications about healthy diets for heart patients, write to:

American Heart Association
7320 Greenville Avenue
Dallas, TX 75231

Psychologically, it may be difficult for the patient to adapt to a new life-style. He may be anxious or nervous about future heart attacks. The care giver can play an important role here. If your patient sees that you are anxious or protective, he may adopt the same attitude. Don't baby him too much. Don't do things he should do for himself. Keep the stress level down, but don't make the household seem like a morgue. During rest periods, keep the noise down, the lights low, and room temperature comfortable.

If your patient is not sleeping, let the doctor know; sedatives may be prescribed. Don't allow the patient to have more than two sleepless nights. If worry is keeping him awake, talk it out together.

Sexual activity may be restricted at this time. When the doctor does allow the patient to have sexual relations, he should avoid strain. The patient should assume a non-dominant position. Avoid sex after exercise or eating. If the patient is taking medications that may cause impotency, talk with your doctor if this becomes a problem.

Your patient may be allowed to work half a day a few times a week and increase his load gradually. If he had a strenuous or stressful occupation, he may be advised to discontinue it. If your patient is a high-pressure person, help him develop some stress-releasing activities. Bicycling is good, even with a stationary bike. Walking or swimming may be recommended. Start all new activities slowly and progress gradually. Avoid exercise in the heat of the day. Stay indoors during hot and humid weather; use an air conditioner on those days.

Angina

Angina is a type of sudden chest pain similar to the pain felt during a heart attack. The difference is that this pain is transient and will subside in a few minutes by itself, or with medication. Angina occurs as a result of spasms in the blood vessels, or when blood supply is briefly inadequate for the heart's increased needs. The pain may be in the jaw, between the shoulder blades, over the heart, and it may or may not radiate down the arm. This pain is a warning signal that the heart is not receiving enough blood.

Nitroglycerine tablets are prescribed for angina; they dilate the blood vessels and allow blood to flow normally. These come in varying strengths and are placed under the person's tongue. The patient usually is told to take nitroglycerine tablets at the first sign of pain and discontinue any activity. The pain should subside in two to three minutes. Report any pain that does not quit.

Ask your doctor about whether the patient should take additional nitroglycerine tablets. Some side effects of the medication are headache; a feeling of faintness; heart palpitations; temporary lowering of blood pressure; face flushing; and nausea. Most of these symptoms occur in patients who have not taken this medication before. After prolonged use, the side effects should diminish.

Some patients use nitroglycerine paste. A patch with nitroglycerine is applied to the chest or upper arm to deliver a slow dose of the drug over an extended period of time (as much as 24 hours). Be sure the patch is applied to a smooth, clean surface free of hair and perspiration. Use a small piece of tape if you have trouble getting the patch to stick. It usually is changed at the same time each day; bedtime is convenient. The patient may shower or bathe with this in place; if it falls off, apply a new one. The patch can cause skin rash or irritation. Side effects will be the same, although more subtle with nitroglycerine patches.

The angina patient initially needs encouragement and reassurance that he is going to be fine. This experience can be frightening and the pain quite uncomfortable. Most patients will adjust with time. Be sure to report any pain not relieved by the medication and rest.

Arrhythmias

The heart has a special nerve conduction system that acts as a pacemaker and helps to keep the heart rhythm in sync. Disorders within that system, diseases, responses to some medications, and other problems can create changes in normal function. Heart rhythm disorders are diagnosed with an electrocardiogram and radiological studies.

In some rhythm disorders, the pulse may be too fast (tachycardia, usually over 100 beats a minute) or too slow (bradycardia, usually less than 60 beats per minute). These values vary depending on the patient's usual pulse and they apply when the person is at rest. When taking your patient's pulse, feel for the rhythm and consistency of the beat. It should be a regular, steady rhythm, almost like the tick of a clock. You may feel a few regular beats, then a few fluttery fast ones, or other variations, possibly indicating problems. Your patient may have tachycardia or bradycardia and still have a regular rhythm.

Major problems occur when this rhythm becomes irregular. Symptoms indicating a change in pulse rate include a change in blood pressure; feeling weak and faint; cold, clammy skin; dizziness; headache; or trouble breathing. Some rhythm disorders correct themselves; others may be life threatening. If you note any of these problems, call your doctor.

Medications or a cardiac pacemaker may be used to treat heart rhythm problems. If the problem is serious, some drugs may be administered intravenously for fast action. In emergencies, a cardiac defibrillator may be used. You've probably seen this treatment dramatized on television. It works by delivering an electrical impulse to the heart. Additional cardiac life support measures may be necessary (cardiopulmonary resuscitation). Learn how to perform CPR if your loved one has a heart condition.

A pacemaker is used to correct some heart rhythm problems. Placement of a pacemaker is a minor procedure, usually done under local anesthesia (the patient is not put to sleep). A small incisional pocket is made in the abdomen or upper chest for the pacemaker, which runs on batteries. These batteries are good for three to five years; some of the newer ones may last for 10 to 20 years. Battery recharging can be done through a simple surgical procedure or externally.

The following problems may occur with a pacemaker: infections at the placement site; other rhythm problems; catheter problems; or a pacemaker malfunction, although mechanical failures rarely occur. Patients are taught to take their pulses daily. They may even be able to feel a rhythm disorder. Symptoms of serious problems include mental confusion or disorientation; chest pain; decreased blood pressure; swelling in the neck; unhealthy skin color; shortness of breath or difficulty breathing; and restlessness. If you note any of these conditions, seek medical attention.

After the pacemaker is implanted, you may be involved in caring for the incision. The edges should be closed; the sutures or stitches may or may not be in place when your patient is discharged. Generally, only a small gauze dressing is used to cover the area, and some patients need no dressing at all. Look for signs of infection: redness, tenderness, discharge, warm to the touch, and drainage. Your patient should wear loose fitting tops. Until the incision heals, activity will be restricted.

Your loved one should carry identification with the following information: the name and type of pacemaker; manufacturer's identification and model number; pacemaker rate; and doctor and hospital where the pacemaker was inserted. Include any special operating instructions. A medallion or bracelet will show that your patient wears a pacemaker if he is unconscious or unable to communicate. For information about bracelets, write to:

Medic Alert Foundation
P.O Box 1009
Turlock, CA 95381

Pacemaker patients should be monitored regularly with an electrocardiogram (ECG). Pacemaker clinics throughout the country have special phone and computer hookups to monitor and test the pacemaker. They are able to pick up the generator's pulse rate and record it on an electrocardiogram. These results are then evaluated by a heart specialist.

Patients with pacemakers should stay away from microwave ovens, some types of electrical generators, or other equipment that is apt to interfere with the pacemaker. Check with your doctor about other areas your patient should avoid. When traveling by air, avoid airline metal detectors. Explain that your patient has a pacemaker and provide identification; he will be allowed to pass around it. It is all right to be checked with a portable, hand-held device.

Postoperative Cardiac Surgical Care

With the evolution of modern technology, there is little that cannot be repaired or replaced with artificial or donor organs. Major heart vessels can be replaced by synthetic ones, or they can be taken from other areas in the body and surgically implanted into the affected area. There are heart transplants and even artificial hearts used to replace a defective heart. Not long ago, patients died from these conditions; many now lead relatively normal lives.

In this section, I will discuss overall postoperative care rather than address each procedure separately. Work closely with the health care team and follow the program recommended for your patient. Before surgery, your patient's health probably was guarded. The recovery period will most likely be long and cautious. Pay attention to some of the possible postoperative complications: infections; bleeding; signs of rejection (if an artificial organ or device is used); heart rhythm problems; fluid retention problems; and kidney problems. The surgical incision will need care. Often, by the time your patient is discharged, the incision is well on its way to being healed and the stitches have been removed. If the incision is still healing, will you need special supplies? Should the technique be sterile or clean? Watch for signs of incision problems; redness, swelling, tenderness, pus or drainage, fever, or pain.

Activities and exercise will be gradually increased. Exercise is important to the heart and cardiovascular system. The patient should not spend too much time in one position. If he is allowed to get up, he should alternate between periods of sitting, standing, and walking. Follow your patient's recommended exercise program faithfully. Avoid exposure to extreme temperatures; an air conditioner may be necessary to keep your patient comfortable.

When your loved one comes home, it may be best that he sleep downstairs until he is allowed to climb stairs. The recuperative process may be anywhere from six weeks to two months, or longer. The patient must have the doctor's permission before he resumes driving or returns to work. If he had a demanding job, he may need to find another line of work.

If your patient has post-surgical pain, pain-killers may be provided. Find out what they are, how they are to be given, get special instructions, and note if there are side effects. Pain medications should be administered at the earliest onset of pain. Do not allow time for the pain to peak, especially if the medications are to be given orally. Most oral medications will take effect in 20 to 30 minutes.

If your patient has pain when coughing or moving, you can help to lessen this pain by using a pillow held tightly in the chest area by the patient. If the patient is having pain, wait until after the pain subsides before having him do any activities. It is important to relieve pain rapidly and effectively because it can also cause stress and added work on the patient's heart. If pain medication does not appear to be effective, report it to your doctor. Keep a record of all your patient's medications; they probably will be numerous.

Be sure to follow any prescribed diet. Most patients will have salt (sodium) restricted. Provide adequate fluid intake, but watch for problems with fluid retention (swollen ankles, decreased urine output). Avoid constipation through diet, medications, or enemas as prescribed by the doctor. If vital signs are to be monitored, be sure you know what the expected values will be and keep an accurate daily record. Provide plenty of rest. You may want to limit visitors at first so your loved one does not overdo or get overtired.

Your patient will need much support and encouragement during this recuperative period. If your attitude is one of confidence and composure, most likely your patient will follow suit.

Care Giver's Checklist

1. Circulatory disorders often require strict attention to diet and exercise; this isn't the time to cheat on diet restrictions. Help your patient learn to adjust to a new, healthier life-style with plenty of positive reassurance.
2. Review your knowledge of vital signs. Know the expected values for your patient's pulse and blood pressure so you can recognize complications at the onset.
3. If your patient has a blood disorder, such as leukemia, or is on anticoagulant therapy for circulatory diseases, pay special attention to bleeding problems. Avoid sharp razors, since a small cut can be difficult to control. Apply added pressure or ice following injections. Nosebleeds can be difficult to control and may require a trip to the emergency room. Watch for subtle signs of bleeding—bleeding at the gums; black tarry stools; or vaginal bleeding.
4. Stroke victims need constant support and encouragement, recuperation can be lengthy and months may pass before you know whether your loved one will fully recover. Gradually increase physical and mental challenges. Learn as much as you can about your patient's disability; perhaps he can understand you, but hasn't the ability to respond appropriately. The stroke victim may sometimes act like a child, but should never be treated like one. Stroke patients still have a need for dignity and understanding.
5. A comatose patient may be sent home when there's no hope of rehabilitation. A comatose patient will be incontinent, unable to eat or drink, move or communicate. He will require 24-hour care which is physically and emotionally demanding for any family. Consider your options carefully before committing to home care of a comatose loved one.

11 The Respiratory System

All living cells need oxygen to carry out activities vital to survival. The body gets oxygen and eliminates carbon dioxide through the respiratory and cardiovascular systems. (You learned about the cardiovascular system in Chapter 10.) The respiratory system comprises the nose, pharynx, trachea, bronchi, and lungs.

Ventilation (breathing) occurs when gases in the atmosphere (oxygen) are drawn down into the lungs and waste gases (carbon dioxide) are expelled back up through the respiratory tract. Since this process is vital to survival, any interference can pose serious consequences for your patient. Processes that can interfere with this vital function include physiological or organic obstruction of the airway passage; some lung disorders; infections; tumors; and chronic respiratory problems. These can be acute, such as having a piece of food caught in the airway, or chronic, usually resulting from years of inadequate ventilation perhaps caused by diminished lung capacity, decreased lung elasticity, or narrowing of the airways. Some examples of chronic respiratory conditions are emphysema, asthma, and chronic bronchitis.

Some signs of acute respiratory problems are choking or gasping for air; wheezing or shortness of breath; or changes in color. A light purple, gray, or ashen color represents airway oxygenation problems. If your patient is black, color may not be a good indicator for detecting respiratory distress. Check the lips or nail beds for signs of cyanosis (dusky purple or blue indicating lack of oyxgen or poor circulation).

Some other common symptoms seen in patients with compromised respiratory function are fever; excess amounts of sputum; changes in pulse; changes in blood pressure; chronic respiratory infections or pneumonia; loss of appetite; mental confusion; restlessness; and easy fatigue.

Acute pulmonary or respiratory problems can be relieved by implementing lifesaving measures such as CPR (cardiopulmonary resuscitation) or the Heimlich maneuver, a sudden thrust to help dislodge an airway obstruction. Other methods include manual clearing of the airway, administering oxygen or medications to dilate the airway passage, performing an emergency tracheostomy, providing artificial breathing apparatus, or through surgical intervention. (Be sure to read Chapter 16 on emergencies.)

Chronic respiratory problems are more difficult to treat since pulmonary damage often has been so severe that no single treatment will cure or reverse the process. In most cases, the symptoms can be treated, and some techniques will help to prevent progression of the illness, but in most cases the patient will have to adapt to living with compromised respiratory function.

Diagnosis can be made through X-rays, blood studies, biopsy, or various respiratory function studies. A special device may be passed down the patient's airway enabling the doctor to inspect the respiratory organs. External factors believed to affect respiratory function include smoking, allergies, chemical or atmospheric irritants or pollutants, and perhaps genetic or inherited tendencies. Testing often is done to determine if irritants are a factor. Asthma and hay fever are pulmonary ailments where irritants are thought to be the cause of the symptoms; some researchers believe irritants are factors in some lung cancers.

The patient with compromised respiratory or pulmonary capacity will require a great deal of emotional support and reassurance. Breathing difficulties can be frightening. Some patients compare it to suffocation. The slightest amount of exercise or activity can make some patients short of breath. For a more severely compromised patient, life begins to consist of bed rest, perhaps sitting up in a chair, and continuous oxygen support.

Caring for Patients with Respiratory Problems

The primary treatment for your patient is to relieve the symptoms, prevent complications and progression of the disease, and help him live with impaired respiratory function. Environment plays a key role. Do you live in an area where weather or altitude contribute to your patient's problems? Some patients are advised to move to a warm, dry, climate.

Your home environment is important, too. Most of these patients should live within a controlled atmosphere, often using air conditioning. Excesses of temperature can make breathing more difficult. A humidifier or air-filtering system may be helpful. If your patient is severely compromised, climbing stairs may be a problem. Can your patient climb to the second floor without shortness of breath? Do you live in an apartment building where there is no elevator and stairs are necessary for access? Changing the patient's indoor environment can make adaptation to the problem easier. Keep your home free of dust, certain plants and flowers, or other irritants that can aggravate your patient's condition. Your patient should be advised not to smoke, and perhaps you should ban smoking in the home. He should avoid areas that are confining or poorly ventilated.

Provide ways to increase pulmonary ventilation. Respiratory equipment and oxygen may be needed. Try elevating your patient's head with pillows to make breathing easier. Your patient may have been taught exercises to strengthen breathing muscles; be sure he does them. Coughing and deep breathing exercises help bring up excess secretions that can sit in the lungs and lead to infection, pneumonia, and other lung problems. If your patient is unable to do this himself, perhaps manual suctioning may have to be done to remove excess secretions (see page 82 for suctioning procedures).

Encourage your patient to drink 10 to 12 glasses of fluid a day to help reduce secretions. Avoid excessively hot or cold fluids, which stimulate coughing, and foods that create mucus, such as milk or dairy products. Avoid gas-forming foods. Give smaller, more frequent feedings to reduce fatigue; avoid large, fatty, and fried meals. Provide rest periods before and after eating.

Patients with respiratory disease experience weight loss due to loss of appetite. You may have to offer high calorie, nutritional supplements. If your patient is losing weight, be sure to report it to your doctor.

Provide frequent and careful oral hygiene since your patient probably does most of his breathing through the mouth. Keep his lips lubricated and his mouth from drying out.

Your patient may be prone to upper respiratory infections. Be sure that he is immunized yearly against flu viruses, if your doctor recommends it. Avoid large crowds or people known to have colds, flu, or other respiratory infections. Fatigue also can lower the patient's ability to combat and fight infection. Check with your doctor about managing upper respiratory infections. Signs of upper respiratory infection are coughing; fever; sore throat; change in sputum or mucus color and consistency; tightness in the chest; fatigue; and difficulty breathing. Report any of these signs to your physician.

The doctor may wish to take a chest X-ray, blood tests, or obtain a sputum specimen to evaluate the infection. Have your patient cough up a specimen into a collection container. If he is unable to cough up the specimen, it can be manually suctioned (see page 83). If you must obtain a sputum specimen, it's best to try first thing in the morning when your patient may be able to produce the largest amount of secretions. Have your patient brush his teeth, rinse out his mouth, and use mouthwash. This will help remove any excess bacteria in the mouth. He should then take a deep cough and spit out any of the mucus into the container. Check with your physician on what you should use to collect the specimen; will a clean jar be sufficient or is a sterile container required? You should have at least a teaspoonful for the specimen to be evaluated. Cover the container and label it with the patient's and doctor's names, the type of specimen, and when it was obtained. Ask your doctor how it should be stored and how soon it must be taken in for evaluation. Various procedures may drain excess mucous secretions from your patient. One method of bringing up secretions is postural drainage, which helps to drain secretions by gravity. Your patient should be positioned so that his head is lower than his chest. (Your physician will tell you how to position your patient.) Sometimes, the patient lies on his abdomen so that he is hanging over the edge of the bed, with his head down toward the floor. While your patient is in this position, he should be encouraged to cough and breathe deeply to raise secretions. Provide a basin for the patient to spit into.

The position and the amount of time the patient can tolerate this procedure will vary depending on his age and physical condition. The procedure can start out gradually until the patient is able to tolerate it for longer periods. It should be done two to three times daily for as long as 20 minutes for best results. Ask someone on the health care team to demonstrate chest percussion, another effective method of raising secretions.

Drug Therapy

Drug therapy for this type of patient may consist of combinations of drugs. Antibiotics may be used to fight infection; bronchodilators to help dilate the vessels in the pulmonary system; steroids or cortisone-like substances to help reduce inflammation and irritation; and diuretics to help reduce excess fluid volume. More than one of these drugs may be used at a time. You should know the names of the drugs prescribed for your patient and what they are used for. How often and by what route should they be given? What is the action of these drugs and what are the side effects? Avoid cough syrups or medications that will suppress coughs and dry secretions.

Bronchodilators (Ephedrine, Aminophylline, Isuprel) probably are the most effective drugs used in relieving the symptoms of pulmonary disease. They can be administered orally, as inhalants, or injected. Some of the side effects are fast pulse rate; elevated blood pressure; headache; nausea; vomiting; nervousness; and agitation. These symptoms may occur immediately following administration of the medication and should disappear shortly. Some occur after the patient's first exposure to the medication and subside following a few doses. If you note any of these, check with your physician; they may indicate other problems. Care should be taken when using these powerful medications on the elderly.

Steroid therapy involves the use of steroids (anti-inflammatory agents) on a gradually escalating basis to reduce some symptoms of chronic lung and pulmonary disease. In most instances, if the patient is taken off this therapy, the dose will be tapered gradually. Your patient should not be abruptly taken off steroid therapy. If there are reasons your patient cannot take his medication (vomiting, nausea), report this to the doctor immediately. If steroids are used, the results will occur rapidly and they can be quite dramatic. Some common side effects are fluid retention; classic moon face (face puffiness); increased appetite; increase in body hair; euphoria and depression (mood swings). Most of these medications should be taken with meals or immediately following to decrease stomach upset.

Diuretics may be used to treat one of the most acute respiratory problems, pulmonary edema. They act by decreasing the reabsorption of salt and water in the kidneys. Be careful when administering these medications as they have a number of severe side effects, such as too much fluid loss; excessive potassium loss (causing muscle spasms or tremors, nausea, weakness, dizziness, numbness, and tingling of the extremities); headache; and palpitations. The patient's urine output should be closely monitored. Follow all fluid restrictions. Potassium may be replaced either with potassium supplements, by diet, or both. Report side effects promptly to your doctor.

Generally, the infections these patients get are streptococcal, which require intensive antibiotic therapy. Antibiotics must be given as ordered, and on time, so their therapeutic levels can be maintained. If your patient is unable to take his prescribed oral medications, report this to your doctor immediately; alternate methods may have to be used. Antibiotics also can be given by intramuscular injections and intravenously. The doctor may place your patient on a broad spectrum antibiotic initially and make changes based on the results of blood and sputum specimens.

Be sure you know if your patient has any allergies to any of these drugs, especially penicillin since some penicillin drugs are referred to by other names. Other medications can interfere with the drugs' effectiveness, so be sure your doctor is aware of any other drugs your patient is taking. Most antibiotics can cause stomach irritation, resulting in nausea, vomiting, loss of appetite, diarrhea, or constipation. This is why it is important that some antibiotics not be taken on an empty stomach. Your patient should avoid sunlight since antibiotics can make him susceptible to sunburn.

It may be important to protect the care giver and the rest of the family from being exposed to your patient's infective organism. Find out if your patient is contagious, and if so, the period of time over which your patient could infect you. Always wash your hands after treating your patient. Do not touch any of his respiratory secretions. If someone usually sleeps with the patient, check with the doctor to see if this should be avoided during this period. Your patient should cover his mouth with his hand or a tissue when coughing. If he is extremely contagious, you may even want the patient to use disposable dishes and utensils. Provide a special container for all of his used materials. Double bag all of his used waste materials and keep them separate.

In some instances, the doctor may advise using a face mask for added protection. If you are wearing a face mask, put it on before going in to see the patient. Leave it in place until you have washed your hands, then take it off and dispose of it with the patient's other contaminated items. Do not carry any of his waste products to other areas of the house. Limit visitors until the doctor tells you it is all right for others to be exposed to your patient.

Oxygen Therapy

Oxygen replenishes and improves tissue oxygenation and is administered to the patient through a catheter, cannula, or mask. The method of administration depends upon what oxygen concentration is required; how often will it be used; patient comfort; and whether high humidity is necessary.

The nasal catheter delivers low-flow oxygen at higher concentrations of 30 to 35 percent and is most often used for short-term treatment. The nasal cannula delivers low concentrations of oxygen at 22 to 30 percent. It is less expensive and more comfortable for patients requiring long-term oxygen therapy. The mask can deliver concentrations up to 100 percent. This is used when the patient requires high, precise concentrations of oxygen or requires humidity, too. It may also be used when the patient cannot tolerate a catheter or cannula placed in his nose, or if he can breathe only through his mouth. The use of a mask may create anxiety or make the patient feel closed in. If this occurs, perhaps another type may be used.

The oxygen source in the home most likely will be the cannister tank. There are large cannisters and small, portable ones. Home respiratory and oxygen therapy companies will supply and assemble all of the equipment you will need. Some home care companies and medical supply centers also supply this equipment. Be sure you keep a close watch on the meter indicating the amount of oxygen left in the tank, and order well in advance. Some suppliers will leave you with a reserve tank. Portable tanks can be used when the patient is out of the house; if your patient is apt to require oxygen, do not forget to take it with you.

Oxygen is an extremely combustible gas, requiring strict adherence to safety rules. There must be no smoking; avoid open flames, some electrical appliances, and improperly grounded televisions, radios, and electric razors. All family members, relatives, and visitors should be notified whenever oxygen is in use. Tape a sign over the patient's bed or on the door stating that oxygen is in use.

Humidity is necessary when administering oxygen because commercial oxygen has no water vapor. The oxygen we naturally take into our bodies contains water in the form of vapor (humidity). Commercial oxygen must be humidified to prevent dryness in the respiratory tract. Special attachments to the oxygen cylinder will add humidity for your patient.

The doctor will determine the oxygen flow rate based on your patient's oxygen requirements. Have your oxygen supplier set up the tank for you, set up all of the appropriate equipment, and show you how to operate it. There will be a flow rate meter on the tank marked in liters, which is the standard measurement for oxygen. The plastic humidity bottle should be filled two-thirds full with sterile distilled water, not ordinary tap water. If you are using a pre-filled bottle, check to be sure the seal has not been broken; you should hear a "swooshing" sound that would indicate you are the first person to break the vacuum. If it appears to have been opened, do not use it. Attach the bottle to the adapter. The water should be replaced every 24 hours. Pour out any leftover water and refill the container. Any commercial containers should be disposed of and new ones used.

Be sure the oxygen valve has been opened. Turn your flow rate meter to two to three liters (by turning clockwise), and check for bubbles in the bottle. This will indicate that the bottle has been applied properly. You should be able to feel air and humidity if you place your hand in front of the faucet. You won't be able to smell anything because oxygen is odorless. This also is a danger, since you will not be able to smell it if the oxygen valve has been left open.

To stop the oxygen flow, be sure to turn the flow rate knob as far as you can counterclockwise; you should also not be able to see anything registering or fluctuating on the flow rate meter. Be sure that the oxygen is closed off tightly. Avoid smoking even when you are sure the tank has been closed off; some slight amounts may still be released, which would be flammable.

Connect all of your tubing to the tank as instructed. To test the mask and tubing, place your hand or face next to the mask or cannula to feel for air flow. Turn the meter to 10 to 15 liters to flush out the tubing and be sure it is open. Set the flow rate meter to the prescribed rate. Gently apply the mask or cannula as instructed; be sure they are not too tight or too loose. You should not see marks on the patient where the elastic has been pulled; but if it is applied too loosely, much of the oxygen will leak out. You can pad any pressure areas with a cotton wad or gauze sponge.

Keep the skin under the mask dry. Whenever necessary, take off the mask and dry the skin. If your patient can tolerate being without oxygen for a few minutes, you can also wash his face with soap and water. The mask should be cleaned regularly with soap and water. The nasal prongs can be cleaned on the inside by using a wet cotton applicator pushed inside; dry them thoroughly. Check with your doctor or respiratory therapist about how often these should be replaced.

Change your patient's position frequently; as often as every two hours if he is not moving on his own. A patient who is short of breath usually is most comfortable if elevated or sitting. Observe your patient for signs of oxygen hunger: gasping for breath, restlessness, increased heart rate, perspiration, yawning, changes in color (cyanosis), and flaring nostrils. Any of these conditions should be reported at once to your doctor.

Increased anxiety or stress also can make it more difficult for the patient to breathe. This can become a vicious cycle; the patient begins to have trouble breathing, becomes frightened and anxious, and the situation gets worse. Your patient should be assured in a calm, soothing manner. This may help him relax and reduce the problem.

Oxygen hunger may indicate that the mask or cannula is not providing effective levels of oxygen or that the flow rate needs to be increased. Do not adjust the flow rate until you have checked with the doctor. Some patients may not be able to tolerate prolonged periods without extra oxygen. If your patient must take off his oxygen mask to eat or drink, perhaps a nasal cannula would provide a better means of continuous oxygen support.

Oxygen is administered on a continuous, or as needed, basis. Some patients become oxygen dependent, and the process of weaning them may be difficult. Whenever taking a patient off oxygen therapy, watch for signs of oxygen hunger and report them to your doctor. Oxygen may have to be restarted. Some patients may show signs of oxygen toxicity, such as changes in blood pressure, heart and respiratory rate, or mental confusion. The lung may even collapse. Oxygen toxicity usually affects patients receiving concentrations of oxygen greater than 60 percent per 24-hour period. Keep a bell or some method of calling for help near your patient. Check with your doctor to see how to take your patient's temperature because oxygen can lower body temperature; if you take the temperature orally, it may be inaccurate.

Tracheostomy

A tracheostomy most often is an emergency intervention performed when the patient has an obstruction in his airway above the level of the trachea. The blockage can be mechanical or pathological, due to severe swelling. Tracheostomy is relatively simple: an incision is made in the trachea (windpipe) and a tube (cannula) is passed down the trachea to provide an artificial airway for the patient. A tracheostomy can be temporary or permanent. If permanent, the trachea is sutured to the skin surface, creating a stoma effect. This will now become the patient's source for breathing.

Two major concerns in caring for a tracheostomy patient are keeping the airway open and free of excess mucus, and keeping the skin clean and free of infection and irritation. Sterile technique will be used in the hospital until the stoma is fully healed, usually four to eight days. When your patient is discharged home, the care will be less intensive and sterile technique usually not required.

Tracheostomy tubes and cannulae come in various sizes, are metal, plastic, or rubber, and are cuffed or un-cuffed. The cuffed tracheostomy has an inflatable cuff on the inside to prevent it from falling out. Cuff-type tracheostomies are used when a patient is on an artificial respirator. If the cuff is properly inflated, you should not be able to hear air leaking and the patient will not be able to speak. Some tracheostomy patients can speak; others cannot, depending on individual medical conditions. The decision to use a particular type of tracheostomy tube will depend on the doctor's personal preference or the patient's condition. The care involved will vary slightly depending on the type used.

There are excess secretions with a new tracheostomy since air is going directly to the trachea, rather than being warmed and moistened by passing through the nose and mouth. The lining of the trachea compensates and reacts by causing coughing and secreting additional amounts of mucus. In time, the body will adapt to this new circumstance and mucous secretions will lessen. Your patient may require extra dressing changes or a bib to absorb some of these excess secretions. In some patients, a suctioning device may be used. It is important to remove excess mucus because it could obstruct airway flow.

Another way of compensating for increased dryness is to provide adequate humidity and moisture. This can be done with a portable humidifier. Some patients also need a special mist apparatus applied directly to the tracheostomy. The use of air conditioners should be avoided at first because they may cause further irritation and dryness.

The patient with a "trach" should be careful bathing or during any other activity involving water; water should not get into the tracheostomy. If water does get into it, it could be as serious as taking water into the lungs. Notify your doctor if you think water may have gotten into the trach. Special precautions should be taken when the patient showers or bathes. Your patient can use special plastic bibs or cover it with his hand. Swimming should be avoided, but other forms of mild recreation and exercise are encouraged.

Your patient's sense of taste and smell may be altered for a short period following insertion of a trach because air is not passing through the body in its usual fashion. This usually is temporary until the body has had time to adjust. Vitamins or supplemental feedings may be offered for patients who are losing weight because of this.

Your patient will need much assurance and support before he begins to feel comfortable, and he will have to be given time to adjust. He may fear being left alone at first; provide emotional security by staying close by.

The bedridden tracheostomy patient should always have a bell to signal for help if he needs it. He may be nervous about performing his own care. Stay with him and help him if he needs it. Have a visiting nurse come in the beginning until he feels comfortable. Your patient may have no problem adjusting if the tracheostomy provided much needed respiratory relief. The stoma site itself is fairly easy to conceal with clothing and most often will go unnoticed. Generally, if the dressings are kept clean of mucous secretions, there will be no odor.

For daily stoma care, wash your hands and put on gloves. Start at the inner surface, wiping away from the stoma area. Use as many sponges as necessary to wipe away mucous and dried secretions. A sterile, cotton-tipped applicator dipped in a recommended cleansing solution may be used to get into small areas. Dry the area thoroughly with sterile gauze sponges. Never remove the cannula completely; it may shut off the airway. However, if your patient has a double section cannula, remove the inner portion by unlocking it, and place it in a container of hydrogen peroxide or other prescribed solution.

Clean the area as described above. Take the cleaned cannula and, using a special sterile brush, scrub the cannula inside and out, removing all mucous formation. Rinse it off with sterile saline. Shake it off and use the sterile gauze sponges to dry the outside; you can wrap a piece of gauze around pipe cleaners to dry the center. The center must be dry before placing it inside the patient. The exterior should remain slightly damp to help slip it back into place. Reinsert the inner piece back into the tracheostomy tube. Be sure that you lock it into place; pull on it gently to check.

It is easier if you use the pre-slit trach dressings. Slip this pad under the stoma. Remove your gloves after you have done this. If this dressing becomes soiled, you can change only that piece without repeating the entire procedure. It is important that this dressing be kept as dry as possible; any moisture can irritate your patient's skin or be a source of infection. Wash your hands afterward.

There are several ways to change the tracheostomy ties that hold the appliance in place; use the method recommended by your doctor. To keep the cannula in place during this procedure, have the patient hold it while you tie the ties, or keep the used one in place until you have fastened the new ones. Do not fasten it too tightly; you should be able to slip one finger underneath. Cut off any excess tie material. Check your patient often to be sure the tie has not become too tight and that the cannula is in place. If cuff inflation or deflation is indicated, follow the procedure your doctor has recommended.

Sometimes, the stoma may shrink and require dilation. If you note any problems or irritation around the stoma, notify the doctor. Also, report changes in the usual color, amount, or consistency of the mucous secretions; it could indicate infection. Watch for signs of increased swelling, which, if unchecked, could close off the patient's airway. Be sure your patient is receiving adequate ventilation and oxygenation through his tracheal airway. Find out if you should have any additional equipment to be used in case of an emergency. Ask your doctor if it is necessary to have equipment to do CPR on this type of patient. If so, you will need the materials and training. If there are signs of respiratory problems, call the rescue squad.

Suctioning a Tracheostomy

This type of suctioning is done by placing a suction catheter directly down the tracheostomy and into the trachea and bronchi. This removes excess secretions and mucus from the patient who is unable to do this on his own. *Get training from a health care professional before you attempt this on your own.* Do not do the procedure too vigorously; it can irritate sensitive mucous membranes and even cause bleeding. Extra caution should be taken if it is a new tracheostomy or the patient is on anticoagulants. This irritation could cause serious bleeding problems. You will need a suctioning device, suction catheters, and standard tracheostomy supplies. Always wash your hands before you begin.

1. Prepare your equipment; the suctioning apparatus can be rented from a medical supply store. Tell even the unconscious patient what you are about to do.
2. The patient should, if possible, be in a semi-sitting position. He should take some deep breaths before you begin. This procedure may cause gagging or coughing so your patient should be prepared for this. In fact, coughing is a good response, as it will help to raise secretions.

3. Place some sterile saline into a container. Prepare the suction catheter; do not contaminate it with anything. If it does get contaminated, you will have to replace it with a new one.
4. Put on your sterile gloves. Take the catheter in your dominant hand and coil it, so that it is not dangling and apt to get contaminated.
5. Turn the suction machine on with your other hand.
6. Dip the catheter into the sterile saline solution to help lubricate it. There should be a device on the catheter so if you cover it with one finger, you initiate suction; if you take it off, suction is stopped.
7. Insert the suction catheter, without the suctioning position on, into the patient's tracheostomy. (If the patient has a cuff on his tracheostomy, it is not necessary to deflate the cuff.) The catheter should be inserted 4 to 5 inches, or until resistance is felt. If you meet resistance, withdraw slightly.
8. Apply suction for five to ten seconds at a time. As you apply suction, gently rotate the catheter around. Turning your patient's head from one side to the other may make suctioning more effective. If you meet any resistance, discontinue the procedure and report it to the doctor. Do not force the catheter.
9. Withdraw the suction catheter, with the suction off.
10. If necessary, wait a few minutes and reinsert and suction again for five to ten seconds, no more. You should continue to repeat this procedure until you have removed all excess secretions and the patient's breathing sounds quieter. Do not continue if the patient appears anxious or seems to be suffering from lack of oxygen.

After this procedure, your patient should rest for 15 minutes. Suctioning should be done as prescribed, or as often as the patient appears to need it. Note the appearance of the mucus; there should be no blood. Blood may indicate you have used improper technique and caused irritation to the mucous membrane lining of the trachea or bronchi.

Artificial Respirators

Most patients requiring artificial means of breathing probably will be hospitalized for this, but a few are treated at home. This therapy is fairly complex and critically important; without it, your patient will not be able to breathe. These patients require continuous care and attention. The patient may be sent home under the supervision of round-the-clock nurses. It is rare when the patient is allowed home on a respirator without 24-hour supervised medical attention. A respiratory therapy team of professionals will most likely be involved.

I will not cover the complete care of the patient on a respirator, but I will describe how it functions and stress some important areas.

The patient usually has an airway established either by a tube (endotracheal tube) passed through his mouth and down into his airway, or a tracheostomy attached to the breathing apparatus. The mechanical ventilator is a positive pressure breathing device that maintains breathing automatically for prolonged periods. The machine can be adjusted so that the patient's breathing can be set at a prescribed pace. Humidified oxygen is pumped into the patient at a designated rate and carbon dioxide is exhaled. The efficiency of the ventilation is monitored by blood tests that show the levels of various blood gases in the body. The patient may be conscious or unconscious. Drugs may be used to suppress the patient's own respiratory system so the machine does not have to fight it.

Your patient may require its use indefinitely; or can be weaned as he is able to breathe on his own. Generally, weaning is done during the day and the patient is placed back on the respirator at night. Signs that the patient may be able to come off the respirator are: the patient is able to cough on his own; he has evidence of gag reflex; he can maintain an adequate airway; he can swallow; or he can move his jaw and clench his teeth. If your patient is off the ventilator, be aware of signs that he may need to go back on: restlessness, air hunger, changes in skin color, increased anxiety, mental confusion, and change in respiratory rate. Report these problems and get help immediately.

The patient may have to be restrained if he is confused, restless, or extremely agitated, so that he does not inadvertently pull out his tubes. Check often to see that all connections are secure. What should be done if there is a power failure? Most machines will run for a limited time on alternative power sources. Become familiar with the respirator, how it works, and how to troubleshoot problems.

One way of verifying respirator accuracy is to count your patient's breaths and compare them to that on the machine setting. Check levels of the humidifier (water) and oxygen supply. All tubing should be changed every 24 hours. Excess moisture should not be allowed to collect in ventilator tubes and you should take care that none of the moisture or water is allowed to enter into the patient's lungs.

Do not neglect other areas of the patient's care. Provide adequate hygiene and mouth care. Your patient should be repositioned every two hours, turning from side to side, and the head of the bed should be moved to different positions periodically. A hospital-type electric bed is best for this type of patient and special pressure mattresses should be used. It is very important that your patient get adequate rest, which may be difficult with the machinery, the various procedures, and people around him all the time. He may fear going to sleep and feel he needs to stay awake to be sure everything is working.

Your patient most likely will have increased anxiety until he sees that he is being cared for and things have settled into some sort of routine. Be sure to provide a way for the patient to communicate (note pads, a blackboard) and offer as much emotional support as possible. You may require it, as well. Get relief when possible, and be sure that you get your much needed sleep.

Care Giver's Checklist

1. Environment can make a world of difference to someone with breathing problems. Weather or altitude may make your loved one's condition worse; consider moving to a better climate, if possible. Indoors, a humidifier, air purifier, or air conditioner might help. Keep the house free of dust, smoke, and plants that cause respiratory irritation.
2. Make sure your loved one receives regular immunization against flu viruses, and avoids large crowds, or friends with respiratory infections.
3. If your patient is on oxygen therapy, follow safety guidelines. Oxygen is a combustible, odorless gas. Avoid smoking even after oxygen is turned off.
4. A tracheostomy may help your patient breathe. Keep the airway open, free of crust and secretions, and the surrounding skin clean and healthy. Learn to suction the trachea and bronchi to remove the secretions that your patient cannot.
5. If your patient has an artificial airway, or needs oxygen or a respirator, be especially sensitive to psychological needs. Your loved one may fear sleep because he thinks he will suffocate if the system fails. Try to maintain a calm, reassuring manner; emotional distress in your patient can dissolve into a vicious cycle of respiratory distress.

12 The Postoperative Patient

Surgery breaks through the body's protective barriers and exposes your patient to numerous risks: bacteria may enter; body fluids leak out; bleeding occurs; chemical imbalance may result; and oxygen is lost. Along with surgical trauma, the body must respond to anesthesia necessary for surgery. Anesthesia puts the body in an abnormal state: temperature may fall; respirations and pulse may weaken; and hypersecretion of mucus and saliva may occur.

Following surgery, the patient's body will need 24 to 48 hours to compensate for the assault; this period is critical for the surgery patient. During the postoperative period, a sterile dressing is placed over the wound; a drain may be put in place to allow excess secretions to escape; lung and breathing exercises are done so fluids do not accumulate; muscles are exercised; fluids are replaced intravenously; blood may be replaced; pain is treated; and healing begins.

Tissues repair themselves through regeneration; if not, a scar forms. The wound is kept clean and free of infection by applying antiseptic ointments or solutions; removing excess debris or dead tissue; using antibiotics; maintaining aseptic or sterile technique; and by enhancing or maintaining blood supply to the wound.

Healing takes place from the inside out, which is why you see the outer healing process last. The circulatory system responds to surgery by sending blood to the area. Infection-fighting white blood cells break down and ingest debris as the process of cell repair (mitosis) begins.

Sutures or stitches are used to stop the bleeding and help the skin and tissues adhere. Some surgical sutures dissolve after healing and need not be removed; others will not dissolve and have to be removed by a physician after healing takes place (usually seven to ten days).

The postoperative patient's recovery will depend on the type of surgery, the hospital experience, complications, patient cooperation, and an adequate rest and recovery period. The care giver can help hasten the patient's recovery by seeing that prescribed exercise is carried out, even if your patient is confined to bed. Promote rest and relaxation. Set limits; don't allow your patient to overdo once he gets home.

The patient's diet is important. If he is on an unrestricted diet, provide well-balanced meals high in protein and vitamin C. You may want to add some fiber to promote proper bowel function.

Pain control may be a problem following surgery, although your patient probably will be free of postoperative pain by the time he is discharged. Some patients may not be, and will require pain management at home. Pain medications most likely will be ordered on an "as necessary" basis at prescribed intervals. Many of these pain medications are narcotic, and addiction can develop from prolonged use. Your patient should take his medication at the onset of pain, provided the appropriate time interval has passed. A patient who tends to be stoic may resist medication. He should not suffer; encourage him to take medication when pain occurs.

Depending on the nature of the surgery, your patient's outlook will vary. If surgery was done to relieve an acute situation, your patient most likely will be on his way to his prior healthy state. If surgery was performed for cancer or some other chronic problem, adaptation and acceptance may be prolonged. This type of patient may not "rebound" quickly, and will require additional time to accept and learn to live with his illness or condition. Rehabilitation may be necessary. Give him lots of emotional support and encouragement.

Postoperative Complications

Factors that may inhibit healing are bleeding disorders; infection; inadequate nutrition; impaired circulation; age; swelling; poor physical condition; some medications; or carelessness with sterile techniques. Most of these complications occur while the patient is still in the hospital, but the growing trend in outpatient surgery (when a patient undergoes an operation and is discharged the same day) has increased the possibility of postoperative complications in home care. Hospitals also are discharging surgery patients sooner than in the past, so they may go home with a need for extended postoperative care. Here are some postoperative complications that you should know about:

Shock results from sudden loss of large quantities of blood or from heart failure. The possibility of this occurring at home is rare; it usually occurs within 24 to 48 hours following surgery. (See Chapter 16 for how to treat shock.)

Thrombophlebitis is a condition of mild to severe swelling of a vein, usually in association with a blood clot in the lower extremities. See Chapter 10 for treatment methods. *Phlebitis* is another type of vein irritation that may occur from the use of intravenous therapy. This usually is not as serious as thrombophlebitis and may not involve blood clots. It is usually treated by changing the IV site and applying ice and then warm soaks to the irritated area.

Disruption, evisceration, or dehiscence all describe the result when surgical sutures give way. This can be caused by excessive coughing, movement, increased swelling, infection, age, poor physical condition, or obesity. It may be seen after abdominal surgery or when extensive surgery has been performed and the incision is quite large. Your patient probably will need immediate surgical repair.

The first sign may be a sudden gush of blood-like fluid, followed by opening of the incision and possibly the spilling of abdominal contents. There will be a great deal of pain and vomiting. Cover the open wound with a sterile dressing. Keep your patient flat and call the doctor. You may be able to anticipate this if you see the edges of the wound spreading apart. All surgical wounds should be close together, much like the seam in a piece of clothing.

An abdominal binder can be used to help keep the incision intact. If your patient is coughing a great deal, the doctor may want to prescribe something to stop the coughing. Whenever your patient coughs, tell him to hold a pillow firmly across his abdomen to support the area. Pay attention to any sudden appearance of drainage or unusual complaints of persistent pain and tenderness.

Wound infection is one of the more common risks following surgery. The hospital environment itself presents a risk because of the sheer numbers of patients suffering from different diseases.

Early signs of a wound infection may be fever; chills; excess drainage or pus; a change in vital signs; tender or swollen site; or the patient may feel tired and weak. The key to treatment is identifying the source of infection and treating it appropriately. Cleanliness can prevent the spread of infection: always wash your hands before touching the patient and after you finish with the patient. Don't touch other areas of your body before you have washed your hands.

Peritonitis is another rare, but serious, postoperative complication affecting the mucous membrane lining of the abdomen. Infectious organisms gain access by way of a rupture of a body organ (commonly the intestines); piercing of the abdominal wall (tumors may cause this); or poor surgical technique. Within hours bacteria breed and contamination occurs. The body swells as fluid and blood cells rush to the area to respond to the infection.

Symptoms may be abdominal pain, a feeling of fullness or bloating, nausea and vomiting, and increase in temperature and pulse rate. Your patient may feel as if something has just given way. If this occurs at home, call an ambulance. Do not move your patient; let him lie flat, elevate his feet on several pillows; turn his head to the side in case he vomits; and do not give him anything to eat or drink. Cover him with a warm blanket. This is a very serious condition; your patient is acutely ill and will be in a great deal of pain.

Surgery will be performed to inspect the abdomen, remove contaminated fluids and damaged tissue, and if necessary, repair anatomical damage.

Pneumonia and other respiratory conditions are apt to occur in the postoperative patient. Limited movement, poor breathing exercises and techniques, excess secretions in the lungs, age and prior physical condition, exposure to anesthesia, narcotics or pain-killers can contribute to respiratory problems in the surgical patient.

The best treatment is prevention. Start breathing exercises before surgery. After surgery, as soon as the patient is allowed, get him out of bed and walking. (See pages 81 and 157 for examples of breathing exercises and treatment of respiratory problems.)

Another type of respiratory problem that may occur after surgery is *atelectasis*, or collapsed lung. It may be caused by obstruction from mucous plugs or excessive secretions or by tumors or enlarged lymph glands compressing the lung. *Bronchitis*, an inflammation of the bronchial mucous membrane, may occur six to eight days following surgery. Watch for a cough with excess mucus, fever, and elevated pulse rate. *Pleurisy* (inflammation of the pleura of the lung) is a fairly common postoperative condition. It has a very classic symptom, that of a knife-like pain in the chest when the patient takes a breath.

Hiccups can occur following abdominal surgery. They usually occur sporadically and do not last long. Some patients may be bothered by persistent prolonged periods of hiccups, causing the patient much distress. Hiccups are spasms of the diaphragm caused in the post-surgical patient by stimulation of the phrenic nerve due to a distended stomach or abdomen; peritonitis, pleurisy, or tumors pressing on these nerves; as a reflex reaction from a tube placed in the body; hot or cold drinks; or from obstruction of the intestines. If hiccups are allowed to persist, they can eventually tire out the patient or put pressure on the surgical incision. If hiccups last beyond one hour, notify the doctor.

Hernias are described as the protrusion or projection of an organ or part through a weakened wall or cavity that normally would contain it. A specific type of hernia can develop following surgery called an incisional hernia. Obese or malnourished patients are prone to this type of hernia. You would be able to see this by noting a slight bulging effect over the surgical incision. Non-surgical treatment involves a truss to stop the hernia from protruding. Whether surgical repair of the hernia is necessary will depend on how much discomfort it causes the patient, or if it is affecting another organ or bodily process. Early treatment and attention are important.

Vomiting is most often seen immediately following surgery as a direct response to anesthesia. Postoperative vomiting can occur as a result of an accumulation of fluid in the stomach, or from taking food and fluids into the stomach too soon after surgery. Anxiety and certain medications also cause vomiting. Infrequent vomiting is not a big problem. Excessive vomiting may deplete the body of valuable nutrients, enzymes, electrolytes, and fluid. A vomiting patient must never be left flat on his back; the vomitus could go into his lungs, causing suffocation. Keep him on his side or sitting.

Your doctor may prescribe anti-vomiting medications (anti-emetics). If you have anti-nausea medication to offer, give it to the patient at the first sign of nausea or stomach upset. Most anti-nausea medications will cause drowsiness and perhaps a dry mouth. Provide frequent oral hygiene, even if your patient is not allowed to eat or drink. He can still brush his teeth, take mouthwash, swish it around, and then spit it out.

If your patient has been vomiting, withhold foods and fluids until the patient feels better. Slowly progress from clear liquids to full liquids, then to soft, bland foods. Immediately following surgery, the action of the stomach (peristalsis) is either sluggish or not functioning; this is why some post-surgical patients cannot resume eating right away. Depending on the type of surgery and the amount of time under anesthesia, the return of peristalsis will vary. Strenuous episodes of vomiting can disrupt the surgical incision; use a pillow or hands to try to splint the incision site, or possibly a special binder.

Constipation is another common side effect of surgery, especially following abdominal or intestinal surgery. Normal intestinal movement can be inhibited for several days following surgery. Constipation can continue to be a problem until the patient is able to get back to his usual diet and activity regime. (See Chapter 9 for symptoms and treatment of constipation.)

Diarrhea (loose, watery, frequent stools) also can be a problem with the post-surgical patient. This can result from infection of the intestinal tract, reactions to certain medications, local irritation of the intestines, an abscess, or as a reaction to special diets or feeding supplements. This can be serious if untreated. Excess amounts of fluid, enzymes, and electrolytes can be lost, rendering the patient dehydrated. Report frequent diarrhea episodes to your doctor.

Abdominal distention is another common postoperative condition caused by slowed intestinal movement that allows gas and excess secretions to become trapped in the stomach and intestines, or by swallowed air. Your patient will feel bloated and may suffer from gas pains.

This can be relieved by walking or movement in bed. If necessary, the doctor or nurse can insert a tube into the rectum in an effort to try to allow passage of gas. A tube may be placed down the patient's nose and into his stomach to help relieve the gas; it probably will remain until the patient's stomach and intestines return to normal.

Urinary retention is a condition in which the patient is unable to urinate. This too can be due to the effect of anesthesia, as well as the slowing down of bodily functions. Sometimes it may be simply that the patient is not used to urinating in a sitting position in a bedpan. Sometimes, running water will help to stimulate urination, or try giving your patient spirit of peppermint to smell. If all of these fail and the patient has gone for six to eight hours without urinating, a health professional may insert a urinary catheter. This is to be avoided, if at all possible, because a catheter puts the patient at an added risk for infection.

Psychosis and other mental and psychological disturbances may be seen in some post-surgical patients. This is often seen in elderly patients or patients who have spent a long time in intensive care, and it is usually temporary. Some patients may become combative and will need to be temporarily restrained. Sedatives or tranquilizers may help. Sometimes narcotics and pain medications may be too strong for your patient; when the dose is lowered or changed, the patient will be more like himself again.

Delirium is often seen when an alcoholic or excessive drug user undergoes chemical or alcohol withdrawal following surgery. A patient accustomed to consuming large amounts of alcohol or drugs should let his doctor know in advance of the surgery. Special precautions may have to be taken. Some form of withdrawal will have to take place before surgery, unless an emergency exists. As a general rule, if regular quantities of any substance or medication are taken routinely, be sure to let the doctor know before surgery.

Wound Care

If your loved one is discharged soon after surgery, you may be responsible for some wound care. Discuss your role with the health care team. Establish whether clean or sterile technique will be required. Should gloves be worn? What cleansing solutions should be used? What type of dressing, and how often should it be changed? Make sure all aspects of care have been explained before you clean and dress your patient's wound.

For wound care, always use a flat, clean, well-lit surface. Gather all equipment and wash your hands before you begin.

1. Prepare your equipment. This will vary depending on whether you are using sterile technique.
2. Gently take off your patient's soiled dressing and discard.
3. Inspect the wound for drainage, redness, inflammation, or any other abnormalities. The incision should be clean and intact.
4. Use a recommended solution; some may cause irritation. Take a sterile cotton-tipped applicator or gauze and, starting from the innermost portion, clean outward. If you clean inward, you'll be carrying bacteria toward the wound. Clean only in one direction (not back and forth). Discard that swab and use another. Keep cleaning until the wound is free of discharge, crust, and debris.
5. After the wound is clean, let it air dry for a few minutes. Do not fan the area; you may bring bacteria to the wound. Apply any needed medications with a sterile applicator.
6. If your doctor has ordered a dressing, prepare it now.

Dressings and Bandages

A wound is covered for many reasons. The dressing keeps it clean; prevents tissue destruction; protects new tissue; decreases the risk of infection; absorbs excess drainage; controls odor; contains medication; and provides comfort. A dressing probably won't be needed to cover a clean, healed, dry incision. The type of dressing will depend on the location and size of the wound. Dressings come in many sizes, and can be cut to accommodate specific areas.

If the procedure and dressing must be sterile, use sterile scissors. You can buy disposable sterile dressing kits. Much of this equipment can be expensive, so check with your insurance carrier to be sure who is paying for it. If you must foot the bill, you may want to compare prices and develop an economical approach. Unfortunately, most of the more convenient, pre-packed, disposable equipment is far more expensive than assembling individual pieces of equipment.

Never touch or contaminate a dressing, even if it does not require sterile technique. Always hold the dressing on the side that will not touch the wound. If ointments, creams, or medications must be applied, use a sterile gauze sponge or a sterile cotton-tipped applicator. Ordinary cotton swabs from the drug store are not considered sterile, nor are all solutions. Never stick a swab into the bottle; pour the solution into a container first or directly onto the dressing. (Check to see if the container should be sterile.)

If there is a large amount of drainage, use extra-absorbent dressing pads. Plastic coated dressings can prevent sticking but are not absorbent. Dressings coated with petroleum jelly are used on burns. Plastic spray coverings used on some patients make it easy to see the wound. Special dressings can be found in pharmacies or medical supply stores. Find out what types of supplies were used when your patient was in the hospital, and get the manufacturer's name, the product number, and the size.

The dressing should be secured with medical tape. If you notice redness or a rash where the tape has been applied, your patient may be allergic or sensitive to the tape. Paper or silk tape seem to be the least irritating, and non-allergic tape is available. Apply tincture of benzoin to the area first to coat the skin protectively and help the tape stick. Try to avoid adhesive tape; it seems to be the most irritating and is difficult to remove. Acetone or nail polish remover will dissolve excess adhesive, but be sure to rinse the area afterward. To remove tape, loosen all edges and pull in the direction of hair growth. Dab some isopropyl alcohol along the edge of the bandage to help lift up hair. Check with your doctor to see if it would be appropriate to shave any areas with excess hair growth.

Special adhesive strips can be cut to various sizes and applied to either side of the wound. These stay on the patient, the dressing is placed in between, and then the two strips are brought together much like the lacing on shoes. Avoid using excess tape whenever possible; use alternative methods of securing dressings. If a dressing does not require regular changing, reinforce it with a little tape to the lifted area. Avoid putting tape on an irritated area; leave it alone and expose it to air to hasten healing.

Some patients may have problems with dressing applications. A patient who is quite overweight, especially one with excess abdominal folds, may need an abdominal binder, which is elastic and fastens with Velcro strips. A binder is helpful for wound incision support, as well as for a patient having frequent dressing changes. You may need an extra binder on hand, so that a soiled one can be washed.

Excess wound drainage requires special attention. Wound drainage can contain blood, pus, mucus, and enzymes that irritate healthy tissue. Some substances (zinc oxide, petroleum jelly, and various ointments or creams) can prevent the skin from absorbing these secretions. Some wounds have drains placed in them after surgery. The drain helps prevent swelling, removes excess fluid, decreases the risk of infection, and reduces the number of dressing changes. Excessive drainage should be reported at once to the doctor. Ask your doctor if the drainage is contagious and, if so, what special protective measures should be taken by you and your family.

Put used wound dressings in a plastic bag, which should be placed in a second plastic bag, secured, and thrown out. If you have an incinerator, burn all waste materials.

Bandages can be cloth, gauze, or elastic, which supplies gentle support. Always wrap the bandage by starting at the farthest point from the wound and work upward to promote circulation. Change the bandage whenever it loosens, or as often as the doctor recommends, but at least every eight hours to check on the wound. Look for signs of adequate circulation.

Swelling can cause the bandage to become too tight. If you are wrapping a leg or ankle, have the patient elevate it for 15 minutes before wrapping so the extremity is in its resting state. If the bandage is wrapped properly, the skin should feel warm to the touch, be healthy looking, and your patient should feel no tingling or numbness (figure 32). If your patient complains or if the extremity gets cold, remove the bandage for 30 minutes; then reapply, but not too tightly. Secure the bandage with metal clips or a safety pin, but not where the patient may be lying on them, causing another pressure point. When the bandage is off, bathe the area, dry it carefully, and apply a lubricating lotion (not too much!).

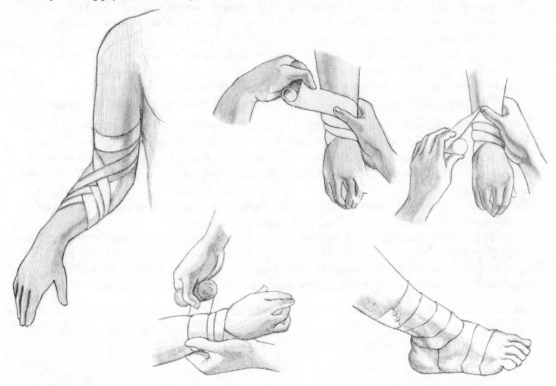

Fig. 32 Bandaging wounds

Wound Irrigation

Your patient's wound may need to be irrigated with an antiseptic or antibiotic solution prescribed by the doctor. This may help prevent premature healing over an abscessed or infected area. Wound irrigation is usually done under sterile conditions. You will need an irrigating syringe and basin, the prescribed solution, a basin to collect drainage (kidney basin), and some plastic or absorbent pads.

Your patient's position will depend on the location of the wound. You will flush the solution into the open wound and excess solution will run out of the wound into the basin. Always wash your hands before you begin.

1. Gather your equipment. Check the label on the irrigating solution to make sure it is exactly what was ordered and that the expiration date is effective. Do not use any solution that has expired or that arrives to you with the seal broken.
2. Position your patient and protect the area surrounding the patient and bed with plastic or absorbent pads. Remove the dressing; don't contaminate it.
3. Ask your doctor whether sterile gloves must be used.
   Prepare your sterile equipment on the sterile field; put on your sterile gloves.
4. Take your syringe and draw up the irrigating solution. Flush the solution into the wound until the syringe is empty. Repeat this process as prescribed. Use a clean, kidney-shaped basin pushed up against the non-sterile portion of the wound to collect excess drainage.
5. Allow the wound to drain for a few moments and keep the patient still. Dry the surrounding skin with sterile gauze sponges; work from the inside out.
6. Provide additional wound care and reapply the patient's sterile dressing.
7. Dispose of used supplies, remove your gloves, and wash your hands throughly.

Your patient may need a wet dressing. This usually is soaked with a prescribed solution, placed inside the wound, and replaced at specific intervals or when it becomes dry. This procedure may be done to clean a wound; promote blood supply; fight against infection; or liquefy dead tissues. This requires sterile technique; use sterile gloves, a sterile basin, gauzes or dressings, and a sterile solution. The gauzes are soaked in the solution, placed on top of or packed inside the wound. This procedure is maintained until the wound appears clean, free of dead tissue, and shows regrowth of healthy tissue.

An open wound may need to be packed with gauze to keep it open until the doctor is sure it is free of infection, dead or damaged tissue. This also may promote internal deep healing when a wound becomes infected or abscessed. This technique is more difficult than other wound care; get training from the health care team before trying to do it alone.

Care Giver's Checklist

1. The growing popularity of day surgery and hospital cost-cutting measures that send patients home soon after surgery mean that you may be faced with postoperative complications that previously were seen only in the hospital. Ask your surgeon to describe trouble signs you should look for following surgery.
2. Vomiting, constipation, diarrhea, and hiccups are common problems following surgery. If untreated, they can present serious problems for your patient. Consult closely with the health care team when any complication occurs.
3. It's important to get your loved one up and moving as soon as he is able after surgery. Movement, whether in or out of bed, will cut down on circulatory, respiratory, and physical complications brought on by inactivity.
4. Wound infection is one of the more common risks following surgery. Always wash your hands before treating your patient's wounds. Watch for signs of wound infection and seek prompt treatment if healing is delayed.
5. Get specific instructions from the health care team on caring for your patient's wound. Learn to prepare a sterile dressing and to wrap a bandage securely without disrupting circulation. Get permission from the doctor before discontinuing wound dressings.

13 The Fracture Patient

There are 206 bones in the human body, bones that provide attachment for muscles, tendons, and joints; provide support and movement; and help to protect delicate parts of the body. Blood cell production takes place within bones, and bones provide storage for mineral salts.

The fracture patient probably will have a long recuperation since bones take time to heal. Some of that time will be spent with the fracture immobilized, and that can mean bed rest. Even if bed rest is not required, the patient's prior activity level may be compromised. The care giver can play an important role in preventing complications and setbacks through good nursing care, exercise, movement, and diet.

How Bones Break and Heal

When a bone is broken, the muscles, joints, tendons, and tissues surrounding the bone are disturbed and possibly damaged. This can cause pain and may expose the body to infection if the bone breaks through the skin. Bleeding and swelling may occur; blood clots can form if circulation is affected. Movement and support are hindered, and deformities can result from a serious fracture.

These are the types of fractures and terms you may hear if your loved one has suffered a broken bone:

Closed (simple): No injury or exposure through the skin surface.

Open (compound): The bone has broken through the skin, causing an open wound that increases the patient's risk of infection.

Comminuted: The bone has been broken or splintered in several places.

Impacted: A portion of the bone is driven into another bone.

Displaced: The two bone ends are separated.

Complicated: A fracture has injured the tissues, blood supply, lymph drainage system, nerves, joints, tendons, or internal organs.

Greenstick: The bone bends and breaks, but not all the way through (like a tree branch that is snapped or twisted). This occurs most often in children because their bones are more flexibile.

Complete: The break goes all the way through the bone.

Pathological: A fracture due to bone disease or a pathological process rendering the bones brittle or fragile; the break usually occurs without trauma.

Compression: A fracture in which a bone has been compressed by another bone.

Spiral: A fracture that twists around the shaft of the bone.

Treatment will depend on the severity and type of fracture and where it occurred. Is it in one of the long bones necessary for weight bearing, or in a small bone that has no weight put on it? What is the patient's age and activity level? Are there other physical problems, medical conditions, or limitations?

First-aid for fractures is standard for all patients and consists of the following:

1. Keep the patient in the position you found her in and do not move her, unless it is

for safety reasons. If you suspect a back or spinal cord injury, do not even allow the patient to lift her head.

2. Keep the patient warm and comfortable. Try to immobilize the fracture. Pillows or a piece of wood can be placed on either side of the extremity.

3. Call for medical help.

4. If there is excess bleeding, make it your first priority. Apply direct pressure to stop the bleeding. *Never* use a tourniquet, except in the case of a severed limb or if bleeding cannot be controlled by any other means. A tourniquet can be a necktie or a piece of rope and it is applied about two inches above the wound.

5. Cut off any clothing in the way. If there is an open wound exposing the bone, keep it covered with a clean towel or sheet.

6. Let rescue workers move the patient. (See Chapter 16 for more information about emergencies.)

Hospital care of the fracture patient will depend on the type of fracture and whether it is repaired with or without surgery. Fractures may be surgically or manually manipulated back into position, or slowly pulled back into place through traction. Diagnosis of a fracture is made by X-ray. After the fracture has been reduced or put back into proper alignment, it must be immobilized. This is done with a cast, splint, surgery, or other devices that keep bones in proper alignment while healing takes place.

Bones heal with time, but the process has many variables: the type of fracture and extent of damage; the type of bone and location; the cause of the fracture; the patient's age and nutritional and general health; and whether adequate reduction and immobilization are made.

Bones actually do knit themselves back together. Blood flows to the area, causing a fibrin network around the break (clot formation usually occurs within 24 hours). This changes into granulation tissue, enzymes are secreted to restore proper pH to the area, and the result is a deposit of calcium, known as callus formation. This usually occurs within six to ten days after the break. The callus will bond the ends of the bones together, but cannot endure strain or weight. The amount of callus formation is directly proportional to the amount of bone damage. Collagen, a fibrous network, is produced after callus formation. This formation, called "osteoid," is what the doctor looks for on an X-ray to determine if healing is taking place. At this time, the patient may be allowed to bear weight on the fracture. It actually takes a full year before the bone returns to its original strength. Bones take longer to heal than do the soft tissues of the body.

In planning your patient's discharge, find out if special orthopedic equipment will be needed. Most of this equipment can be bought or rented from a medical supply store. Where the patient will recuperate at home is important, especially if movement will be a problem. A hospital electric bed is very useful with an orthopedic patient because of its ease in providing various positions. An overbed trapeze will help the patient lift herself up. Fracture bedpans are smaller and easier for the fracture patient to use; urinals for both men and women may be of help, as well. A bedside commode can be used as a portable bedside toilet for the patient who cannot walk. Be sure special equipment is sized for your patient, including wheelchairs, and make certain the equipment will fit into your home.

If physical therapy is needed, a number of agencies will send therapists to your home, or your loved one may use a nearby rehabilitation center. If exercise is prescribed, help your patient carry it out as ordered.

If your loved one is unable to get out of bed on her own, provide a bell or a means to call for help. Make an emergency exit plan.

The fracture patient will need diversion because, in most cases, she is not acutely ill and may become bored or depressed. If she is allowed to get out of bed or use a wheelchair, take her outdoors or for rides in the car.

Fracture Reduction

Fracture reduction is the setting of the bones back to their prior state. The goal is to return proper alignment to the fracture, restore function and movement, and correct impaired circulation or tissue damage. The longer the interval before the fracture is set, the more difficult it may be to bring the fracture into proper alignment.

One method of fracture reduction is by manual manipulation (closed reduction). This will depend on the amount of bone displacement, tissue damage, and how much manipulation will be necessary. There can be a tremendous amount of pain. Most patients will be placed under anesthesia for this type of reduction. Muscle relaxants may be given to relax muscles and spasms. An X-ray will establish whether proper alignment has been made; then a cast or splint may be used to immobilize the area.

If the bone is protruding through the skin, or the fracture cannot be reduced manually, a surgical procedure known as open reduction will be performed. A surgical incision is made and the fractured ends are brought into place, if possible. With some fractures, surgical pins, rods, nails, plates, screws, or wires may be used to hold the bones or bone fragments in place. This is called internal fixation.

Traction may be used to help bring the bones into proper alignment. Traction is the process of using weights to exert a gentle force on the bones. The treatment of fractured ribs, some pathological fractures, clavicles, and fingers and toes may involve only temporary immobilization. Slings, splints, bandages, or elastic belts may be used for support.

Care of the fracture patient will vary depending on the method used for fracture reduction. On *all* fracture patients, the injured area should be observed for adequate circulation; the area should be elevated, if possible, to reduce swelling; pain-killers and muscle relaxants may be offered; fluid and blood replacement may be necessary; patient's vital signs may need to be monitored; and active use of the nearby muscle groups should begin as soon as possible.

Cast Management

Your patient's type of cast will depend on the area it covers, the function it provides, and whether the patient will use it for weight bearing. Some casts are bivalved (split in half) so they can be opened or removed, if necessary. This type of cast may be used when the patient needs a cast only for walking; if the doctor wants to be able to see the area; or if increased swelling is expected.

Casts immobilize and support the fracture. At first, circulation is especially important when the cast is in place and swelling has not yet subsided. Swelling may obstruct circulation. Feel her skin for warmth; check for a healthy skin color. Can you feel a pulse in the area? Look for signs of tingling or numbness, foul odors from the cast, or swollen fingers or toes. Pay close attention to your patient's complaints; they could be important.

Occasional elevation may prevent swelling. Place the limb or extremity on pillows (above the level of the heart). Have your patient lie flat in bed several times a day to help promote complete fluid drainage of the injured area. You should be able to place a single finger inside the edge of the cast. It will take 24 to 48 hours for a plaster cast to completely dry. The cast must be left uncovered to dry. If the cast must be lifted, use the entire palm of your hand so individual fingerprints aren't left on the wet cast. Some doctors recommend using a hair dryer to help dry the cast (check first with your doctor). Always place a damp cast on pillows, not directly on the hard bed. Use plastic or absorbent pads to protect the pillows. The cast can be cleaned with a slightly damp cloth (no soap) or brightened with white shoe polish.

An open weave fiber glass cast may be used on some patients. It takes just five to ten minutes for the cast to harden. This type of cast is lighter, provides for more ventilation, and some patients may be allowed to get it wet.

Generally, casts should never get moist or wet. If your patient's cast does get wet, tell the doctor. Your patient may not be allowed to shower or bathe while the cast is in place. If the doctor does allow the patient to bathe, protect the cast with plastic. Someone may have to help the patient so the cast stays dry.

Even though your patient may have itching inside the cast, objects should never be placed down the cast. Patients devise all sorts of ways to get to the itch, but the danger is that you may drop something into the cast. Ask your doctor about ways to relieve itching. If there are signs or complaints of pressure in a specific area, report this immediately. If the patient complains of such pain or pressure, do not administer pain medications until the source is established.

Some patients will be allowed to get up and move around immediately following application of the cast. The doctor may recommend the use of crutches. The patient who has a cast but will not be moving on crutches needs special assistance. If she is allowed to get out of bed into a chair, support the cast so it remains elevated.

To turn a patient in a cast, gently support the cast as the patient turns on her own, if she can. Be sure the cast is placed on pillows and not on top of another extremity. The patient may need help eating if the cast is on her arm. If your patient is walking with an arm cast, use a sling for support and to help promote circulation (figure 33). Fingers and toes should be exercised often during the day (hourly is best). Muscle toning exercises can be done without moving the affected limb. Have the patient contract and relax her muscles to maintain strength.

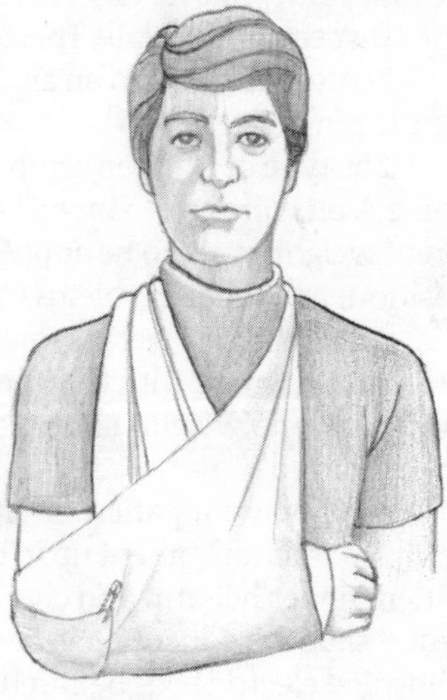

Fig. 33 Arm sling

A cast is removed when the doctor feels adequate healing has occurred. This is a simple, painless procedure involving a cast cutting device. The skin underneath will be dry and should be washed with mild soap and water. Apply some cream or lubricant to keep the skin moist. Don't let your patient scratch skin just out of a cast; it will be delicate and easily irritated. Sometimes a second cast is applied if additional time is needed for healing.

Your loved one may feel discomfort, weakness, and stiffness when the cast is removed, but after a period of exercise and muscle strengthening, the area should return to normal. Anti-embolism stockings or support hose may be used to enhance sluggish circulation (see page 84). Muscles may appear atrophied or shrunken from disuse. Weight bearing may or may not be allowed at this time. The doctor may want the patient to keep using a cane, crutches, or a walker for awhile.

Traction

Traction is the application of force in a horizontal position to help align two bones properly, reduce muscle spasm, immobilize the fracture, and regain the normal length of the extremity (usually on the lower part of the body). Traction can be accomplished by applying force directly to the skin (skin traction) or directly to the bone (skeletal traction). Your patient will have a special orthopedic bed and traction setup with a weight and pulley system.

Skin traction involves a series of straps, bandages, or girdles to attach the traction to the skin. Surgery is not required. Watch for circulatory problems, skin irritation, and pressure areas. Your patient will need frequent skin care and daily reapplication of bandages. Be sure your patient's foot is adequately supported and that there is no excess pressure on the heel. Regular skin care and heel massage will help. A sheepskin blanket placed under the feet can help to prevent pressure and friction. Keep the foot in proper alignment; if you don't complications such as foot drop can occur (figure 13).

With skeletal traction, a metal pin or wire is inserted into the bone or joint. This usually is done under local anesthesia and sterile conditions. The traction is attached with the ropes, weights, and pulleys. Pay special attention to the insertion site where there is a risk of infection. Inspect the site daily for signs inflammation, drainage, or odors. Clean the area with sterile cotton swabs and an antiseptic solution; the doctor may prescribe a cream or ointment for the pin sites.

The type of traction setup will depend on the patient's circumstances. If your patient is at home, you will need to know how the system works; the desired traction weight, and if different weights need to be applied; proper patient positioning, and how to move your patient's position; and what problems to expect.

Follow these general principles in caring for a patient in traction: the limb should be in straight alignment with the traction being applied; all ropes should be in the wheel grooves of the pulleys; no weights should touch the floor; and the weights should hang free and unobstructed.

Position your patient so she doesn't slip down in the bed, diminishing the traction effect. To pull a traction patient up in bed (she can help you if she has the use of one leg) support the patient under her arm and chest; have her bend the unaffected leg, and on the count of three, gently slide the patient up in bed. If possible, lower the head of the bed for this. If you are using a hospital electric bed, be careful not to interfere with the traction weights when the bed level is moved up and down.

Make sure traction ropes are intact and properly secured. The way the knot is tied is important; learn how to tie a proper knot. Weights should never be adjusted or removed unless you are told to remove them, or if there is an emergency.
If weights are removed, the whole purpose of traction is defeated. Don't bump into the patient or the weights; this can be painful for your patient.

The patient in traction will have to stay in bed. Intermittent traction techniques are used for some patients, allowing them to get up and move around when the traction is off. Avoid development of pressure areas and use a pressure mattress, if possible. Your patient will be spending all of her time on her back, so back care should be given often. The patient can change her position and avoid pressure sores by lifting up her buttocks periodically. This can be done by performing a push-up with both hands placed firmly on either side and lifting up off the mattress; this also is a good form of muscle strengthening. An overbed trapeze is useful for changing positions. Lowering the head of the bed may redistribute pressure, as well. The patient may turn slightly from side to side, provided her leg doesn't move out of alignment. Report pressure areas (red, broken, irritated skin) when they are discovered and reposition your patient frequently.

The patient should be taught exercises that can be performed in bed to maintain and strengthen muscles. Deep breathing and other respiratory exercises may prevent respiratory complications due to inactivity. (See Chapter 7 for more information about caring for a patient confined to bed.)

To bathe a patient in traction, have her clean all of the areas she can reach on her own. You will most likely have to clean her back and buttocks. Clean the genitals by placing the patient on a bedpan and pouring warm water through.

This type of patient will have to use a bedpan. Have your patient lift up her bottom while you slide the bedpan under. You may want to put absorbent pads underneath to keep linens dry. Be careful not to let urine get onto the cast. Sprinkle talcum powder on the edges of the bedpan to make sliding easier.

To change the bed, you'll have to use the top-to-bottom method described in Chapter 3. Put the top of the bed down flat, take all of the sheets down to the buttocks, put the new ones in place at the top, and bring them down to the buttocks. The patient must lift herself up as you slide all the linens underneath. Now pull the linens beneath the traction area to the bottom of the bed. Make any adjustments at this time. Once the linens are under the patient's buttocks, she may lie back on the bed. Be sure to remove all wrinkles. Put a piece of sheepskin under the buttocks to help relieve pressure.

Internal Fixation

A patient with internal fixation has had surgery to immobilize the fracture with a nailing or plate attachment, pins, rods, wires, or prosthetic devices surgically placed in the fracture site. These may be temporary or permanent. Since a surgical incision is made, the patient is treated like any other postoperative patient, although special attention is given to the fracture site. Internal fixation may involve manipulation of the bone and surrounding tissues. Large amounts of bleeding may occur. Blood and blood products may have to be replaced following surgery. Your loved one will most likely have a great deal of postsurgical pain, which can be treated with pain-killers.

The patient's postoperative course will vary depending on the type of procedure and the patient's age and physical condition. One advantage of internal fixation is that the patient may be allowed to start walking shortly after the procedure; rehabilitation will follow. Some patients are immobilized for ten to 12 weeks and then allowed to start some form of partial weight bearing on the limb. Full weight bearing may not be permitted for up to six months, usually when fractures have occurred in the large, weight-bearing bones. The patient allowed to get up and move at the earliest opportunity will most likely do much better than the patient who is bedridden.

Internal fixation may be used to repair fractured hips, which often occur in the elderly. The elderly patient's health may already be compromised, presenting an added surgical and postsurgical risk. These patients should be moving as soon as possible. If walking is allowed, encourage your patient to use a walker. Walkers are the safest device for the elderly patient, provided they are used correctly.

If your patient is able to get up in a chair or wheelchair, see that this is done three to four times a day. Provide support for the affected limb; it may be important to elevate it.

Consult with the health care team for tips on moving or turning your patient. Generally, you may place a pillow between her legs and slowly turn the patient to her side. You may help her by gently holding the affected limb as she turns on her own. The affected limb should be in proper alignment and supported by pillows. The legs should always be separated by pillows and never left one on top of the other.

For the patient who has an artificial hip prosthesis, keep the leg straight; lift it only straight up, about four to six inches. Don't let the leg rotate outward. This can be prevented by using pillows, rolled up blankets, or sand bags to keep the leg and hip in alignment. Ask the doctor if exercises are recommended.

Prosthetic Devices

Damaged joints may be surgically repaired with prosthetic devices. This often is done when some form of degenerative process has damaged the joint; arthritis is a common cause of these problems. If this is a problem for your loved one, the doctor may recommend total hip replacement. Following surgery, the hip is held in abduction (slightly out). Your patient must lie flat for a prescribed period of time; she may be allowed to turn only 45° to the unoperated side. She must not abduct or flex the operated hip at this time.

Your patient will be at risk for infection, blood clots, and respiratory problems due to lack of movement. Deep infection at the site of the prosthetic implant is a possible complication, and can occur even years after the implant surgery. Most of the risk for infection occurs at the time of surgery.

Shortly following surgery, active exercises of the foot and surrounding area are done to promote circulation and maintain muscle strength. Pain management is important; pain medication usually is given 30 minutes before exercises, if needed. When the patient is out of bed, it is important to keep the affected hip abducted; use a splint or pillows between the legs to maintain this position. To maintain abduction after she is up and about, your patient should avoid stooping, excessive bending, twisting, and the lifting of heavy objects. Sleeping on the unoperated side with a pillow between her legs may help prevent hip dislocation. Your patient should avoid crossing her legs and sitting or standing for a long time.

Your patient may be taught to use a walker, with most of the weight-bearing going onto her hands and arms. She may then progress to crutches. Her age, pre-surgical condition, and postoperative outlook will determine how long this will take. Crutches probably will be needed for at least six weeks. Then your patient may begin using a cane. Walking is the best exercise for this patient. If you are unsure of your loved one's steadiness, walk beside her and offer support. Report any falls to the doctor.

Complications in Fracture Patients

Fracture reduction techniques and lengthy recuperation periods put some fracture patients at increased risk of a host of complications. Here are some common complications; many can be avoided with preventive measures.

Pressure sores. These can develop from bed rest, restricted circulation, or inadequate movement. The best treatment is prevention. See Chapter 7 for information about how to prevent pressure sores or treat them if they occur.

Fat emboli. This is a condition that develops following a fracture when fat deposits are released into the bloodstream, possibly causing blockage of blood vessels. It usually occurs within 48 hours after injury, generally in patients who have multiple fractures in the larger, long bones of the body. Some symptoms of this condition are mental confusion, restlessness, or bizarre behavior; all of these are signs that the blood supply to the brain has been blocked. Other signs may be respiratory distress, chest pain, and noisy, rattling breathing. This is a serious complication requiring prompt medical intervention.

Shock/Hemorrhage. This usually occurs immediately following an injury when there has been excessive blood loss. See Chapter 16 for information about treatment of shock.

Blood clots. Blood clots and other clotting disorders may occur due to massive tissue damage and bleeding; bed rest; immobilization of a limb; slow bleeding into tissues; use of an intravenous feeding catheter; or as a complication of surgery. Treatment will vary, but any clotting problems or bleeding disorders represent serious complications and require prompt medical attention. Some symptoms are bruising; bleeding on the cast or dressing; fever; redness over a vein; leg cramps; increased swelling; the area is warm to the touch; respiratory difficulties; or decreased urinary output.

Infection. If a bone breaks through the skin, infection can occur. The wound must be carefully cleaned in the hospital and your patient probably will be placed on antibiotics. The wound will most likely be left open for cleansing and drainage. A sterile dressing will be placed over the wound and wound irrigations may be done. A permanent cast probably won't be applied. This care may be continued at home and you will have to know how to care for the wound and recognize complications.

Kidney stones. The combination of local decalcification and bed rest may leave excess calcium salts to be excreted through the kidneys, which can cause kidney stones. This can be prevented in most patients by providing increased fluids (eight to 12 glasses a day, but avoid large quantities of milk) and increasing exercise and movement. Patients with a tendency toward kidney stone formation should drink cranberry juice to keep the urine pH level less acidic. An acid environment is believed to promote kidney stone formation, so avoid acidic beverages such as orange juice. Some signs of kidney stones are flank pain; blood in the urine; pain during urination; spasms; nausea and vomiting. Treatment involves spontaneous passing of the stone, mechanical destruction, or surgery.

Delayed union or non-union. These conditions are caused by improper alignment of the bone pieces, ineffective traction technique, infection, or impaired blood flow. The type of fracture and the location may contribute to this problem. In delayed union, the healing process has been unusually slow. In non-union, the callus formation does not occur and another approach will have to be taken to promote healing.

Musculoskeletal problems. Most of these occur as a direct result of immobilization. Muscles can shrink, become flaccid and weak from disuse; joints can lock or become arthritic. A serious complication known as foot drop can occur in which the muscles and tendons cannot hold the foot in place. These side effects may be prevented with proper body alignment and positioning, and bed exercises. (See Chapter 7 for prevention tips.)

Pain. Pain is common in the fracture patient because of bone, muscle, tendon, and tissue damage, as well as surgical manipulation. Your loved one should have adequate pain medication, while respecting the risk involved with using narcotic analgesics. Pain from swelling or pressure may indicate other problems. Evaluate all of your patient's pain complaints and report them to your doctor. Most pain should subside within four to eight days following the injury.

Constipation.   This usually occurs as a result of bed rest or as a side effect of prolonged use of narcotic pain medications. Prevention is possible through diet or stool softeners. (See Chapter 9 for complete information.) Consult with your doctor if constipation seems to be a problem.

Urinary tract problems.   Most of these problems are caused by bed rest. Your patient may experience urinary retention; kidney stones; infections; inability to void; or urinary incontinence. Most of these problems are prevented through diet and offering plenty of fluids. Some patients, especially men, have trouble using a bedpan at first. Elderly male patients may have problems with prostatitis, which makes urination difficult. (See Chapter 9 for information about urinary disorders.)

Necrosis.   Necrosis (tissue death) may occur when the bone loses its blood supply as a result of traumatic injury or massive infection. If not corrected, the bone will weaken and become useless. Artificial implants may replace necrotic bone.

Respiratory problems.   These are a complication of bed rest. The patient is unable to aerate her lungs and mucous secretions build up, possibly followed by pneumonia and other upper respiratory illnesses. Your patient should do deep breathing exercises and change her position often. (See Chapter 11 for more information.)

Movement for Fracture Patients

The doctor will order your patient to get up as soon as it is medically possible. At first, your patient may be allowed only to sit in a chair or wheelchair with no weight on the affected limb. Your patient will need the limb supported while she is transferred into the chair. Be sure the limb is elevated and secured so it cannot be bumped out of place.

A transfer board may help you slide the patient from bed to chair or wheelchair. If a wheelchair is used, be sure the wheels are locked and turned inward before taking a patient in and out of it. Some wheelchairs have an adjustable leg pedal to elevate a limb; it should be properly secured, too. Put pillows under the cast and use old neckties or a belt to secure it. If your patient is to be outside in the wheelchair, fasten her safety belt. Accidents have occurred where the wheel of the wheelchair has struck a grate or bump in the street, causing the patient to be thrown from the chair.

If your patient is allowed to walk, the type of weight bearing allowed (none, partial, or full) and her physical condition will most likely determine which apparatus she will use; crutches, canes, or walkers. Make sure your patient is shown how to use them and that these aides are fitted individually. (See Chapter 3 for additional information about sizing and use of crutches, canes, and walkers.)

There are two types of crutches; standard and forearm, which are aluminum. All crutches should be measured to your patient. A properly-sized crutch will allow 1 ½ to 2 inches of space between the top and the patient's armpit. Some patients begin training for crutch use while still in bed, doing special exercises to strengthen muscles that will be used. Have your patient flex and extend her arms; push up to a sitting position with her arms; do push-ups from a sitting position in bed; or squeeze a rubber ball to gain upper body strength.

There are several crutch gaits, depending on the severity of the disability and the patient's physical condition. Crutches should be advanced no more than eight to ten inches at one time. The crutch gaits are:

Swing through, when both crutches are advanced at the same time and the patient swings through to the point where the crutches are placed. This gait is used when there is lower paralysis or weakness and weight bearing is limited.

Two point, when the right crutch is advanced along with the left leg, weight is shifted, then the left crutch and right leg come through.

Three point calls for advance of both crutches. The patient brings the weaker leg through while placing weight on the stronger leg. This gait is used when one extremity cannot bear weight.

Four point gait is when the crutches and feet get placed one at a time: the right crutch; the left leg; the left crutch; the right leg. This is used when weight bearing is allowed on both legs and only slight support is needed.

To go down stairs on crutches, position your patient as close to the step as possible. Have her put both crutches onto the next step, bringing the weaker leg down first and then the stronger one. If only one crutch is being used, she should hold the crutch on the stronger side, then put the crutch down on the next step; place the weak foot down first and then the stronger one. To go up stairs, reverse the process. The stronger leg goes first, then the crutches, then the weaker leg.

If you are unsure of your patient's balance, stay close by her or even follow her with a chair in case she becomes tired and needs to sit down quickly. Walk beside the patient calling out placement to help her remember which crutch and which foot goes where and when.

To sit down on a chair or the toilet, she should walk to the chair, then turn and back into it. She should not sit until she feels the presence of the chair behind her. She should transfer the crutches onto the stronger side, or lean them against the wall, and slowly ease downward, holding the arms of the chair for support. Getting up may not be as easy (there are elevated toilet seats and chairs available). Have your patient put the crutches in her stronger hand, provide a base between her feet of eight to ten inches, and pull herself up. Consider installing handrails in the bathroom.

All crutches should have rubber tips on the base and fit properly. Weight should never be put directly on the armpits, even when resting. Your patient should wear rubber-soled, flat shoes; bedroom slippers are not safe. Keep objects out of the patient's way. Use caution with area rugs and slippery floors.

If your patient is using a cane, it should be placed in the hand of the stronger or unaffected side. Your patient should keep it close to the body and advance it at the same time as the affected leg. Many canes are adjustable, but still must be individually fitted for your patient. Some canes come with a "quad" base (four legs) for added support. To go up stairs with a cane, have your patient place her stronger leg on the stair, then the cane, and then the weaker leg. To go down, reverse the process. A patient using a cane may find that stair railings are safer than using the cane on stairs.

Walkers have four legs, are adjustable, and should be sized for your patient. Some models have wheels, but they are less safe than walkers with rubber tips on the bottom of the legs. To use a walker, have your patient plant it a short distance in front of her and then walk up to it. A walker should not be used for the non-weight bearing patient, and should never be used on stairs.

Don't let your patient become dependent on these devices. Some patients continue to rely on them long after their use is required. This may cause a problem because muscles will not get exercise. If your patient is fearful of going it alone, she can begin by walking around the house and building up her confidence. She may slowly explore the neighborhood with your help, and then be encouraged to venture out on her own. This is a gradual process and large, crowded areas should be avoided.

Care Giver's Checklist

1. Plan carefully for your loved one's return home after hospitalization for a fracture. You may need an electric bed, orthopedic equipment, a fracture bedpan, or an appliance to raise your toilet seat. Wheelchairs, walkers, crutches, and canes should be individually fitted. Narrow doorways, slippery floors or throw rugs, and lots of stairs can be obstacles in home care of fracture patients.
2. Keep your patient's cast dry. Watch for numbness, swelling, or foul odors from the cast. Keep the cast elevated to reduce swelling. Drugs may be prescribed for pain.
3. Traction—either skin or skeletal—is a lengthy process involving an orthopedic bed and a series of weights and pulleys. Your loved one will be at risk for all complications of bed rest; skeletal traction carries the additional risk of infection where pins are surgically implanted in the bone. Ask your home care team for training in traction management.
4. Not all fractures heal as planned. Your patient may experience delayed union or non-union, so ask how soon to expect results and report delays in healing to your physician.
5. Movement is essential to recovery from a fracture. Begin exercises while the cast is in place. Get your patient fitted for a cane or crutches, and then get her moving! As her strength returns, don't let your patient develop a dependency on these devices; help her gain the confidence needed to eventually throw aside her crutches.

14 The Diabetic Patient

Diabetes mellitus is a metabolic disorder in which there is some degree of insulin insufficiency that results in the body's inability to metabolize carbohydrates, fats, and proteins. Put simply, the diabetic patient's cells lose their ability to take in and use sugar. Because of this insufficient amount of insulin, abnormal amounts of sugar accumulate in the blood and eventually the urine. If this excess of sugar is left uncontrolled, the patient can suffer numerous complications.

Diabetes is a very complex disease to manage. Control can be obtained by balancing diet, hypoglycemic agents, and exercise, while testing urine and blood for excess sugar to determine whether control has been established. Patient education is extremely important because the patient should bear the responsibility of managing his diabetes.

The diabetic patient should understand the disease; dietary management; proper administration of medication; be able to do his own urine or blood testing; be aware of symptoms of hyperglycemia and hypoglycemia, and know how to treat them.

No age group is exempt from diabetes, and it is felt that it is an inherited disorder. Symptoms will vary, depending on the severity of the disease, but common signs are excessive thirst or urination; elevated blood sugar; feeling hungry much of the time; and periods of the skin feeling cold and clammy. This all is directly related to the metabolic process of the body being unable to metabolize glucose (sugar) properly.

Encourage your diabetic patient to exercise. Unless he is acutely sick and confined to bed, the diabetic can take part in almost any activity. Keep in mind his altered needs for insulin if he plans to increase his activities.

Diabetics should carry some form of identification at all times, including the patient's name, his doctor's name, telephone numbers, and what medications or form and dose of insulin the patient requires. This ID card also is important if the patient will be traveling and carrying insulin and syringes. The American Diabetes Association provides special ID cards that explain emergency measures to be taken if a diabetic appears to be in trouble.

Diabetes and Diet

The most effective way to treat this condition is through diet. Controlling the amount and types of food taken into the body is the main basis for all treatment of diabetes. In the past, there was much more emphasis on carbohydrate restriction, but the current feeling is that fat content is more important. Studies have shown a low fat diet has a positive effect on levels of serum triglycerides (a neutral fat) and vascular disease. Diabetics with high cholesterol or triglyceride levels are at a greater risk for heart disease and associated vascular problems.

The regulation of diabetes through diet must be balanced. For example, increased food intake usually requires increased levels of insulin. If the diabetic exercises or eats less, there may be decreased blood glucose levels requiring less insulin. The diet must be contoured to each patient, usually through modifying eating habits. Consult with the nutritionist on your health care team if your loved one is diabetic.

The recommended diet for diabetics is:

1. Protein: 1 gram for each kilogram of ideal body weight (60-100 grams per day).
2. Carbohydrates: 150-250 grams per day.
3. Fats: These must be carefully calculated because they provide the most calories per gram; if not used, the body stores them. The dietitian will determine the amount based on the patient's desired weight.

The ratio of calories should be carbohydrates 40%; proteins 20%; and fats 40%.

The diabetic patient will be given a list of the foods he will be able to eat, and will be allowed to make exchanges from each category. Here are some guidelines for feeding the diabetic patient:

1. Spread food intake throughout the day. If you don't, insulin will be inadequate, increasing blood sugar (glucose). Divide daily intake into portions of one-fifth of allotted calories at breakfast; two-fifths at lunch; and two-fifths at dinner, with small snacks in-between and at bedtime. Make adjustments according to activities and exercise.
2. The diet must provide balanced proportions of carbohydrates, fats, proteins, and other elements essential to good nutrition.
3. The diet should provide the same amounts of food each day to maintain stability, except when extra energy is needed.

Many patients who develop diabetes in middle and late life retain some ability to manufacture insulin. This amount of insulin, although inadequate, may be enough if the patient's diet and activity level are adjusted. This is why each diabetic diet requires individual calculation, taking into consideration the patient's daily activities, current weight, and desired body weight, since many diabetic patients are overweight and require calorie restrictions.

The stress of illness can influence the diabetic patient in many ways. If your loved one is being treated for a problem unrelated to his diabetes, the doctor who oversees his diabetic care should be notified. The doctor may want to make changes in the current regime due to effects of illness such as decreased activity, fever, nausea and vomiting, or inability to eat.

I am assuming that diabetics have received extensive teaching from the health care team, so I have stressed only the main points of diabetic diets. If you want to know more, write to:

American Diabetes Association
505 Eighth Avenue
New York, NY 10018

The association has a number of teaching guides, lists of recommended readings, and diet information.

The Joslin Clinic in Boston specializes in diabetes and distributes *The Joslin Diabetes Manual*, edited by Leo Krall. This comprehensive reference book covers all aspects of diabetic care and is written for the lay person with diabetes. For more information, write to:

Joslin Clinic Diabetic Foundation
1 Joslin Place
Boston, MA 02215

Oral Medications

If diet alone cannot control diabetes, oral medications may be prescribed. Oral medications (Orinase, Diabenase, Tolinase) are not insulin, but they may eliminate or decrease the need for insulin by stimulating the pancreas (where insulin is produced) to secrete more insulin. For oral agents to work properly, the patient must have cells that are capable of responding to this form of direct stimulation. Oral agents usually are used on patients with a mild form of diabetes.

Insulin and Diabetes

Insulin injections are prescribed when the disease cannot be controlled through diet alone or the use of oral agents. (Some patients wear portable insulin pumps; ask your doctor about them.) Insulin is believed to increase the transport of glucose into the cells to be metabolized. Insulin is destroyed in the stomach, so it cannot be taken orally. Remember that it is not a cure for diabetes; it is merely an effective means of controlling the disease.

Insulin comes in two different strengths, U-100 and U-500, which is prescribed for insulin-resistant patients. You must use a needle and syringe sized specifically for U-100 or U-500 insulin. Insulins are categorized according to the onset, peak, and duration of action. Know the different properties of the insulin prescribed for your patient. Some can act within 30 minutes; others may take six to eight hours. Some have a duration period of eight hours; others last as long as 36 hours. The doctor will determine the insulin type and dosage for your patient through a series of blood sugar tests. This may continue to be evaluated in some patients who test their own blood or urine and administer insulin based on the results. This is known as giving insulin on a "sliding scale" basis.

If you must give insulin injections, follow safety guidelines for injectable medications listed in Chapter 8. Never use a bottle of insulin that appears to have been opened. Most insulin should be refrigerated after it has been opened, but never freeze it; freezing decreases its potency. Be sure to warm the insulin for 20 to 30 minutes before you inject it. Check the insulin for proper labeling and consistency; some insulins are supposed to be cloudy, others clear. Keep adequate supplies on hand at all times.

Always keep a bottle of "regular" insulin on hand for emergencies. It is a rapid acting form of insulin that can be used if your patient needs quick treatment, *but never use it without direct orders from your physician.*

Other medications can interfere with insulin. This is particularly important if several doctors are treating your patient; every physician should be told that your patient also is taking insulin. Some drugs known to interfere with insulin and blood sugar levels are steroids (cortisone); some diuretics (fluid or water pills); oral contraceptives; some antibiotics; anti-gout medications; some anti-hypertension drugs (high blood pressure pills); thyroid medications; aspirin; some cough syrups; heart medications; anticoagulants; some sleeping medications; antihistamines (cold pills); and drugs for

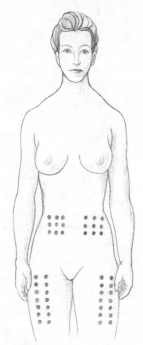

Fig. 34 Self-injection sites

Parkinson's disease. Vitamin C and increased amounts of caffeine or alcohol also may interfere.

Insulin can be injected in many sites, but if the patient will be injecting himself, he will be limited to areas he can reach (figure 34). It is important to rotate sites as the skin will become thickened, scarred, and lumps may appear, possibly leading to delayed absorption or abscesses. Do not use any area that appears overused or inject directly into a lump or hardened spot. If you are using all available sites, you should be able to allow one month's interval before you have to inject in that spot again.

Insulin injections should be given as ordered and on time. If there is any reason you cannot, or feel you should not, give the medication, call the doctor immediately.

Disposable syringes are convenient, but expensive. Some patients prefer to save money with reusable syringes and needles, but extra effort must be made to maintain sterility and to keep the needle sharp. If you are using this method, learn how to sterilize and maintain your equipment. Never sterilize a disposable needle and syringe; they are not meant to be reused.

Injecting Insulin

Before giving an insulin injection, prepare a clean work surface, gather your equipment, and wash your hands. If the insulin is refrigerated, take it out 20 to 30 minutes before the injection so it can warm to room temperature. Gently mix the insulin solution by rolling it between your palms. Do not shake it up.

1. Clean the top of the insulin bottle with an alcohol sponge.
2. Take the appropriate insulin syringe and draw up the same amount of air as the amount of insulin you will be removing from the vial.
3. Insert the needle into the vial and inject the air.
4. With the needle still in the vial, invert the vial, and bring it up to eye level.
5. Take the plunger and pull back until you have a little more than the prescribed amount of medication. Then slowly push the plunger in until you have arrived at your patient's exact dose.
6. Take out the syringe. Flick away tiny air bubbles by tapping the side of the syringe with your finger. Recap the syringe and take it to your patient.
7. Rub the injection site with an alcohol sponge and let it air dry. Uncap the needle, taking care not to contaminate it.
8. Steady the skin with your non-dominant hand.
9. Insert the syringe with your dominant hand, using a firm, swift motion. The needle should enter the patient at a 15 to 20 degree angle. You cannot inject insulin too deeply since the needle is not long enough.
10. Gently pull back on the plunger to check for any blood in the injection site. This will occur rarely, mostly when the injection has been given improperly. If you see blood, withdraw the syringe, prepare another fresh one, and give the injection in another area. If you do not see blood, push down on the plunger and slowly inject the medication.
11. Withdraw the needle and gently pat the injection site with the alcohol sponge.

The stresses of illness may have an effect on the patient's usual insulin dose. Fever, infections, surgery, or fractures may antagonize the insulin effect, raising the body's requirement for insulin. Never omit an insulin dose for this reason, since the patient probably will require more insulin rather than less at this time. To compensate, your patient may have to switch to regular insulin, which is the faster-acting form.

Your patient may suffer from side effects if he doesn't get enough insulin, or if he gets too much. A lack of insulin can cause hyperglycemia, noted by the following symptoms: confusion, mental changes; weakness; irritability; loss of appetite; nausea and vomiting; flushed face; increased respiratory rate; acetone breath (sweet smell); dry mouth; drowsiness; rapid and weak pulse; dry skin; or coma. Death is possible if not treated immediately. Treatment consists of administration of regular insulin and prompt medical attention.

Insulin reaction (hypoglycemia) can occur if too much insulin is given; if exercise is increased; or if your patient isn't eating enough. Blood glucose levels are usually below 60 mg when this occurs. The onset of this problem usually is sudden, associated with the following symptoms: moist and cool skin; pale color; weakness; sweating; headaches; tingling of mouth and fingers; hunger; nausea; mental confusion; and unconsciousness if treatment is delayed.

Give prompt treatment by administering anything sweet—four ounces of a soft drink, apple juice, or orange juice; hard candy; honey or corn syrup, sugar, or chewable glucose tablets. Most patients should start to respond immediately. Don't give additional sugar; this can inhibit absorption and delay reversal of the symptoms. Report this occurrence to your doctor. If the patient is unconscious, do not try to feed him anything; call the doctor immediately.

There is an antidote (Glucagon) that is injected like insulin. Your doctor may want you to keep this on hand and use only after consulting with him or her. Results should be seen within five minutes, but some patients may require an additional dose.

The state of unconsciousness seen in extreme cases of diabetic coma and insulin reaction may be confused with other causes of unconsciousness occurring in the elderly patient. The patient may have had a stroke or heart attack. A good indicator is that if the onset is sudden, you can assume it is related to the diabetes.

In the unconscious patient, check to be sure the patient is breathing; turn his head to the side if vomiting occurs. Be sure an adequate airway is established. If breathing and pulse have ceased, start emergency cardiopulmonary resuscitation (CPR, see Chapter 16) and seek prompt medical attention.

Blood and Urine Testing

There are a variety of commercial diabetic testing products available for testing blood and urine for the presence of sugar. During illness, it may be necessary to test more frequently for sugar. Some testing products are fully automated with digital readouts. Most diabetic equipment can be found in pharmacies or medical supply stores.

Urine testing for sugar should be done as often as prescribed by your doctor. Avoid using the first urine sample of the morning, or a sample taken after long periods of not urinating. Discard the first urine sample, have your patient drink a glass or two of water, and collect a second urine sample. A test tape or pill comes with the testing kit; ask your health care team to recommend a brand and follow directions carefully.

If the urine tests positive for sugar, check for acetone, too. When there is a shortage of insulin, the body breaks fats down into ketones that include acetone. Significant amounts of ketones in the diabetic patient may indicate problems and can be an early indicator of diabetic coma or ketoacidosis. Never ignore this occurrence; double check the acetone test to be sure.

Acetone testing is done by putting a drop of urine on an acetone tablet. A color change indicates acetone is present. Check the chart with your test kit to verify acetone content. Do not adjust the insulin dose; call the doctor for instructions. This condition also may exist if the timing of the insulin is off in relation to the serving of the patient's meal. The onset is slow and can occur in hours or even days.

Checking for sugar in the blood is the most accurate and common way of testing for excess sugar because urine tests lag behind by several hours. Sugar usually appears in the blood 30 minutes to one hour after eating. To test blood, have the patient wash his hands and clean one finger carefully with an alcohol sponge. Prick the finger with a lancet and put a drop of blood on a test strip. Consult directions on the package to read the results.

Your patient may want to use an Autolet, a spring-loaded lancet that allows you to take blood samples with minimum discomfort. The Glucometer will test the blood sample and give a digital readout of the results. Alternate fingers for blood tests and be sure to clean with alcohol before and after every puncture.

Daily Care for Diabetics

Diabetics often have impaired circulation. Many of the reasons for this are not known, but one cause may be an increased thickening of the walls of some of the blood vessels, which can impair circulation, especially to feet. As a result, one of the leading causes of disability in the diabetic patient is poor foot care. Clean your patient's feet daily. Some doctors feel that diabetics should never soak their feet, and that cleaning should be done only with a washcloth. Check with your doctor to see what he or she recommends.

If your patient is allowed to soak his feet, do so for no more than five minutes. Soak feet in a mild solution of soap and water no hotter than 105 °F (40 °C). Test the water before offering it to the patient. After soaking, rinse and carefully dry the feet; be sure to dry between each toe!

At night, apply a lanolin lotion (but not between the toes), if your doctor allows. Try to prevent dry, cracked feet, and watch the feet and toes for cuts; signs of infection; swelling; redness; and healthy skin temperature. Report any problems.

Never cut the diabetic's toenails; file them straight across. Nothing should be cut away on the diabetic patient; let the doctor take care of it. If your patient has thick nails, corns, or calluses, you may wish to have a podiatrist take care of his feet. Use mild antiseptic solutions to prevent infection. If tape is used, be sure it's non-allergic tape. Powder can be used to prevent excess moisture.

Diabetics should avoid shoes that add pressure or promote swelling. Socks and stockings should not wrinkle or bag at the ankles. Nothing should interfere with circulation to the feet and lower extremities. Have your patient elevate his feet when resting, especially if he has foot problems. If dressings are applied, they should not be too tight, and should be applied only after the foot has been elevated for 20 minutes. Do not use ointments, creams, or other medications unless they have been prescribed by your doctor. If diabetes is under control, and if problems have been reported promptly, your patient should be at no greater risk than any other non-diabetic patient.

Oral hygiene also is important for diabetics; poor control of diabetes is associated with gum disease. This area is sometimes neglected when a patient is sick or has other prevailing problems. Do not overlook it; provide proper oral hygiene and report any red or irritated gums and any bleeding around the gums.

Complications and Diabetes

Illness, surgery, or injury may alter your patient's usual diabetic program. If the patient is on insulin, adjustments in dosage or diet may have to be made. If your patient is vomiting or unable to take food orally, report this at once to the doctor. Offer broth, tea, or plain rice to replace lost body fluids and salts. Intravenous feeding may be needed. Do not omit or alter insulin doses on your own; do so only after consulting with the doctor.

Wounds from trauma or surgery may require that insulin be adjusted and wound healing may be delayed due to circulatory and vascular problems. Careful attention should be given to the use of sterile technique in providing wound care for this patient. The following complications may be seen in a diabetic patient:

Infection. Diabetics are believed to have a greater susceptibility to infection. The lower extremities are extremely vulnerable to infections because of diminished circulation. Fungus infections can occur between the toes, boils and carbuncles can develop, and abscesses and cellulitis can be a problem. Promptly report any complaints of pain, irritation, or signs of impaired circulation. Gangrene can result if proper attention is not given, perhaps resulting in the loss of toes or the entire foot. Treatment consists of finding the source of the infection, proper adjustments of insulin, and the use of antibiotics. Use sterile cleaning and dressing techniques and elevate the extremity to improve circulation.

Neuropathies. Disorders of the nervous system and nerves are often seen in the diabetic patient. The cause is not precisely known, but all nervous tissue in the body can be affected. Diabetics may have difficulty distinguishing between hot and cold, which is why you must check to see that bath water is not too hot, or that electric heating pads are at a safe temperature. Your patient may complain of leg pains or cramping, tingling or numbness, often at night. This may dissipate if your patient gets up and walks around a little bit. This process occurs in some diabetics, but may be relieved with proper control of the diabetic condition. Once it occurs, it usually cannot be reversed, only alleviated.

Visual Problems. In some diabetic patients, tiny blood vessels in the eye may break, causing hemorrhaging and eventually scar formation. This is a subtle process taking place internally over a period of time and the patient may not even be aware of it until he starts to complain of eye problems. This condition can cause blindness. Some of these problems can be prevented by adequate control and management of the diabetes.

If your patient has eye complaints (pain; blurred, patchy vision; red lines in the eye; or even red spots) report them at once. Early treatment can help to prevent permanent eye damage. The doctor may be able to control or stop eye hemorrhage. Annual visits to the eye doctor are recommended for the diabetic patient. Those with complaints and problems should go more often.

Vascular or Circulatory Problems. These can occur in the diabetic patient as a result of narrowing of the blood vessels and an inability to metabolize fats. Arteriosclerosis, elevated fat and cholesterol levels, heart attacks, or strokes are possible. Control of diabetes through diet may help to prevent or lower the possibility of these complications. Avoid anything that can constrict or confine circulation. Use properly fitted shoes and frequently elevate the legs.

Renal/Kidney Problems. The glomeruli, the vascular structure of the kidney that serves as the filtering system for the urinary tract, can be affected by diabetes, resulting in chronic renal problems. Problems with urine retention, blood pressure, or renal failure may result. The syndrome usually occurs only when the diabetic patient has had diabetes for a long time or has had problems keeping it under control.

Another problem that may occur in the urinary tract is with the nervous system; the diabetic patient may not be aware his bladder is full and requires emptying. There may be problems with urinary incontinence or urinary retention. These problems will affect the bladder tone necessary for bladder control and may also make the patient more prone to urinary tract infections. Pay close attention to the patient's urine output and fluid intake. Any problems in this area should be reported to the doctor at once.

Care Giver's Checklist

1. Diabetes is an insulin deficiency that renders the body helpless in its efforts to metabolize sugar. It is a complex disease that can be difficult to manage. Your loved one will need to understand his diabetes and adhere to the regimen required to control it.
2. Diet is the first line of defense against diabetes. The dietitian on your health care team will prescribe a regimen contoured especially for your patient. Stick to the list of recommended foods or exchanges allowed in the plan.
3. Oral medications or insulin injections may be necessary if diet alone cannot control the disease. Neither will cure your loved one, but they may make it possible to live an active life. Make sure your patient understands that changes in his routine (strenuous exercise or long periods between meals) can increase his need for insulin.
4. Diabetics often have impaired circulation, especially in the lower extremities. Poor foot care can cause disability for your diabetic patient. Clean his feet daily and watch for signs of infection. Have a professional deal with corns or calluses.
5. Illness can affect your patient's insulin needs, and diabetes sometimes can retard healing. Be sure all doctors treating your loved one know about his diabetes and consider the effects of various drugs interacting with insulin.

15 Kidney Dialysis at Home

The urinary tract (two kidneys, bladder, two ureters, and urethra) controls the body's concentration and volume of blood by removing or restoring selected amounts of water and dissolvable substances. The kidneys act as a filtering system and remove wastes from the blood in the form of urine. Urine passes out of the kidneys, via the ureters, to the bladder, where it is stored. The bladder is a muscular organ containing nerve tissue that releases urine from the body. This happens when the bladder reaches a capacity of 200 to 400 ml of urine (the total capacity is 700 to 800 ml). Nerves are stimulated carrying messages to the brain signaling the urge to urinate. Muscle contraction and relaxation take place allowing urine to empty out of the bladder, pass through the urethra, and out of the body.

Kidney dialysis becomes necesssary when chronic or acute kidney damage prevents proper filtering of the blood and the extraction of waste products. The urine may appear normal in amount, but not in quality. The kidneys can shut down completely. When this occurs, urinary output ranges from nothing to 200 ml per day and is highly concentrated, indicating inadequate filtering by the kidneys.

Dialysis does the job of the kidneys on a temporary or permanent basis, but it will not cure your patient's condition; dialysis merely compensates for the loss of kidney function. Dialysis patients can be maintained for years. Almost all patients, regardless of age or income, will qualify for Medicare reimbursements if they are "end stage" renal patients, meaning dialysis or a transplant is necessary for life. The government pays 80 to 90 percent of dialysis costs, which can range from $15,000 to $30,000 a year. Some patients use dialysis while waiting for a valuable kidney transplant, which is the only way kidney disorders can be reversed.

Home dialysis can help to maintain your loved one's life-style. It can be scheduled around a patient's other commitments, whereas if he must go to a clinic, he may be assigned a specific time slot. Home dialysis may even be initiated at bedtime so as not to interfere with daily activities.

Your patient most likely will develop a regular routine, and he and the family will adjust to this intrusion over a period of time. It will not be easy on any of you, especially the patient. In most cases, it will be a lifetime commitment that regularly consumes your patient's time.

Although home treatment may be more convenient, if your patient does not go to a dialysis treatment center he may be cut off from some of the support that comes from being around other dialysis patients. If there is a need for additional emotional support, it can be found; there are well over 50,000 dialysis patients today. Your doctor, social worker, or dialysis center will be able to provide you with additional information. (See the Appendix for a resource list.)

Not all patients are candidates for home dialysis. Some limiting factors include the patient's physical condition; home environment; patient compliance; dialysis needs; and finances. Be sure to check with your insurance provider about coverage. There also may be financial assistance available. Contact these associations for details:

American Kidney Fund
P.O. Box 975
Washington, DC 20044

National Kidney Foundation
Two Park Avenue
New York, NY 10016

The National Association of Patients
on Hemodialysis and Transplantation
505 Northern Boulevard
Great Neck, NY 11021

The association publishes a newsletter for patients and their families.

If you are considering home dialysis, be sure to check what types of electrical outlets are available in case of power failures. You may have to adapt your electrical or plumbing system for this procedure to be done at home.

Care of the Home Dialysis Patient

If home dialysis is to be successful, you must be trained in the dialysis procedure; all patients, if possible, should participate in their dialysis care. The patient must adhere to dietary regimes and prescribed fluid restrictions. The patient and care giver must know how to assemble and use all equipment, administer medications and solutions, and be capable of handling emergencies or problems.

Diet is very important for the dialysis patient because his condition and the treatment may cause the loss of valuable nutrients. His diet may have to be supplemented with high protein foods; vitamins and minerals may have to be replaced; and fluid balance maintained. Sodium (salt) usually is restricted because it retains body fluid. Potassium (found in fruits and tomatoes) may be restricted as well. Often, once dialysis is started and the patient begins to exhibit renal compensation, some dietary restrictions may be lifted.

The diet will be tailored to your patient's needs. Know your loved one's dietary regimen and see that it is followed closely. If the diet cannot be maintained, report to your physician. Daily weighing may be necessary to monitor patient progress. Accurate intake and output records may need to be kept. The fluid balance of the dialysis patient should be about even or may show a slight fluid loss at the time of dialysis. Before dialysis, excess fluids may be retained, which can mask actual weight loss in your patient.

The diet may be limited to carbohydrates and fat. It is often difficult to get the desired fat into the patient without protein. Fatty meals may cause stomach upset, nausea, or vomiting, creating a vicious cycle for your patient. Meals should be spaced in an effort to curb this syndrome—perhaps six small feedings instead of three large meals a day. High carbohydrate snacks or drinks can be offered in between to maintain weight.

Frequent mouth care should be given, especially for a patient on fluid restriction. The doctor will most likely allow hard candies for the patient to suck.

No medications should be taken without the physician's permission, since most medications are excreted via the kidneys. Patients with impaired renal function may not be able to efficiently get rid of medications. If your patient is taking other drugs, their effects may be diminished, particularly with hemodialysis. Consider scheduling medications around dialysis. Be sure your doctor is aware of other medications the patient may need and the schedule established for them.

Encourage moderate activity and exercise if your patient is up and about between treatments. Strenuous activity should be avoided to protect the shunt or catheter and guard against excess fluid loss through perspiration. Avoid extremes in temperatures, especially heat. During dialysis, the patient should be made comfortable. He may sleep, watch television, or enjoy any other form of quiet diversional activity during treatment.

There are two basic dialysis methods: *hemodialysis* requires some form of access to the patient's circulatory system, and *continuous ambulatory peritoneal dialysis (CAPD)* uses a catheter inserted into the peritoneum, a mucous membrane that lines the cavity of the abdomen.

Hemodialysis

In hemodialysis, the patient's blood is circulated through a dialyzer to be filtered, purified, and returned to the body. The process consists of a reservoir filled with tap water to which essential electrolytes and salts are added (dialysate). Plastic coils or other devices that serve as a semipermeable membrane are immersed in the reservoir. The patient's blood is redirected through these coils and the membrane permits the exchange of water and ions (electrically charged particles) through its walls. It does not allow proteins, blood, or bacteria to pass. The flow is created by an external pump that regulates and maintains passage of blood through the system.

Hemodialysis requires some form of access to the patient's circulatory system. During hemodialysis, blood leaves the body via a cannula (tube) or needle and circulates through the dialysis machine. Blood returns to the body via another cannula or needle. Access is established during a minor surgical procedure creating an external shunt (arteriovenous shunt) or an internal fistula (arteriovenous fistula). A shunt or fistula usually is placed in the patient's forearm, groin, or upper thigh.

Daily care of the shunt or fistula will depend on what type is used, and whether your patient's condition is temporary or permanent. A shunt or fistula can last a few months or a few years, as long as it remains patent (open). Either type will require surgical revision if it becomes clotted or if the original procedure was inadequate.

An external shunt should be inspected frequently for signs of infection (swelling, irritation, tenderness, or drainage). To determine adequate arterial flow, place your hand over the area: You should feel a rushing, pulsating feeling (do this several times a day). The blood color in the shunt should be bright red; any darkened color may indicate clot formation or an obstruction.

Don't use an arm with a shunt for taking blood pressures or drawing blood, and avoid heavy lifting with that arm. Avoid restrictive clothing, handbags, or jewelry on that arm. This type of shunt should not be immersed in water; protect it with plastic when bathing. The shunt and dressing should be handled carefully and caution should be taken not to bump it or allow trauma to the area.

An external shunt requires frequent assessment for patency and daily sterile cleansing of the shunt area. *Ask the health care team for specific instructions on cleansing the shunt area. If your guidelines differ from those below, use only the method recommended by your health care team.*

Always wash your hands before you begin. If your doctor wants you to use sterile gloves, gather all supplies before putting on your gloves.

1. Remove the clamps from the gauze dressing. These clamps should be attached at all times. If a bleeding emergency occurs, the patient will be able to clamp the shunt and stop the bleeding.
2. Carefully take off the gauze dressing and the gauze sponges under the shunt. Never cut off the bandage or use scissors near the shunt.
3. Don't touch the area with your hands. Look for adequate blood flow and check the skin for signs of inflammation or infection. When the dressing is exposed, check to see that the connections are secure and that separation does not occur. If it does, clamp both sides immediately and seek medical attention. Your doctor may have secured the shunt with a piece of tape; do not remove it unless told to do so.
4. Using whatever antiseptic solution your doctor has prescribed, clean the area and exit sites with sterile cotton-tipped applicators and sterile gauze sponges. Start from the inner portion and wipe outward. Use a different applicator or sponge each time. Continue until the area is clean.
5. Allow the area to dry for a few moments. Place a dry sterile gauze sponge under the shunt so it cannot irritate the skin.
6. Place another sterile gauze sponge over the exit sites, and apply a strip of non-allergic tape to secure the gauze.
7. Gently apply an elastic bandage over the shunt site. Leave a small area of the shunt exposed for easy viewing. Don't wrap it too tightly. Reapply clamps to the top of the bandage.

An internal fistula (arteriovenous fistula) surgically joins a vein and artery, and usually is placed for permanent use. During dialysis, needles are inserted through the skin and into the fistula; this causes slight pain, but an internal fistula may last two years or longer, and it is less restrictive and poses a lower risk of infection. Your patient may have an arteriovenous graft if there is insufficient vein in the area where the fistula is needed.

If your loved one has an internal fistula, you must still feel for adequate circulation over the shunt area, just as you would for an external shunt. Avoid constriction or trauma to the area; don't take blood pressures or draw blood from that arm. However, your patient may bathe as usual.

Both procedures involve a surgical incision. The incision probably will be covered with a sterile dressing when your patient is discharged from the hospital. You may be instructed to clean the area with an antiseptic solution and maintain sterility until the sutures are removed. Ask your doctor for instructions in post-surgical care. Don't bathe the area until your doctor gives approval.

Hemodialysis procedures vary depending on the type of equipment, the venous access, and the solutions used. To avoid confusion, I will emphasize only general principles of home dialysis. *Consult closely with your health care team for specific instructions in caring for a patient on home dialysis. Never attempt dialysis at home until you have been trained in the procedures. This procedure must be done correctly; mistakes or machine malfunctions can result in serious complications, even death.*

Most hemodialysis devices use one of three principles. The ***coil dialyzer*** (most common) uses coils as a semipermeable membrane. Blood passes through the coils and the system pumps dialysate between the coil layers. The *flat plate dialyzer* has two layers of semipermeable membranes bound by a rigid structure. Blood ports are located at each end of the dialyzer between the membranes. The blood flows between the membranes and dialysate flows between the supporting structures and one of the membranes. The *hollow-fiber artificial kidney* contains fine capillaries with the semipermeable membranes enclosed in a plastic cylinder. Blood flows through the capillaries as the system pumps dialysate in the opposite direction on the outside of the capillaries.

The frequency of hemodialysis will depend on your patient's condition. The patient usually is connected to the hemodialysis equipment for about six hours, or as long as he is able to tolerate the procedure.

Know how access is obtained into the shunt or fistula. Always follow sterile technique; do not use any equipment or solutions that have been opened or contaminated. Weigh your patient before and after treatment to establish that adequate filtration has occurred. Some patients lose up to four pounds after a single dialysis treatment.

Take your patient's vital signs as prescribed. Fever may indicate infection, solution contamination, or that the dialysate is too hot. During treatment, the patient, the dialyzer, and the dialysate bath must be carefully monitored. Check all alarms and make sure correct limits are set on the thermostat, and on arterial, venous, and dialysate pressure monitors.

Before starting, check for adequate blood flow in the shunt and fistula; watch for signs of inflammation, irritation, or excess drainage with an external shunt. Make sure all points of attachment are secure. Never start dialysis if you suspect problems of any kind; consult immediately with your doctor.

If too much fluid is removed too fast, your patient may experience muscle cramps, confusion, backaches, headache, or possibly seizures. Excessive removal of fluid during ultrafiltration can cause a sudden drop in blood pressure, cardiac arrhythmias, or an angina-type of chest pain. Electrolyte and sugar imbalance can occur. Watch for signs of hyperglycemia: confusion, mental changes, nausea, vomiting, flushed face, dry skin or mouth, and drowsiness. Hemorrhage can occur if the blood lines separate or if the dialyzer membrane ruptures. If there are bleeding problems with the shunt, clamp the area immediately and call your doctor.

One common problem with home hemodialysis is air embolism. Never allow solutions to run dry because air will enter the lines. Other problems include hepatitis; inadequate or excessive ultrafiltration; blood leaks; infection; shunt or fistula complications; and clotting problems. You will be using heparin (an anticoagulant) to avoid clotting problems, so be sure to report any excess bleeding. Watch for nose bleeds, rectal or vaginal bleeding, or blood seen in vomitus, stool, or urine. Heart attacks and heart disease, strokes, and peripheral vascular disorders may be seen with prolonged dialysis. *Ask the health care team for advice on what to expect and how to handle any emergencies during dialysis.*

Continuous Ambulatory Peritoneal Dialysis

Continuous ambulatory peritoneal dialysis (CAPD) is another means of providing dialysis and usually prescribed when the patient's condition is acute, or when his body cannot tolerate hemodialysis. The goal is the same, but instead of a dialysis machine, the peritoneum (membrane lining the abdomen) filters the blood. The process takes 36 to 48 hours to achieve what hemodialysis can do in six hours, but the advantages over hemodialysis are that it can be done effectively in the home; it can be easily learned; it is relatively safe; it affords the patient a more natural life-style; and it is less expensive than hemodialysis. However, all renal dialysis patients are not candidates for this type of therapy.

For CAPD, a special catheter is inserted into the peritoneum to allow introduction of the dialysate. The dialysate absorbs waste products from the blood and is subsequently drained. During CAPD, sterile technique is required; the patient's weight, fluid balance, and intake and output are monitored. Watch carefully for signs of infection; peritonitis (inflammation of the peritoneum from infection) is a possible serious complication of CAPD, usually caused by carelessness with sterile technique. Observe your patient for the following: abdominal pain; cloudy dialysate return; fever; and excess drainage (yellow discharge). Antibiotic therapy usually solves the problem, but scarring may occur that decreases the effectiveness of CAPD.

The patient should follow a strict time schedule for fluid exchanges in an effort to maintain optimal effects. Time the beginning and end of each exchange. Record the amount of solution infused and recovered, the number of exchanges done, and the patient's weight before and after dialysis. The fluid balance should be about even or show a slight loss. The duration of dialysis will depend on the patient's weight, severity of the condition, and physical ability.

There should be no pain with CAPD; if pain occurs, it may be because the dialyzing solution is not at body temperature; the catheter is irritating the peritoneum; there is incomplete drainage; or the peritoneum is infected. There should be no bleeding; presence of blood may indicate irritation of the peritoneum, or the addition of heparin to the solution.

Protein depletion may occur following treatment, as well as dehydration owing to excessive fluid loss. This can occur as a result of improper management of dialysis and poor diet and fluid intake before therapy. Report any of these problems to your doctor.

Your health care team will give you specific instruction in the administration of peritoneal dialysis. Do not attempt this procedure until you have been trained by a professional and are confident about the method. You must be thoroughly familiar with sterile technique (see Chapter 3). All solutions should arrive unopened; check the label for expiration dates and storage instructions (most are refrigerated). You may also have to add other medications to the solution, also using sterile technique (see Chapter 8). Make sure the solution is warmed to *body temperature* before you begin.

As with hemodialysis, observe the catheter site for signs of infection (pain or tenderness). You'll be instructed in sterile cleansing of the site before administering the solution, which flows by gravity. If the flow is impaired, it may indicate blood clotting or catheter problems. Repositioning sometimes relieves flow problems.

CAPD is lengthy and can be tiring for the patient. Watch for signs of fluid overload or respiratory problems. When the process is complete, you'll cleanse the area again, disconnect the solution administration tube, and reapply a sterile catheter dressing.

Care Giver's Checklist

1. If you're planning on home dialysis for your patient, make sure the house is suitable. You may have to make electrical or plumbing changes.
2. Adhere to all diet and fluid restrictions. The diet will be tailored to your loved one's condition; once dialysis begins, some restrictions may be lifted. You may need to weigh your patient daily and keep fluid intake and output records.
3. Make sure the home care team gives you ample instruction on home dialysis and how to handle complications or emergencies.
4. The dialysate temperature must be accurate. Watch for complications during hemodialysis such as muscle cramps, headaches, seizures, and cardiac or blood pressure changes.
5. Home dialysis can give your loved one control over his schedule, rather than planning his life around a clinic schedule, but he may miss out on support systems developed at dialysis treatment centers. Seek out emotional support so your loved one knows he is not alone in coping with kidney dialysis.

16 Medical Emergencies

Even with the best care and planning, medical emergencies can occur at home. While you can't anticipate every crisis, there are ways to prepare for critical situations. For example, know all of the expected side effects of your patient's medications and find out if she has any drug allergies. Write down all emergency telephone numbers and keep them by the telephone. Does your fire department or police department provide trained personnel and lifesaving equipment? Some departments offer only transportation to the hospital. Make sure your hospital has a 24-hour emergency ward or trauma center. Know as much as you can about your patient's condition, what problems to expect, and how to handle them. Should you have special training or certain equipment on hand? All homes should have a basic first aid kit containing bandages, dressings, antiseptics, tape, scissors, thermometer, an elastic bandage, and some safety pins.

Have all medical equipment checked and be sure your household electrical system can accommodate it. What should be done if the power fails? How will the patient escape from a fire? Sit down and answer these questions now, before an emergency occurs.

In any crisis, stay calm, call for help, think clearly, and provide emergency care until help arrives. If there is another person in the house, someone should stay at the patient's side while you seek help. When you call emergency services, give the dispatcher the telephone number you are calling from and the address where the emergency has occurred. Give as much information as possible; tell the dispatcher whether your patient is breathing or has a pulse and what type of first aid is being given. This is valuable information that can save rescue workers time when they arrive. Never hang up before the dispatcher does; you may be asked for additional information.

Cardiopulmonary resuscitation (CPR) basic life support is a rescue approach that can be performed by non-medical professionals until emergency medical services (EMS) arrive. Community hospitals, the American Red Cross, the American Heart Association, and some fire departments offer CPR training and certification. The following CPR instructions are from the American Heart Association *Heartsaver Manual*, which has been used in CPR courses to teach this lifesaving technique to thousands of Americans. ***These instructions are included as a reminder for persons trained in CPR; they are not a substitute for professional training. Do not attempt CPR without training from a certified instructor.***

Artificial Respiration and Cardiopulmonary Resuscitation (CPR)

Cardiopulmonary resuscitation (CPR) is a holding action for sudden cardiac or respiratory arrest until more advanced life support care can be made available. CPR involves a combination of mouth-to-mouth rescue breathing (or other artificial ventilation techniques) and chest compressions. It keeps some oxygenated blood flowing to the brain and other vital organs until appropriate medical treatment can restore normal heart action.

Cardiac arrest causes the victim to lose consciousness within seconds. **If CPR is started promptly** after the pulse stops and if advanced life support is available quickly, the person has a chance to survive.

Cardiopulmonary resuscitation includes three basic rescue skills, the ABC's of CPR: Airway, Breathing, and Circulation.

Airway. The first action for successful resuscitation is immediate opening of the airway. It is important to remember that the back of the tongue and the epiglottis are the most common cause of airway obstruction in the unconscious victim. Since the tongue, directly, and the epiglottis, indirectly, are attached to the lower jaw, tilting the head back and moving the lower jaw (chin) forward lifts the tongue and the epiglottis from the back of the throat and usually opens the airway.

Breathing. When breathing stops, the body has only the oxygen remaining in the lungs and bloodstream. It has no other oxygen reserve. Therefore, when breathing stops, cardiac arrest and death quickly follow. Mouth-to-mouth rescue breathing is the quickest way to get oxygen into the victim's lungs. There is more than enough oxygen in the air you breathe into the victim to at least partly supply his or her needs. Rescue breathing must be performed until the victim can breathe on his or her own or until trained professionals take over. *Remember:* If the victim's heart is beating, you must (1) maintain an open airway and (2) breathe, for an adult victim, once every 5 seconds (12 times per minute). *If the victim's heart is not beating, you will have to perform mouth-to-mouth rescue breathing* plus *chest compressions.*

Circulation. The third skill of CPR is chest compressions, which replace the heartbeats of the victim. They thus maintain some blood flow to the lungs, brain, coronary arteries, and other major organs. Anytime chest compressions are performed, mouth-to-mouth rescue breathing (or a suitable alternate method of artificial ventilation) must also be performed.

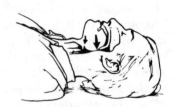

Fig. 35 Positioning the victim

Remember, CPR, like any skill, needs to be practiced every now and then to keep the important steps straight. That way, if any emergency arises, you may be able to help save a life. Refresh your skills at least every two years by contacting an American Heart Association office and taking a refresher course. A yearly refresher course is even more desirable. It will only take a little of your time to review these steps and skills, and you will feel good knowing that you are still able to do CPR. A refresher course also keeps you informed about advances in CPR technique.

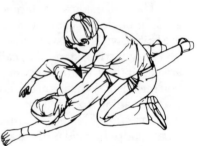

Never rehearse or practice these skills on another person! Reading material does *not,* by itself, constitute a CPR course. It is necessary to practice on manikins, with certified instructors to guide you, to gain the skills of CPR.

1. Assessment: Determine unresponsiveness. Get help if possible. Tap or gently shake shoulder. Shout "Are you OK?" Call out "help!"

One concern about teaching people CPR is the risk of possible damage from unnecessarily resuscitating sleepers, fainters, etc. Call for help will summon nearby bystanders.

2. Position the victim (4-10 seconds). Turn on back as a unit, if necessary, supporting head and neck (figure 35).

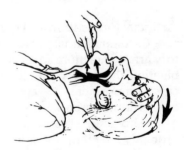

Fig. 36 Opening airway

Frequently the victim will be facedown. Effective CPR can be provided only with the victim flat on back. The head cannot be above the level of the heart or CPR is ineffective.

3. Open the airway (head-tilt/chin-lift, figure 36). Kneel beside the victim's shoulder; lift the chin up gently with one hand while pushing down on the forehead with the other to tilt the head back. The chin should be lifted so that the teeth are brought almost together. Avoid completely closing the mouth.

Airway must be opened to establish breathlessness. Many victims may be making efforts at breathing that are ineffective because of obstruction by the tongue.

4. Assessment: Determine breathlessness (3–5 seconds). Maintain open airway. Turn your head toward victim's chest with your ear directly over and close to victim's mouth.

Look at the chest for a moment. *Listen* for the sounds of breathing. *Feel* for breath on your cheek.

Hearing and feeling are the only true ways of determining the presence of breathing. If there is chest movement but you cannot feel or hear air, the airway is still obstructed. Accurate diagnosis is important; rescue breathing should not be performed on someone who is breathing.

5. Give 2 full breaths (1 to 1½ seconds per breath, figure 37).

Pinch off nostrils with thumb and forefinger of upper hand while maintaining pressure on victim's forehead to keep the head tilted.

Open your mouth wide, take a deep breath, and make a tight seal.Breathe into victim's mouth 2 times with complete refilling of your lungs after each breath. Watch for victim's chest to rise.

Rescue breaths are given at the rate of 1 to 1½ seconds each, allowing the lungs to deflate between breaths.

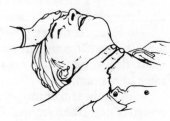

Fig. 37 Rescue breathing

If you cannot give rescue breaths to a victim, start the obstructed airway sequence (see The Choking Patient, page 208).

When you are beginning rescue breathing, it is important to get as much oxygen as possible to the victim. If your rescue breathing is effective, you will:

- feel air going in as you blow
- feel the resistance of the victim's lungs
- feel your own lungs emptying
- see the rise and fall of the victim's chest and belly.

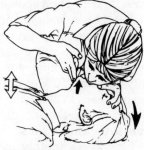

6. Establish pulselessness (5–10 seconds). Place 2–3 fingers on the Adam's apple (voice box) just below chin. Slide fingers into the groove between Adam's apple and muscle, on the side nearest you. Maintain head-tilt with other hand (figure 38). Feel for the carotid pulse.

This activity should take 5 to 10 seconds because it takes time to find the right place, and the pulse itself may be slow or very weak and rapid. The victim's condition must be properly assessed.

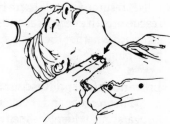

Fig. 38 Checking pulse

7. Activate the EMS system. Know your local EMS or rescue unit telephone number. Send second rescuer to call. Notification of the EMS system at this time allows the caller to give complete information about the victim's condition.

8. Begin first cycle of rescue breathing *with* chest compressions (figure 39).

To begin first cycle: Move your hands to the victim's chest. Run the index and middle fingers up the lower margin of the rib cage and locate the sternal notch with your middle finger. With index finger on sternum, place heel of the hand closest to the head on the sternum next to, but not covering, the index finger. Place second hand on top of first. Precise hand placement is essential to avoid serious injury.

Position body. Compress with weight transmitted vertically downward, elbows straight and locked, and shoulders over hands. Between compressions, the pressure must be released and the chest allowed to return to its normal position, but the hands should not be lifted off the chest.

Say mnemonic at proper rate and ratio. (Count aloud to establish rhythm: "one-and-two-and-three-and-four-and...".) Fifty percent of compression/relaxation is downward to empty the heart; 50% of compression/relaxation is upward to fill the heart. With each compression, you want to squeeze the heart or increase pressure within the chest so that blood moves to the vital organs.

Compress smoothly and evenly, keeping fingers off victim's ribs. The rescuer must apply enough force to depress the sternum 1½–2 inches (4–5 cm), at a rate of 80–100 compressions per minute.

9. Fifteen compressions (9 to 11 seconds) and two ventilations (figure 40). Ventilate properly: After every 15 compressions, deliver two rescue breaths. Adequate oxygenation must be maintained.

10. At the end of four cycles (52–73 seconds), check for return of pulse for 5 seconds (figure 38). Check pulse. If no pulse, resume CPR. If there is a pulse but no breathing, give 1 rescue breath every 5 seconds (12 per minute). This is done to establish whether there is a spontaneous return of pulse or breathing.

Entrance of a 2nd Rescuer to Replace the 1st Rescuer

First rescuer ends cycle with 2 breaths. Second rescuer appears and 1) identifies self: "I know CPR; can I help?" 2) checks pulse for 5 seconds.

If no pulse, second rescuer starts one-rescuer CPR with two breaths. First rescuer assesses the adequacy of second rescuer by:

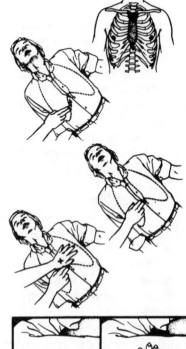

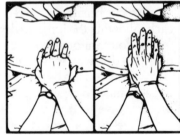

Fig. 39 Giving chest compressions

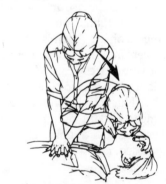

Fig. 40 Compression and ventilation

- watching for chest to rise during rescue breaths
- checking the pulse during chest compressions.

Here are a few other tips for rescue breathing and CPR:

Try to be certain that you are getting air into the lungs. Sometimes air goes into the stomach and may cause vomiting, which can be fatal to an unconscious person. The stomach will begin to bulge if it's filling with air. To avoid forcing air into the stomach, make sure your patient's head is tilted properly, don't give the breaths too quickly, and pause long enough for the lungs to empty. Don't breathe too hard or too fast into your patient.

If your patient has a tracheostomy in place, pinch her nostrils and close off the mouth. Look, listen, and feel over the stoma, instead of the mouth. Breathing is done directly over the tracheostomy or stoma, not into the mouth. (If the tracheostomy cuff is inflated, you will not have to close off the nose and mouth.) Don't tilt the head back when performing rescue breathing on someone with a tracheostomy. Never block the stoma; it is the patient's only source of air.

The breathing and chest compression count and technique will remain the same if you must administer full CPR to a tracheostomy patient. Talk with your doctor about how to handle such an emergency if your patient has a tracheostomy.

If your patient vomits, turn her on her side right away so she won't choke on vomitus. If you cannot breathe through her mouth, you will have to use mouth-to-nose ventilation. Tilt back her head, close off the mouth, pull the jaw forward, take a deep breath, and seal your lips around the patient's nose. Between breaths, open the patient's lips to allow for passage of air out. Then continue to repeat this cycle.

I recommend you make up a small sheet of CPR and rescue breathing instructions and keep them by the patient's bed. The technique is slightly different for infants and children; if you are caring for a child, get training in infant-child CPR.

If your patient is known to have breathing problems, your doctor may recommend some other valuable pieces of equipment available at a pharmacy or medical supply store. One of them is an artificial airway; a disposable piece of equipment that is inserted through the patient's mouth and into the airway. Not only does this provide an adequate airway for the patient, but it is a more hygienic means of providing mouth-to-mouth resuscitation. Most pharmacies have them on hand or can order one for you. They are not expensive and are an important safety item to keep at your patient's bedside.

The artificial airway is made of plastic or rubber and is curved to fit into the mouth, compress the tongue, and pass down into the patient's airway. If there are dentures in place, remove them. Your patient should be flat on her back, with her neck gently pulled up and extended for easier insertion. Open her mouth and pass the airway back over the tongue and down; some gentle rotation may be required. The mouth portion of the airway should be resting between the patient's teeth and lips (figure 41). If the patient starts to gag as the airway is being inserted, stop for a moment and then continue (gagging is an automatic response). Coughing or gagging may indicate that the patient has resumed breathing; if so, remove the airway.

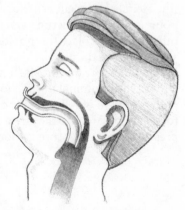

Fig. 41 Artificial airway

You may want to get a breathing bag, which comes with a face mask attached. The mask is placed tightly over the patient's nose and mouth and the breathing bag is compressed manually. This item is more expensive than an airway, but very effective. A small pocket mask with a nozzle to breathe into also is sold. These items are not mandatory, but you should know they are available. Get training before using this equipment on your own.

Advanced life support represents the type of CPR that is seen in the hospital, when other sophisticated life-support machinery is available. Advanced life support measures consist of drugs, airway devices, cardiac defibrillator, electrocardiogram monitor, and other breathing aids.

The Choking Patient

If your patient appears to be choking on something and cannot speak; is unable to cough up an obstruction; or appears to have trouble breathing, he will need your help. Signs of respiratory distress include difficulty breathing; gasping for air; loud, noisy respirations; choking; and skin color changes.

Airway obstruction often occurs during mealtimes. Cut your patient's food into small pieces, don't rush the meal, and don't offer beverages until food has been swallowed.

The following guidelines from the American Heart Association *Heartsaver Manual* may be used to help a patient with an airway obstruction.

Obstructed Airway: Conscious Adult

1. Rescuer asks, "Are you choking?" Victim may be using the "Universal Distress Signal" of choking: clutching the neck between thumb and index finger. Rescuer must identify complete airway obstruction by determining if victim is able to speak or cough.

In the conscious victim it is essential to recognize the signs of an airway obstruction and take action immediately. If the victim is able to speak or cough effectively, do not interfere with his or her attempts to expel the foreign body. Continually check for success.

2. Perform the Heimlich maneuver (subdiaphragmatic abdominal thrusts) until the foreign body is expelled or the victim becomes unconscious.

SUBDIAPHRAGMATIC ABDOMINAL THRUSTS (the Heimlich maneuver): Stand behind the victim and wrap your arms around victim's waist. Grasp one fist with your other hand and place thumb side of your fist in the midline slightly above the navel. Press fist into abdomen with quick inward and upward thrusts (figure 42).

Each abdominal thrust should be delivered decisively, with the intent of relieving the obstruction. Such thrusts can force air upward into the airway from the lungs with enough pressure to expel the foreign body.

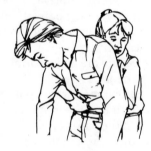

Fig. 42 The Heimlich maneuver

3. *For victims in late pregnancy or who are obese, perform* CHEST THRUSTS: Stand behind victim and place your arms under victim's armpits to encircle the chest. Grasp one fist withother hand and place thumb side on the middle of the breastbone. Press with quick backward thrusts (figure 43).

Chest thrusts are more easily done than abdominal thrusts when the abdominal girth is large, as in gross obesity or in advanced pregnancy.

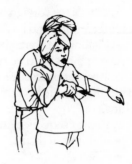

Fig. 43 Chest thrust

Obstructed Airway: Conscious Adult Who Becomes Unconscious

1. Position the victim and get help. Activate the EMS system.

Turn victim on back as a unit, if necessary, supporting head and neck. The victim must be properly positioned on his or her back in case CPR becomes necessary (figure 35).

Call out "Help!" Activate EMS; or if someone responds to call for help, send them. It is vitally important to gain access to advanced life support.

2. Foreign body check. Perform tongue-jaw lift. Sweep deeply into mouth to remove foreign body. This can be done only in the unconscious victim (figure 44).

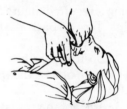

Fig. 44 Foreign body sweep

3. Open airway and attempt to ventilate. Use head-tilt/chin-lift. Attempt rescue breathing (figure 37). Complete airway obstruction by a foreign body is assumed present, but at this point an attempt must be made to get some air into the lungs just in case the victim's fall has dislodged the foreign body.

4. Airway remains obstructed? Give 6–10 abdominal thrusts.

SUBDIAPHRAGMATIC ABDOMINAL THRUSTS (the Heimlich maneuver): Straddle the victim's thighs. Place heel of one hand on the abdomen in the midline slightly above the navel and well below the tip of the xiphoid (tip of the sternum). Place the second hand directly on top of the first hand. Press into the abdomen with quick upward thrusts. Perform 6–10 thrusts. Such thrusts can force air upward into the airway from the lungs with enough pressure to expel the foreign body.

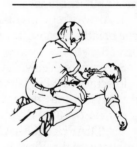

Fig. 45 Abdominal thrust for bedridden patient

Continually check for success. Each abdominal thrust should be delivered with the intent of relieving the obstruction (figure 45).

(CHEST THRUSTS: Same hand position as that of for applying external chest compression. Exert quick downward thrust (figure 46). Chest thrusts are preferred in the presence of large abdominal girth (advanced pregnancy or obesity). Downward thrusts generate effective airway pressure.

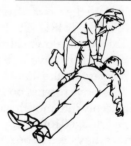

Fig. 46 Chest thrust for bedridden patient

5. Check for foreign body using finger sweep. Turn head up, open mouth with tongue-jaw lift technique and sweep deeply into mouth along cheek with hooked finger (figure 44).

A dislodged foreign body may now be manually accessible if it has not been expelled. Dentures may need to be removed to improve finger sweep.

6. Reattempt rescue breaths (figure 37). Open airway by the head-tilt/chin-lift maneuver, and attempt rescue breathing. By this time another attempt must be made to get some air into the lungs.

7. Repeat sequence until successful. Alternate the above maneuvers in rapid sequence:
- abdominal thrusts
- finger sweep
- attempt rescue breathing

Persistent attempts are rapidly made in sequence in order to relieve the obstruction. As the victim becomes more deprived of oxygen, the muscles will relax and maneuvers that were previously ineffective may become effective.

Obstructed Airway: Unconscious Adult

1. Establish unresponsiveness, call for help, and position victim. Allow 4–10 seconds if turning is required (figure 35). Tap, gently shake shoulder, shout "Are you OK?" Call out "Help!" Turn on back as a unit, if necessary, supporting head and neck. This initial call for help is to alert bystanders.

2. Open airway. Establish breathlessness. Kneel properly. Head-tilt with one hand and chin-lift with other hand (figure 36). Ear over mouth, observe chest: look, listen, and feel for breaths.

3. Attempt to ventilate (figure 37). Attempt rescue breathing. Complete airway obstruction by a foreign body is assumed present, but at this point an attempt must be made to get some air into the lungs.

4. Airway remains obstructed? Reattempt ventilation. Reposition head; attempt to give rescue breaths because improper head-tilt is the most common cause of airway obstruction (figure 36).

5. Activate the EMS system. If unsuccessful, and a second person is available, he or she should activate EMS system. Know your local EMS or rescue unit number. Advance life support capability may be required.

6. Give 6–10 subdiaphragmatic abdominal thrusts.

SUBDIAPHRAGMATIC ABDOMINAL THRUSTS (the Heimlich maneuver): Straddle the victim's thighs. Place heel of one hand on the abdomen in the midline slightly above the navel and well below the tip of the xiphoid. Place the second hand directly on top of the first hand. Press into the abdomen with quick upward thrusts (figure 45). Such thrusts can force air upward into the airway from the lungs with enough pressure to expel the foreign body.

(CHEST THRUSTS: Same hand position as that for applying external chest compression. Exert quick downward thrusts.) Chest thrusts are preferred in the presence of large abdominal girth (advanced pregnancy or obesity). Downward thrusts generate effective airway pressure (figure 46).

7. Remove foreign body. Turn head up, open mouth with tongue-jaw lift technique and sweep deeply into mouth along cheek with hooked finger (figure 44).

A dislodged foreign body may now be manually accessible if it has not been expelled. Dentures may need to be removed to improve finger sweep.

8. Attempt to ventilate (figure 37). Reposition head using head-tilt/chin-lift. Attempt to

give rescue breaths. By this time another attempt must be made to get some air into the lungs.

9. Repeat sequence until successful. If the airway remains obstructed, alternate the above maneuvers in rapid sequence:

- abdominal thrusts
- finger sweep
- attempt to ventilate

Persistent attempts are rapidly made in sequence in order to relieve the obstruction. As the victim becomes more deprived of oxygen, the muscles will relax and maneuvers that were previously ineffective may become effective.

If the patient vomits, turn her to her side so she does not choke or swallow the vomitus. Turning her also may help to dislodge an object. These measures may not work and prompt medical attention will be necessary. If there is full obstruction of the airway, mouth-to-mouth resuscitation will not help since air will not pass beyond the obstruction. All you can do is continue with the various maneuvers listed above in hopes that they will dislodge the object.

If there is partial airway obstruction, your patient may be getting some air into her lungs. Try to keep your patient calm; anxiety will only make breathing more difficult.

Physiological conditions in the patient's body may cause swelling (edema) in the airway, closing it partially or completely. Some probable causes of this are drug allergies; increased mucous secretions lodged in the airway; or spasms. These can not be relieved by manual maneuvers. Artificial respiration may help, but only if the airway is not totally obstructed. If suctioning equipment is available, you could try to suction the patient in an effort to clear the patient's airway. Seek prompt medical attention at the earliest sign of distress.

Bleeding

The first step is to stop the bleeding! Apply direct pressure over the area for a few minutes. A gauze sponge or dressing held over the wound will help to promote clotting. Some parts of the body are more vascular—have a greater blood supply—and tend to bleed more than other areas. The head and face are vascular areas; a very small wound can cause a lot of bleeding. If you feel added pressure is necessary, use several gauze sponges, a sanitary pad, or a clean towel secured with tape, a bandage, or even hosiery. Do not pull off the dressing, as you can disturb the clot.

Factors that can affect bleeding are the type of wound, its location and severity; certain medications; or some blood disorders. Excessive blood loss, or bleeding that will not stop, present life-threatening complications that require prompt emergency medical attention.

One method of stopping bleeding is by applying pressure to one of the arterial pressure points in the body. The arteries are the vessels pumping blood away from the heart, and almost all bleeding can be stopped by applying direct pressure over one of them (except when a major artery has been severed). Apply direct pressure to the nearest pressure point using dressings or a towel firmly held over the area (figure 47). Never use a tourniquet, except in the case of a severed artery or limb. If a tourniquet is used, apply it tightly just above the wound and get immediate medical attention. Note the time that you applied the tourniquet; it can cause irreparable nerve and vascular damage if left on too long.

The bleeding patient should be flat on her back, with her feet elevated slightly. Cover your patient with a blanket to keep her warm. With excessive blood loss, a patient may go into shock (hypovolemic shock) caused by the sudden decrease in blood volume. Signs of shock are cold, moist skin; pale skin color; increased, weak pulse initially; mental confusion; decreased blood pressure; and possible cardiac arrest. In this case, stop the bleeding, call for emergency attention, and initiate CPR if your patient has stopped breathing and has no pulse. Your patient will need further medical care that you will not be equipped to offer.

Nosebleeds can occur from injury, as a side effect of certain medications, and from some physical conditions or disorders such as high blood pressure. They can occur after a minor trauma, or spontaneously, without apparent reason. If nosebleed occurs for no reason, notify your doctor, who may wish to pursue probable causes.

Try to control the bleeding by applying direct pressure to the person's nostril. Have your patient sit up and lean forward, so the blood does not drain back into the patient. Ice can be applied to the nose. If bleeding does not stop after a few minutes, or appears profuse, put a piece of gauze into the nostril, continue to maintain pressure, and seek medical attention. Serious nosebleeds are usually seen with anticoagulants, anti-cancer drugs, and certain blood disorders. These patients may require special nasal packing and clotting procedures performed by a professional. Some form of blood replacement may be required if bleeding has been excessive.

Some minor wounds will not need medical attention, but you should report the incident to your doctor in case additional medical attention is needed. Sutures or stitches are used primarily to stop bleeding, and prevent infection, as well as for cosmetic reasons. Simple cuts, scrapes, and abrasions do

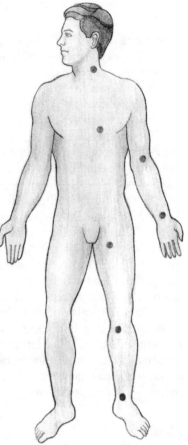

Fig. 47 Controlling bleeding

not require sutures. Ask your doctor what you should cleanse the wound with; hydrogen peroxide usually is a good cleansing agent and should not cause discomfort. Use sterile dressings and avoid placing tape directly over the wound. To remove tape, pull it up gently in the direction of the hair growth. A dressing is required until a scab forms. Some types of wounds should not be covered, and your doctor will specify when a dressing would not be indicated. Be sure to report any non-healing or infectious process to your doctor.

Seizures

If your patient is known to have seizures, take steps to protect her. If there are bed railings, pad them with blankets or pillows and put them up during the seizure. When a person is having a seizure, the most important thing you can do is to protect her from injuring herself. Cradle or place something soft under the patient's head. Get your patient onto the floor, if possible, and clear the area of any objects that could injure her. During a seizure, your patient is unconscious and unaware of her environment; when the seizure is over, she may not recall the incident. Some patients can tell a seizure is coming and prepare for it. As the seizure begins, muscles go into severe spasms, followed by jerking movements, changes in face color (flushing), possible drooling or foaming at the mouth, and sometimes loss of bladder and bowel control.

Try not to touch your patient or restrict movement; you may injure her. One area of controversy involves whether to place a padded seizure stick into the patient's mouth so she does not bite her tongue, or let it fall back into the airway. Some professionals feel more injury is caused by trying to get this device into the patient's mouth during a seizure. The care giver can be bitten, or the patient's teeth broken. If your patient is apt to have seizures, check with your doctor on this issue. If the patient begins to vomit, try to turn her to her side. If she stops breathing, begin rescue breathing.

Try to record the time the seizure started, when it finished, and what occurred during the seizure. Stay by the patient's side and report to the doctor when it is through. Clean the patient following the seizure. Your patient will most likely be exhausted and require rest. Most seizures are not life-threatening, and usually nothing can be done to prevent them, although some can be controlled by medications. Do not try to feed anything to the patient until the seizure is over. If there are repeated attacks, or if the seizure lasts more than ten minutes, take your patient to the doctor immediately.

Fainting

Fainting occurs when the blood supply to the brain is reduced, resulting in a temporary unconscious state. This can result from various medical conditions, hypoglycemia (low blood sugar), fatigue, after prolonged periods of bed rest, or low blood pressure. The patient usually can feel it coming on; she may feel light-headed, weak, nauseated, dizzy, or experience tingling or numbness in hands and feet.

To prevent fainting, have your patient lie in bed or place her head between her knees. Cool, fresh air may help, as well as a glass of orange juice with an extra spoonful of sugar. If your patient has been confined to bed, she should never get up quickly.

If your patient has fainted, get her into a lying position (on her back) either in bed or on the floor. Turn her head to the side in case she vomits. Allow fresh air to circulate and loosen the patient's clothing. Do not offer any food or drink at this time. Apply a cool cloth to the face and forehead. If your patient has fallen, she may have injured herself. If a bone is broken, make her comfortable and seek medical advice. If possible, do not leave her alone. In simple fainting, consciousness may not be lost and the patient should feel better in a matter of moments. If your patient does not feel better, it may indicate that something else is wrong. If so, seek prompt medical attention, and administer appropriate first aid.

Heart Attacks

Most heart attacks occur when one or more of the major blood vessels has been blocked off, decreasing the blood supply to the heart. The patient may or may not experience pain. The classic sign of a heart attack is chest pain, usually felt in the center of the chest, and radiating down to the patient's left arm. Your patient may feel fullness or tightness in the chest behind the breastbone. Depending on its severity of the attack, your patient may have some respiratory difficulty; her color may become quite pale and her lips and fingernails may appear bluish. Some patients also complain of intense jaw pain, nausea, indigestion, sweating, and shortness of breath.

It is imperative that the patient receive prompt medical attention. Do not hesitate, even if it turns out there was no heart attack. Either call an ambulance or take your patient to the local emergency department. If breathing and pulse stop, initiate CPR. Do not feed your patient; try to keep her comfortable. She may sit up, but should avoid exerting herself. If your patient has a heart condition and takes nitroglycerine, or a similar medication, offer this as your doctor has directed. See Chapter 10 for more information on heart attacks.

Strokes

A stroke occurs when the blood supply to the brain is cut off. A stroke usually is quite sudden, resulting from release of a clot or hemorrhage caused by rupture of a blood vessel. This condition requires prompt medical attention; damage will depend on how severely blood flow was impaired.

The symptoms of stroke are weakness or numbness on one side; difficulty swallowing; visual problems; dizziness; loss of consciousness; severe headache; loss of understanding or speech; or mental changes.

First aid consists of having the patient lie flat, her head turned to one side so that her tongue cannot obstruct the airway and so excess saliva and mucus can drain out. Do not move the patient, except to protect her from further injury. Movement may further dislodge blood clots. Seek emergency assistance. Stay with the patient, keeping her warm and comfortable. Do not offer food or medications. See Chapter 10 for more information about stroke patients.

Drug Overdose

All medications are potentially dangerous substances if abused, or if bodily functions prevent proper exit from the body. Whenever medications are used, store them safely out of reach of children.

If your patient is unconscious but breathing, report what drug you believe was taken, and the amount, to emergency rescue workers. If your patient is unconscious, not breathing, and has no pulse, administer CPR while someone calls for help. Some medication overdoses can be treated by inducing vomiting or through gastric lavage (stomach pump). If there is time, check with your local poison control center or hospital emergency room to see if there is an antidote that could be administered right away. Toxic substances must be removed from the stomach before they are absorbed into the bloodstream. If you know when the overdose was taken, tell rescue workers; they may use different procedures based on that information. Bring any suspected medications to the hospital; they will be of tremendous value to the doctors.

Applications of Heat and Cold

Hot or cold applications are sometimes prescribed following injuries to decrease the damage or make the patient more comfortable. Cold (ice) helps to constrict blood vessels to stop bleeding and slow swelling. Cold applications usually are used 24 to 48 hours following an injury. Cold can be applied either in a moist/wet or dry form; moist application appears to penetrate better than a dry application.

A moist cold application consists of crushed ice placed inside a plastic bag, rubber glove, towel, pillowcase, or hot water bottle, or the area can be immersed directly in a container that has water and ice in it (59 °F/15 °C). Get your physician's permission to use this type of application; find out how often and how long the treatment should be given. Dry cold packs contain a special chemical that becomes cold when activated. Any cold application should be covered before applying it to the patient. Cover only the treatment area and keep the rest of the patient warm.

Most cold applications last 20 to 30 minutes and never longer than one hour. Watch for complaints of chilling; numbness; color changes (grayish/bluish); blistering; and discomfort.

Use special care when this procedure is prescribed for a patient with circulatory problems or who is neurologically impaired; she may not be able to feel the treatment and will be unaware of any problems. Following treatment, dry and cover the area.

Heat applications are used for a number of therapeutic reasons. Heat causes vessel dilation, which in turn promotes circulation or blood supply to the area. This aids the healing process by bringing blood, with its important infection fighting cells, to the area. Heat also can help to relieve muscle spasm or pain as a direct result of vessel dilation.

Heat can either be applied in a moist/wet or dry form. Heat devices include hot water bottles, heating pads, warm compresses, disposable hot packs, or direct immersion into warm water (no hotter than 125°F/50°C, even lower for some patients). Moist/wet heat allows for deeper penetration, but there is a greater risk of burning your patient than when dry heat is used. Use heat only when indicated by your doctor. Heat should not be used when bleeding may occur, in conditions where increased swelling may occur (sprains), or to relieve or conceal any acute condition, such as abdominal pain. Be careful using heat on a patient with circulatory problems or impaired sensations.

The frequency and duration of the treatment should be prescribed by the doctor. If your patient has any complaints or if you note any problems, such as excessive redness, blistering, pain, or swelling, stop the treatment. Don't apply heat directly over scars, stomas, or new incisions. A heat treatment usually lasts 20 to 30 minutes. If a heating pad or other heating device is used, apply a piece of tape over the control knob so that it cannot slip and get set to a higher level. Never apply the heat directly on the extremity unless you are using a moist/wet application; use a flannel covering or a pillowcase over hot water bottles and other heating devices.

If you are applying a moist, warm pack, you can use a warm towel, wring it out and apply it directly over the area. One way of maintaining that heat is to wrap it in plastic wrap so that the heat cannot escape. Use a plastic absorbent pad under the area when using either hot or cold applications to protect the bed from getting wet.

Care Giver's Checklist

1. Make an emergency plan *now*. Investigate the capabilities of your community's emergency services and make a list of all important telephone numbers.
2. Discuss your loved one's illness or disability with the health care team to determine whether you can anticipate any medical emergencies based on her physical condition.
3. Take a certified course in cardiopulmonary resuscitation and get first aid training in emergency health care. Call the American Red Cross or the American Heart Association for information about courses in your community.
4. Assemble a basic first aid kit containing bandages, dressings, antiseptic solutions, tape, scissors, thermometers, an elastic bandage, and safety pins. Find out what additional equipment is recommended for your patient, such as an artificial airway, breathing bag, or a padded seizure stick, if your patient is prone to seizures and your doctor recommends one.
5. Hot or cold applications may be prescribed for certain types of injuries or medical conditions. Find out how long and how often to apply these and whether applications should be moist or dry. Make sure the temperature will accomplish the medical goal without injuring your loved one.

17 Rehabilitation at Home

A home rehabilitation program is aimed at restoring a person's physical and emotional well-being. Your patient may need to adapt to some physical limitation, but the focus should not be on limits; it should be on what she *can* do. Set specific goals and give your patient an active role in the process. Some disabilities may be progressive, but efforts can be made to halt or diminish long-term effects. The goal is to help your patient live as independently as possible.

In most cases, rehabilitation begins when the patient enters the hospital. This is a team effort involving the patient, her family, her physician, nurses, physical and occupational therapists, social workers, and other health professionals. With any major illness there is the risk of disability. Prolonged bed rest can complicate your patient's full recovery. Sometimes complications can cause more problems than the initial injury or illness.

The goals of each patient must be recognized. Is this a temporary or permanent disability? What are her physical limitations, and what can be done to correct them or make her more functional? Rehabilitation affects your patient's whole life: her home, her job, and her sense of self-esteem. The work that must be done extends from that point on. Can your patient return to her job, or must changes be made? Can she manage independently in her own home, or must adaptations be made? Can she get around outside the home, or will she need help?

Consider the answers to these and other questions before rehabilitation begins at home. Some hospitals have units delegated for rehabilitation that serve as a step between the hospital and home. The patient is encouraged to do as much of her own care as possible and is helped with anything she cannot accomplish alone.

Talk to your social worker or discharge planner about nursing assistance or physical therapy. Your patient may require regular or daily visits, or even some form of continual care. She may need to return to the hospital outpatient department for therapy. Not all patients are candidates for rehabilitation at home; some need extensive rehabilitation in a hospital or extended care facility.

To determine whether your loved one is a candidate for rehabilitation at home, consider the following: What is the physical setup of the home? Will there be someone to assist with the patient's needs? Is it feasible? What is your financial commitment? Can the rehabilitation program realistically be maintained at home? The entire rehabilitation team should be involved in this decision. Try to be sure that your commitment to rehabilitation at home is a realistic, rather than emotional, decision.

Preparing Your Home

Members of the rehabilitation team can help you and your family adapt your home to your patient's needs. What equipment will be needed? Must structural changes be considered? Some companies specialize in adapting homes for people with physical disabilities (see Appendix for resources). Before making permanent changes, consider your patient's needs and how long the disability will last. Keep potential costs in mind, including the impact of permanent adaptations on the resale value of the house.

Your home may have useful rehabilitation aids that you've never thought about. A swimming pool is very useful for some types of therapy; gym equipment can be adapted for a home rehabilitation program. Your local "Y" or community center may have rehabilitation classes in the pool.

If rehabilitation equipment will be used on a permanent or long-term basis, it may be cheaper to buy than to rent from a medical supplier. Check with your insurance provider to see what reimbursement will be allowed.

If your loved one is in a wheelchair, it should fit through all doorways. Have other family members spend an hour in the wheelchair navigating around the house; not only will they get insight into the patient's new life, they also will see some of the obstacles she faces when toys or sports equipment are strewn about the house. After such an experience, family members take extra care to keep things off the floor and out of the way.

Don't forget about transportation. You will need to know how to help your patient into and out of the car. Can your car carry a wheelchair? Carriers are available to hold the wheelchair on the back of the car; they work like a bicycle rack. Some wheelchairs are collapsible. A motorized lift can be used to lift the patient and wheelchair into the van.

If your patient can't get up and down stairs, electrical chair devices can be installed so your patient can get from one level to another. The federal Department of Health and Human Services has a number of directories and services available to assist disabled individuals. Write to:

The Superintendent of Documents
Government Printing Office
Washington, D.C. 20420

Although much has been done to meet the needs of the disabled, continued efforts are necessary. Report observations to your local governing body or to:

Office of Human Development
Architectural and Transportation Barriers Compliance Board
Washington, D.C. 20420

Check with your state's motor vehicles department about getting special license plates that will enable you to take advantage of parking areas for the handicapped. Look into community resources. Some will provide transportation or make equipment loans free to families in need. Call your local chapter of these agencies (Multiple Sclerosis Society, United Way, American Cancer Society) for information.

Transferring Techniques

The home health care team can teach you lifting and transferring techniques. Some will require strengthening exercises so the patient's muscles are strong enough to support her weight. A good deal of movement must be done using the upper extremities; often they have not been used to bearing weight.

Special equipment also is available to assist the patient and care giver in moving the patient. A transfer board is a sturdy, flat board used between the patient and the area to which she wishes to move. The board must be smooth and strong enough to support your patient's weight. Place it so the patient can slide across the board onto the other area. The two areas should be of equal or similar height. A transfer board can be used to help the patient get from the bed to a chair or wheelchair; from a wheelchair into a car; or from one chair to another. Most patients, when strong enough, use this piece of equipment to get about on their own.

The overbed trapeze is attached to a special bed frame over the patient's bed. It helps your patient raise herself in bed and adjust her position on her own. She also can use it to help to raise herself out of a wheelchair and into bed. Hang it at the proper height; your patient should be able to grasp the bar with both hands, arms straight, while lying flat in bed. This piece of equipment can be purchased or rented from a medical supply store.

A mechanical lift (Hoyer lift) can help you get the patient out of bed and into the bathtub or wheelchair. This is done by using slings under the patient's buttocks and back to hoist her up. Some even include a scale so you may weigh the patient at the same time. Get instructions in using this equipment before trying it with your patient.

The hospital staff will recognize most of your patient's needs for special equipment; some won't be apparent until your loved one is at home. If you find you need help or have an idea about something that will make life easier for your patient, consult with your hospital's physical or occupational therapy department. Look through home care catalogs for ideas, too.

Wheelchairs

Many different types of wheelchairs and ambulatory devices are available in today's market. Your patient may find that more than one is necessary to meet her needs. Even if she will use a wheelchair for an extended period of time, it might be best to rent before buying one. This way your patient will have a chance to determine what her specific needs may be and choose the best chair. Some chairs recline, the side pieces can come off, foot pedals can be moved into various positions, and some even convert into a portable commode.

The wheelchair must be fitted to your patient. Most medical supply stores carry wheelchairs, but not all of them have personnel qualified to help you make the right choice. Ask the home health care team to recommend a dependable supplier. Two leading manufacturers of wheelchairs are:

Everest & Jennings, Inc.
3233 Mission Oaks Boulevard
Camarillo, CA 93010

Invacare
P.O. Box 4028
Elyria, OH 44036

Write to either of these companies for information about wheelchairs and what to look for when buying one. It is often possible to trade in a used wheelchair when purchasing a new one, or it can be donated to a local community group.

Electric wheelchairs may be recommended, but they are not for every patient. They are more expensive than standard wheelchairs, and usually larger and heavier, making maneuverability more difficult. The motorized attachment makes it impossible to fold this type of chair. An electric wheelchair is most useful for a patient who will be using the chair full-time.

Another type of motorized transport, the Amigo, is a three-wheeled scooter that is much narrower than a standard wheelchair, making movement around the house somewhat easier. All patients are not candidates for this type of device, as it offers less support to some areas of the body than the standard wheelchair. For information, write to:

Amigo Sales, Inc.
6693 Dixie Highway
Bridgeport, MI 48722

Don't forget wheelchair safety. Make sure there's a safety belt in the wheelchair and that your loved one uses it. Many patients in wheelchairs have limited movement in their lower extremities, which makes them top-heavy. It is not uncommon for a patient to reach down for something and topple out of the chair and onto the floor.

Use wheelchair brakes whenever moving a patient into or out of a wheelchair, and turn the wheels inward. Patients who have lost feeling in their legs tend to be at a greater risk for leg fractures. They have brittle, fragile bones that are easy to break. Use caution when moving your patient; always be sure her legs are supported and never dropped into place. Some wheelchairs have special heel supports and straps to keep the legs in proper alignment. These also help your patient with balance.

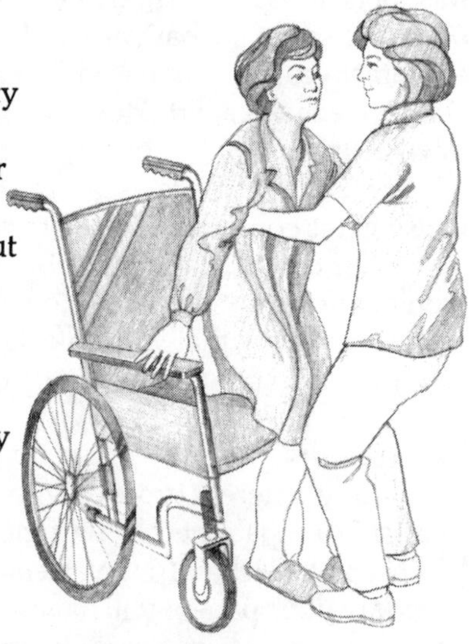

Fig. 48 Lifting someone from a wheelchair

If you will be helping your patient into and out of a wheelchair, you should be shown how to do this properly, both to protect your patient as well as your own back (figure 48). The patient should do much of the transfer herself and be helped only when she is unable to manage on her own. You should also be shown how to properly wheel a patient; it's not as easy as it looks. Learn how to take a wheelchair up and down curbs, or up and down stairs. If not done correctly, you can easily tip your patient out of the chair or injure yourself. Always have both hands in place and look ahead for sidewalk cracks. Don't push the chair too fast; you may frighten your patient.

Make your home accessible to the wheelchair patient. Can she be wheeled in close to the dining room table, or pull in close to the sink? Can she reach her own clothes, or are her things placed up too high? What about access into and out of your home; will you need ramps? What about the bathroom? Toilet seats are somewhat easier to use if their height is raised. This is easily done with a raised toilet seat that can be purchased from any medical supplier or home care outlet.

I recommend that the patient live in the home for a while before making any changes. Keep a list of problem areas and what alterations may be needed. For the homemaker, most traditional kitchens are impossible to use with a wheelchair. Some patients find that a low work table or even a portable tray attached to the wheelchair provides an adequate work area. Your patient can use long-handled tongs to reach things at a higher level.

Another consideration is your patient's wardrobe. Clothing should be comfortable; many wheelchair patients prefer loose, easy to remove clothes. Keep in mind that the patient may need to get clothing up and down to use the toilet. Jogging suits, perhaps an extra size larger, with elastic waistbands are preferred by many wheelchair patients. Skirts, dresses, or pants should be worn somewhat longer since the patient will be sitting. Have your loved one dress before she gets into the chair. Smooth out all clothing as she is positioned in the wheelchair; even wrinkles can cause pressure sores! Feet tend to swell when a patient is in a wheelchair; you may want to buy shoes one or two sizes larger. If the patient will be wheeling herself, leather gloves will protect her hands and give her a firm grip.

Life in a wheelchair will be frustrating as both the patient and family adjust, but you'll find many ways of adapting to these limitations. You may need the help and resources of others. Experience can be gained by talking to someone who has been there. Your doctor or therapist may give you the name of another patient who would be willing to share her experience.

Complications

Because a patient undergoing physical rehabilitation has limited movement, there are increased risks of complications. Your loved one may suffer pneumonia, pressure sores, contractures, joint immobility, infections, and bladder and bowel problems. Both the patient and care giver can play an important role in preventing troublesome, debilitating complications that can impair the course of recovery.

Exercise is perhaps one of the most important areas in rehabilitation. Exercise provides movement of muscles, joints, tendons, bones, and nerves, as well as allowing the heart and respiratory system to work at capacity. All parts of the body, if inactive, will begin to function less efficiently. Muscles will shrink and shorten; the circulatory system will become sluggish; breathing will be impaired; tissues will be malnourished, resulting in skin and tissue breakdown; and bowel and bladder function may become impaired. It is imperative that a daily exercise regimen be established and maintained. Even the patient who is unable to move on her own can be helped or have exercises done for her. See Chapter 7 for information about exercising and positioning of patients who are confined to bed or have limited movement.

The disabled patient's diet should be balanced, high in protein, and include plenty of fluids. Protein helps to restore and rebuild body tissue and aids in the healing process. If the patient is not eating or appears to have a decreased appetite, consult your nutritionist. One probable cause may be from lack of exercise and activity.

An immobilized patient often has problems with weight gain, which will only make movement and lifting more difficult. Talk to your doctor about ways to limit your patient's weight. See Chapter 5 for information about nutrition and healing.

Bowel and bladder problems are frequently seen in the disabled, especially those with neurological impairment. Diminished muscle tone and a loss of sensitivity will make it difficult for some patients to control these functions; they may be unaware of a need to urinate or move their bowels. Consult closely with the health care team, especially if your patient is incontinent. Urinary tract infections and skin problems are common with these types of patients. Make sure your loved one gets ten to 12 glasses of fluid daily. There's a tendency to limit fluids if urinary incontinence is a problem, but this is a mistake because adequate fluids are needed to flush the urinary tract and lower the risk of bladder infections. See Chapter 9 for more information about bladder and bowel problems.

Psychology of the Disabled

The newly disabled person will require psychological support. Your patient may pass through a number of phases in adjusting and learning to cope with her disability. She may feel she has lost her sense of independence. Perhaps she feels she is being a burden, particularly to her family. Her disability may mean a loss of income; she may have been the family's sole provider. She may need to learn to live with a long-term medical condition that will deteriorate as time goes on. All of these factors will play a major role in how well she will adapt to her physical limitations.

You may be able to predict how your patient will cope and what mechanisms she will use based on her prior means of dealing with serious problems. Common coping mechanisms are anger, withdrawal, depression, and denial. She may express grief and a deep sense of loss. Even the patient who has been known throughout her life as a pillar of strength may find this beyond her ability to cope.

Your patient may be frustrated by her lack of control over the situation. In many cases, it has emerged suddenly and leaves no possibility for planning. Sometimes your patient's ability to cope will be directly affected by how others react to her. If she sees that she is being accepted as the same mother, wife, or business associate, she may respond positively. It's important to allow your patient to take responsibility for herself.

Anger is perhaps the most difficult of all emotions, both for the care giver and the patient. It is your loved one's form of self-defense against a situation she cannot control. Your patient, subconsciously, has found a way to make someone else feel powerless or inadequate, thereby sharing her feelings of helplessness. For example, your patient may express dissatisfaction with all of your efforts and complain constantly, no matter what you do to please her. If you stop trying, your patient may believe you no longer care, but continuing in the same fashion will only leave you frustrated and exhausted. It is important to recognize the forms of patient defense and deal with them through regular communication between the patient, family, and the medical team. Uncontrolled anger can be wasted emotional energy directed against an unalterable situation.

Listen to your loved one. Pay attention not only to what she says, but to the message behind her actions. For example, if your patient is constantly calling someone into her room to make insignificant requests, you may find that there's more than a pillow that needs fluffing. She may really be trying to tell you that she is afraid to be alone, or that she is uncertain that you still love her.

Watch for forms of non-verbal communication. Restlessness, hand wringing, insomnia, general disinterest, or withdrawal all can be indications that something may be bothering the patient. Try to draw her out by talking about what's bothering her. For instance, in the morning you may casually remark that she did not appear to have slept well. Ask her about it, and use leading questions that require a complete answer. Show her that you care how she feels and that you want to help.

If your loved one cannot cope with her disability, she may need professional help if the problem has persisted beyond a reasonable period of time or if it interferes significantly with her capacity to function. Investigate individual or group counseling; groups may be helpful if the patient feels she is alone in coping with her problem. Some doctors recommend anti-depressants, tranquilizers, or sedatives to help patients through the process of adapting.

Sexuality

Recognizing and dealing with sexual concerns is very important, although many patients and their families are reluctant to discuss this with others. Consequently, concerns about sexuality often go unresolved, resulting in feelings of frustration, inadequacy, and lost sexuality. These problems can be intensified by an inability to communicate openly between spouses or with medical professionals.

Male impotence can occur as a result of a nerve or spinal cord injury, psychological disturbances, or from medications and disease processes. Some problems of male impotence can be corrected, others may not. You will need to know if this is a temporary or permanent condition. Is the source of the problem physical or psychological? What was your patient's prior sexual interest and ability? Seek out specific information from the patient's physician about physical limitations and how they may affect sexuality. What is your patient allowed to do, and are there alternatives? If your patient must refrain from sexual intercourse for a period of time, when can she resume? Are there risks involved? Is family planning a consideration? Is there any reason why it would not be appropriate, or possible, to start a family at this time? What about sperm banks, if therapy includes anti-cancer or radiation treatments?

Make a list of all of your questions and take it with you when you visit your physician. Some doctors may appear insensitive because they are uncomfortable discussing sexuality. If so, ask for a recommendation of a counselor or therapist who will be more knowledgeable and helpful.

There are a number of cosmetic and surgical procedures done today to correct a variety of sexual dysfunction problems. Some procedures, such as penile implants, may not correct the disorder, but they help the patient feel sexually whole again. Ask if your loved one may be a candidate for this type of treatment.

A non-disabled spouse or sexual partner may have fears. He or she may not fully understand the effects of the patient's illness or disability on sexuality. It is important that the patient's need for love, nurturing, and sexual being not be forgotten. However, the care giver may have problems separating the role of nurse and provider of bedpans from that of a sexual partner. If so, seek counseling.

Care Giver's Checklist

1. Help your disabled loved one do as much as possible for herself. Allow ample time for a task; let her struggle, if need be. The sense of accomplishment will be complete when she finally succeeds.
2. Adapt your home for rehabilitation. Work closely with the health care team so you have the proper equipment on hand when your patient comes home. Make sure the home is accessible to the disabled.
3. Your patient may have the same complications seen in bedridden patients. Stick to prescribed plans for exercise and diet. Deal with complications such as urinary incontinence so your loved one may feel comfortable and confident.
4. Physical disability, especially when it is permanent, takes a deep psychological toll. Understand your loved one's defense mechanisms against this bitter disappointment so you can better deal with her anger and grief. Don't be afraid to seek counseling; this is a heavy burden to carry.
5. Disability can affect your patient's sexuality, and the sexual feelings of the care giver. Discuss your patient's physical limitations with the doctor and what may be causing sexual dysfunction. If the reason is medical, perhaps it can be corrected. If sexual impotence results from psychological concerns, counseling for both parties may ease the problem.

18 The AIDS Patient

AIDS (Acquired Immune Deficiency Syndrome) is caused by a virus that has been labeled in various ways as medical researchers search for the key to defeating this deadly new disease. The virus, known world-wide as Human Immunodeficiency Virus (HIV), also may be called Human T-Lymphotropic Virus Variant III (HTLV III) or Lymphadenopathy-Associated Virus (LAV) in the literature you find about AIDS.

The AIDS virus attacks the body's white blood cells (T-Lymphocytes), which combat infection. Once this protective immune system is compromised or destroyed, the patient is vulnerable to numerous viruses, bacteria, and fungi that ordinarily present no problem to a person with a healthy immune system.

If your loved one has AIDS, he may have many of these common complaints: fatigue; chills or feeling cold; night sweats; weight loss; swollen glands in the neck, groin, and underarms; fevers; chronic diarrhea; flu and cold-like symptoms; and skin rashes. AIDS victims are susceptible to opportunistic infections, rare cancers, and central nervous system disorders.

Overall management of AIDS probably will be handled by an infectious disease specialist. Other specialists are involved with your loved one's care as needed; a gastrointestinal specialist, internist, medical oncologist, hematologist, vascular surgeon, opthalmologist, dermatologist, or allergist may be involved with treating your patient.

Patients experience an often turbulent course with this disease. There may be periods when it appears to be under control, and then times when the patient contracts one infection after another, wearing him down physically and emotionally. I will discuss some of the more serious infections seen with AIDS later in this chapter.

Caring for Someone with AIDS

Before you undertake home care of the AIDS patient, it's important to understand how one contracts the disease. *Caring for a loved one with AIDS does not put you at risk of contracting the disease as long as you follow some safety guidelines and avoid high-risk behaviors that are known to spread AIDS.* Since AIDS is virtually incurable, it does cause panic in many people. But you cannot contract AIDS by sitting in the room with an AIDS patient, or by touching or caring for him.

AIDS is spread by the exchange of body fluids from one person to another through semen, blood, and other secretions. The majority of AIDS sufferers contracted the disease through sexual contact, by sharing of contaminated needles, or through contaminated blood products. Homosexual or bisexual males, intravenous drug users, hemophiliacs or blood transfusion recipients—and the sexual partners of persons in those categories—are considered at a higher risk of contracting AIDS. The statistics are constantly changing and *no one is immune to AIDS.* Blood supplies in the United States now are screened for presence of HIV virus, dramatically lowering the risk of contracting AIDS from blood products.

The relatively small number of persons reported to have contracted AIDS in the workplace were contaminated either by a needle puncture, by spills of contaminated blood directly onto skin with a cut or abrasion, or were already in the high risk category. Studies of family members living with AIDS patients have found no evidence of transmission to persons who are not sexual contacts of the infected patient.

Pregnant women are not known to be at any greater risk of contracting AIDS, but if a pregnant woman is infected, the unborn fetus also is at risk. Because of this, pregnant women should be familiar with all procedures and precautions when caring for someone with AIDS.

AIDS care in the United States is being carried out primarily in the home, except when the patient is acutely ill or if the home environment is inadequate. Confer with all members of the health care team about your patient's condition and how you can care for him at home. The American Red Cross in some communities offers a home care course on nursing someone with AIDS.

In general, there is no added risk to family members if a person with AIDS is cared for in your home, but special precautions must be taken when handling blood and body secretions or fluids. Always wear rubber gloves when in contact with any of these.

If you accidentally stick yourself with a contaminated needle, or if contaminated blood or other contaminated body fluids get into your eyes, mouth, or broken skin, medical researchers recommend the following:

1. Immediately wash the contaminated area with soap or antiseptic cleanser and water.
2. Contact the doctor and report the exposure; ask what steps he or she recommends.
3. Get your blood tested for the AIDS virus and retested periodically over the next year.
4. Get professional counseling about the risk of transmission of the virus to allay your fears. The chance of contracting AIDS through an accidental needlestick is 1 percent.

If you will be giving your patient injections, ask your doctor about whether you should be immunized against hepatitis, which could be contracted from a needlestick. It is impossible to immunize yourself against AIDS.

Use extreme caution when handling contaminated needles. Never bend, break, or recap used needles. Dispose of them in specially provided impenetrable needle containers. Never throw needles or contaminated items directly into the regular trash. Ask the health care team about waste services that will pick them up and dispose of them appropriately.

Living in an AIDS Household

In caring for a loved one with AIDS, you will have two goals: limiting your own exposure to the virus, and the equally important task of limiting your patient's exposure to viruses and bacteria that will bring on debilitating infections. Personal cleanliness is important in the AIDS household, both for the patient and care givers.

Never share or touch body secretions, particularly blood and semen. Bathe regularly and wash hands after using the bathroom or coming into contact with body fluids (such as a cough or sneeze). Persons with AIDS should cough or sneeze into a disposable tissue and discard it separately in their own trash container.

Do not share toothbrushes, razors, enema equipment, or sex toys. Towels and washcloths should not be shared unless laundered in between; add chlorine bleach to the wash cyle. Washing machines and dishwashers are adequate to decontaminate linens, clothing, dishes, glassware, and utensils. If you don't have a dishwasher, soak your dishes in a 1:10 bleach solution (one part chlorine bleach to ten parts water) and then wash as usual with hot, soapy water. Use the 1:10 bleach solution to clean the shower and bathtub, too; it will kill any fungus lurking there.

Normal street clothing can be worn when caring for someone with AIDS. If you will be handling blood or body secretions, wear rubber gloves and an apron or smock that can be easily washed in case of spills. Some additional accessories, such as protective eye goggles or face masks, may be recommended by your physician.

Always wash hands before preparing food; people with AIDS can safely cook and prepare food for others if they wash their hands first. Don't give unpasteurized milk or milk products to an AIDS patient; it puts him at risk of contracting salmonella. Don't give him uncooked organically-grown foods. Peel and wash all fresh fruits and vegetables.

Family members may share the kitchen and bathroom. Use normal sanitary practices to protect the AIDS patient from infections. In the kitchen, clean counters with scouring powder to remove debris and food particles. Sponges used to clean the kitchen should not be used elsewhere, and sponges should be changed regularly.

Clean the inside of the refrigerator with soap and water to control mold formation. Mop the kitchen floor at least weekly and clean up spills as they occur. For spills involving body secretions, put on disposable rubber gloves and clean with a 1:10 solution of chlorine bleach and water. Use extra-absorbent paper towels or other disposable cleaning cloths or sponges. Floor mops can be disinfected by soaking them in a 1:10 bleach solution for five minutes.

Except for disposal of contaminated needles, your trash disposal is much the same as for any household. Anything contaminated with blood or body wastes should be double bagged in plastic and tied securely before it is thrown away. Wastes may be flushed down the toilet, and the toilet bowl cleaned with a 1:10 bleach solution.

Wear gloves when cleaning bird cages, cat litter boxes, tropical fish tanks, or doing other other pet care tasks. This is to protect your patient from the diseases animals may carry, such as toxoplasmosis (often found in cat feces). If possible, someone healthy should do pet care. Some researchers feel tropical fish tanks may contain organisms not well tolerated by persons with AIDS.

Keep your home well-ventilated. Airborne organisms and diseases are less likely to be a problem when diluted by lots of air. Avoid large crowds whenever possible. Anyone with a cold or flu should not visit the AIDS patient. Someone with a cold who lives in the same household could wear a face mask to protect the AIDS patient.

Treating the AIDS Patient

AIDS patients today are surviving longer and have a better quality of life as researchers develop new drugs and treatments for AIDS-related infections and symptoms. Most of these problems are treated as they occur, usually with an array of oral, intravenous, and topical medications. As a care giver, you can help by making your patient more comfortable when some of them occur. AIDS sufferers may complain of night sweats, feeling cold and tired, and having diarrhea.

Night sweats sometimes are associated with fever, but other times are unrelated since AIDS patients often have fluctuations in body temperature for no apparent reason. Low grade fevers (99 °F to 100 °F) are often seen in AIDS patients; these may signal the presence of an infection elsewhere in the body. Report all fevers to the patient's physician. Most doctors recommend these fevers be treated with non-aspirin drugs. Watch for other indications of infection, especially if the fever does not respond to anti-fever medications or if the patient experiences other symptoms. Don't share his thermometer with anyone else.

Your patient may wake up and find his bed cold and wet. Give him an extra blanket and put dry sheets on the bed; flannel sheets will provide added warmth and absorbency. AIDS sufferers often feel cold. Avoid cold, drafty rooms and keep extra blankets on hand, even on warm days.

Chronic fatigue is another common problem for AIDS patients. Help your loved one conserve energy, and assist him whenever you can; perhaps a wheelchair would help. Plan activities indoors such as renting videos or playing board games. Invite friends to call, but don't let the patient overdo. Try to avoid placing undue stress on your patient; some physicians believe this further weakens the immune system.

Diarrhea is a chronic problem for many AIDS patients. Its cause may be related to the virus itself or to other forms of bacteria or parasites seen in the immunocompromised AIDS patient. Any prolonged episodes of diarrhea should be reported to your doctor; this may indicate more serious problems that require prompt medical attention.

Treatment usually consists of oral anti-diarrhea and parasite medications. Many of these patients already suffer from chronic hemorrhoids that are further irritated by the diarrhea. Warm sitz baths every few hours may help to soothe inflamed hemorrhoids. Discuss this with the doctor.

Diarrhea also can cause weight loss and dehydration. This is easily compounded by the fact that many of these patients already suffer from loss of appetite and taste distortion. Intravenous feedings may be prescribed to rest the intestines and hydrate the patient. Make sure the patient's diet doesn't make the stools more liquid (roughage, caffeine).

If weight loss continues to be a problem, consult with a nutritionist. Canned nutritional supplements to maintain body weight and nutritional health may be prescribed. It may be difficult to get added pounds to stay on your patient or to get him back to his pre-illness weight, but you should try to keep him from losing any more weight.

Skin problems are frequently seen in AIDS patients, especially skin rashes. Some may be caused by allergies to AIDS medications, others—such as psoriasis or viral warts—invade when the immune system is compromised. Many of these skin problems are treated with prescription creams and lotions, but some are fairly complex and may require treatment by a dermatologist. Wear gloves when you are applying creams or lotions to skin rashes.

The treatment of AIDS usually requires a number of medications, often all at the same time. Be sure you know what each one is used for and what the side effects may be. Many treatments for AIDS symptoms involve intravenous therapy. Because of this, many AIDS patients will have venous access devices implanted so that long-term intravenous therapy can take place. (See Chapters 5 and 8 for additional information on medications and intravenous therapy.)

Azidothymidine (AZT), an orally administered drug, has shown some promise in improving the depressed immune system and decreasing some AIDS symptoms and the incidence of opportunistic infections. However, this drug is not helpful for all AIDS patients and it has serious side effects. AZT is toxic to bone marrow and may cause blood counts to drop. Sometimes lowering the dose helps, or blood transfusions take care of the problem. However, AZT may cause such bone marrow toxicity that it must be discontinued. Close monitoring of the blood count is necessary and will be ordered by the doctor on a regular basis.

Opportunistic Infections

Because your loved one's natural defenses against infection are being destroyed, he will be susceptible to many opportunistic infections that take advantage of his weakened state. *Cytomegalovirus* (CMV) is in the herpes virus family and seen in many AIDS patients. The symptoms will depend on what area of the body the virus invades; the retina of the eye (CMV retinitis), the intestines (CMV colitis), or lungs (CMV pneumonitis). CMV also may spread to the adrenal glands, the brain, the urinary tract, or the blood, causing serious infection. There is an experimental intravenous drug, DHPG (Gancyclovin), used to prevent CMV retinitis and associated blindness. This usually is given at home.

The *herpes simplex* virus is found in almost all AIDS patients, usually as sores on the mouth, lips, and genitals. Herpes simplex is contagious and you should not touch an infected area. There are a number of fairly successful anti-herpes drugs available, but they are expensive. *Herpes zoster* is commonly known as shingles and the virus usually settles along the nerve pathway and often occurs along the upper back, upper arms, buttocks, and thighs. It can be extremely uncomfortable, even requiring pain medication. These herpes conditions usually are chronic and treatments, although helpful, are not curative.

Candida, known as thrush, is one of the most common ailments in AIDS patients. It usually occurs in the mouth or tongue, but can invade the throat, causing extreme discomfort and making swallowing difficult and painful. Candida appears as a thick, white coating. It is not life-threatening and usually is treated with oral lozenges and medications.

Common bacterial problems are *shigella* and *salmonella*, which infect the intestines. When these occur, the patient usually is very ill and can have severe episodes of diarrhea. Both conditions are treatable, but the treatments are fairly toxic, rendering the patient even sicker. Often the patient is so sick that hospitalization is necessary.

Pneumocystis carinii pneumonia (PCP) is commonly seen in AIDS patients, but otherwise rare. The patient has upper respiratory symptoms, difficulty breathing, coughing, fatigue, and most likely fevers. This form of pneumonia is treatable, especially if the patient seeks early treatment. Intravenous therapy may be started in the hospital, but if the patient does well, he may be allowed to come home to continue therapy there. PCP can reoccur; report any symptoms when noted.

Cryptosporidiosis is caused by a parasite that invades the intestinal tract, causing severe diarrhea. Intravenous feeding often is prescribed to combat problems with dehydration and malnutrition. There may be severe abdominal cramps associated with explosive diarrhea.

Toxoplasmosis is another parasitic infection that usually invades the nervous system (often the brain). New drugs are being worked on to treat this condition. Early symptoms include forgetfulness, mental confusion, gait disturbances, imbalance and problems with coordination, severe headaches, fevers, and possible seizures. *Cryptococcal meningitis* also invades the brain and causes inflammation. The symptoms include severe headaches, visual disturbance, and high fevers. Treatment usually involves highly toxic drugs administered intravenously. If the patient does well in the hospital, he may continue this therapy at home.

Leukoencelopathy is usually fatal and difficult to treat. Early symptoms include headaches, fevers, possible paralysis, loss of memory and coordination, hallucinations, disorientation, and child-like withdrawn behavior. It is felt this may be caused by a number of AIDS related viruses acting at once.

AIDS patients may contract *mycobacterium tuberculosis*. The symptoms include fatigue, fever, appetite loss, weight loss, and increased coughing, possibly with blood or pus in the sputum. *Mycobacterium avium intracellulare (MAI)* is a natural environmental contaminant found in household dust, soil, and water. Fever, sweats, weight loss, coughing, severe diarrhea, or abdominal pain all are common symptoms of this debilitating condition, which is seen in 20 percent of AIDS patients. Someone with a healthy immune system is not at risk of developing MAI.

AIDS and the Central Nervous System

The AIDS virus may also attack the nervous system and damage the brain. This damage may take years to develop and symptoms may show up in the form of memory loss, loss of coordination, paralysis, and other neurological symptoms. AIDS patients often suffer from short-term memory loss. Because of this, encourage your loved one to write things down and keep notes; you should also write things down that you want him to remember.

AIDS-Related Cancers

Kaposi's sarcoma is a rare form of cancer seen in conjunction with AIDS. Not all persons with AIDS will have this type of skin cancer. It first appears as a purplish, reddish discoloring on the skin, usually on the extremities but also in the mouth, anus, nose, and throat. The majority of physicians feel that chemotherapy and radiation should be used only in cases where certain vital organs have been invaded and treatment is necessary to shrink lesions. Chemotherapy is known to suppress the immune system and may render the patient even more susceptible to other AIDS-related infections. Many physicians feel the side effects are so toxic that if the growths are small, nothing should be done. These lesions can become quite large.

If your patient has Kaposi's sarcoma and you will be treating lesions, be sure to wear rubber gloves if the lesions are open and draining. Ask your physician how to treat them; a sterile, dry gauze bandage or dressing usually is recommended.

AIDS-Related Complex

AIDS-related complex (ARC) is a condition in which the patient has been exposed to the AIDS virus, but has not developed any of the diseases now associated with AIDS. The ARC patient should be closely monitored; he may later develop AIDS diseases, or he may never get AIDS. Symptoms seen in ARC patients are similar to those in early AIDS cases; fatigue, night sweats, swollen glands, recurring flus or colds, diarrhea, weight loss, or skin conditions.

Being an AIDS Care Giver

Nursing a loved one with AIDS is an awesome task; you may not be able to do this alone and still have a life of your own. Seek out help, discuss your needs with the patient's social worker, or contact community organizations for help. Subscribe to newsletters from AIDS organizations that will keep you informed about current treatments, trends, and AIDS information. (See the Appendix for support groups.)

Some agencies have volunteers that serve as care partners who help out with light housekeeping, errands, marketing, or meals. Support groups may even offer legal aid or estate planning to AIDS patients and their loved ones. See if your community has an AIDS hotline for up-to-date information on local services. Home health services specializing in AIDS care are growing. These provide everything from nurses to supplies and medications.

Care givers who have the love, courage, and conviction to take on this tremendous challenge will most likely experience great satisfaction. It won't always be easy, and if it's too much to handle, take a break and try to get away for a bit. You, too, need your rest. Try to share care-giving responsibilities. Join a care givers support group where you can share both your frustrations and what you have learned. Most of all, don't give up hope. Medical researchers are working toward the day when we no longer have people dying from AIDS.

Care Giver's Checklist

1. AIDS is virtually incurable and contagious, but caring for a loved one with AIDS does not put you at risk of contracting the disease. AIDS is spread through contaminated blood and body secretions or fluids. Always wear rubber gloves, and a protective smock or accessories, if recommended, when handling your patient's blood or body secretions.
2. If you accidentally stick yourself with a contaminated needle, clean the area and notify your physician. Periodic blood tests are recommended to determine whether the AIDS virus has invaded your body. Seek professional counseling to allay your fears.
3. Cleanliness, always important in health care, is especially critical in caring for the AIDS patient. Protect him from opportunistic infections by keeping your home clean and well-ventilated. A 1:10 bleach solution (one part chlorine bleach to ten parts water) can be used to disinfect clothing, dishes, and the shower, tub, or toilet.
4. The AIDS virus compromises or destroys your loved one's ability to fight disease. He will be vulnerable to infections and rare cancers, and his central nervous system may be affected, causing loss of memory and coordination. Treatment will vary and may consist of a wide array of medications to combat numerous complications.
5. Nursing a loved one with AIDS is a tremendous challenge. Seek out care givers' groups for emotional support; community organizations with volunteers to share your burden; and home health care agencies that specialize in AIDS cases. See if your community has an AIDS hotline to help you find local resources.

19 Nursing a Dying Loved One

The words "terminal," "incurable," "untreatable," all conjure up feelings of loss and hopelessness. When a patient and his family learn he has an incurable condition, they must cope with the inevitable. A number of important decisions must be made at this time.

Should your loved one be told he is dying? Many families want to protect the patient from the diagnosis. They feel if Grandpa knows he is dying, he won't be able to handle it and will give up. It's not easy to tell someone he is dying, but there are practical, positive reasons for sharing this sad fact. Knowing the diagnosis allows your patient to deal realistically with a limited future; get his affairs together; settle unresolved conflicts; and come to terms with dying. When a family asks the physician not to tell the patient, it puts the doctor in an awkward position and the patient-physician relationship becomes one of deception. The patient often is already aware of what is happening, but feels compelled to play his part in the charade.

One important reason for sharing the diagnosis is so the patient may make his own decisions regarding treatment: Does he want to be at home or in the hospital? Does he want life-sustaining measures used? If you keep the truth from him, you may further isolate him at the time of his greatest need. If you are unsure about how to relate to your loved one, consult with your doctor or a counselor on the health care team. There may be some cases when it is not wise to tell the patient that he has a terminal illness, but many deal amazingly well with the truth.

Should other family members know their loved one is dying? They should not be denied the chance to be with him at this time. Don't overlook the children; they may be acutely aware of what is going on around them. Children who are denied the truth often experience feelings of guilt and self-blame for a long time following the loss.

Most patients and families want to know how long the patient will live. Doctors can be only reasonably sure of the probability of death and how it may occur. To a physician, "terminal" means the patient has less than one month to live. Most physicians are reluctant to speculate; they make predictions based on prior medical data.

Many doctors are reluctant to strip a patient of all hope for a cure and will continue to treat the symptoms or even try new medical treatments that are under trial. Such treatments lack extensive human testing and usually are offered first to patients who fail to respond to traditional treatments. The patient and his family will have to decide if the risks outweigh the possibility of a response to treatment.

It is not uncommon for families to lose their entire fortunes traveling all over the world searching for cures or promises of cures. Before you go chasing after one of these promises, I recommend a full discussion with the family physician or another doctor. Some organizations, such as the American Cancer Society, offer a list of unproven medical treatments. Many so-called cancer cures that you read about are difficult to substantiate. Watch out for profit-making organizations that take considerable amounts of money from desperate families seeking a cure for their loved one at any price. This does not mean all of unproven medicine is bad, but I do recommend that emotions be put aside while you carefully investigate claims for miracle drugs or cures.

Consistency is important. If the doctor tells the family the patient is going to die, and Aunt Bessie is busy denying it and believes she has found a cure in crushed peach pits, it will only make things more difficult for everyone. Hope is important, but it's not fair to get the patient involved every time someone thinks he has found a new cure. Accept any advice relatives and friends have to offer, but check things out first with your doctor before raising your loved one's hopes.

Your doctor may be aware of treatments available in other countries and can discuss the pros and cons with you. Sometimes new treatments are available first outside the United States, but any experimental treatment with merit usually will be offered here. In considering whether to travel for medical treatment, consider the following: What is your patient's physical condition? Is he able to make the trip? What will it accomplish? Are you being realistic? Have vital organs already been irreversibly damaged? Who will benefit, you or the patient? Will this mean that your loved one will be separated from his family, and perhaps die away from home? Answer these questions carefully before making your decision.

If your loved one wants to die at home, the family, patient, and health care team must realistically discuss options. Much support is available for families that take their loved one home to die. Hospice services, visiting nurse agencies, counseling services, and home care companies help make home care of the dying possible.

Hospices now exist in most communities. What is hospice? Hospice is an organization that emphasizes care of the dying, rather than the illness itself. Most patients must be in the terminal phase of an illness to qualify for hospice care. Hospices usually have support units with or without inpatient facilities and a staff consisting of nurses, doctors, social workers, therapists, and clergy. A hospice works with the whole family to make dying as easy as possible for all concerned. For information, contact:

National Hospice Organization
1901 Fort Myer Drive, Suite 307
Arlington, VA 22209

Ask your physician or social worker for information about hospices in your community. Check your insurance policy to see if hospice care is covered.

If you decide to take your loved one home, this decision will affect the entire family. When your patient comes home, family members will need to know what is expected of them, both physically and emotionally. Establish a general plan of care, which most likely will change as the patient's condition deteriorates. You may find family members will not be able to handle the prognosis and will withdraw. You may have to put your own life on hold while you wait for death. This period is difficult for everyone. The family should try to carry on with daily activities, taking it one step at a time.

Accepting the Prognosis

Much research and study has gone into the subject of death in recent years and today the emphasis is on what can be done to make this a time of peace and spiritual fulfillment. Elisabeth Kubler-Ross, in her noted book *On Death and Dying*, discusses how patients may respond to dying by passing through predictable emotional stages. It's important to be aware of some of these coping mechanisms, but also to realize that not all patients will experience them. She defines them as denial, withdrawal, anger, bargaining, depression, and acceptance.

To some degree, *denial* is a healthy coping mechanism that allows a patient to carry on without the constant reminder of the grim reality of his illness. It is seen as unrealistic only when the denial is so great that the patient refuses to deal with his limited future. *Withdrawal* is an unhealthy form of coping; the patient closes himself off from his family and loved ones and loses interest in things that ordinarily would bring joy. *Anger* is perhaps the most difficult emotion for the patient and those around him. Anger is a response to a situation that makes the patient feel threatened, helpless, and outraged. The patient is really saying "Why me?" Expression of this anger is healthy and should be acknowledged.

Bargaining is a form of "striking a deal" with the patient's God, doctor, or a significant other. In this phase, the patient appears to accept his destiny, but only if he perceives a benefit in return—living long enough to attend his son's wedding, or being assured of a pain-free death. If possible, it's important to fulfill these wishes. *Depression* is nearly a universal response to major illness. Your patient may be unable to sleep, eat, or socialize. Severe cases can be treated by anti-depressants; professional psychiatric counseling may help. In many patients, depression precedes *acceptance.* In this final phase, the patient quietly reviews his life, his accomplishments and failures, and is ready to die. He has come to terms with his life and is at peace with himself and the world.

Your patient also may experience regression, displacement, anxiety, or guilt. Anyone facing death must adapt to a painful reality, but much can be done to make it more than just a time to grieve. There can be dignity and peace in dying. What can the family do? Provide time and space for your loved one to go through his own grief process. Be there for him, offer your support, and let him know he is not alone. Give your patient a chance to talk about his illness; he may fear alienating others by discussing his feelings and needs. The hardest part of all may be just to sit with the patient and do nothing but listen. Be honest and open with your patient. Tell him how you feel, that you are sad he is dying and angry, too.

Don't isolate your patient from family activities. Many patients remain vital until the end; they want to know what's going on, hear a good story or joke, or even join a noisy row now and then. Encourage visitors and activities that keep him from becoming totally occupied with his illness. Let him maintain as much of his prior role in the household as possible.

Preparing for Death

If your patient needs to dwell on the past, let him; it is part of his need to get things in order. If he has personal matters to settle, or funeral arrangements to discuss, do not prevent him from doing so. If your patient does not want to talk about his death, what should you do? Perhaps ask a leading question and slowly introduce the subject. Choose a time when the patient is not medicated and can give you his attention. For example, ask whether he wants to stay at home, or go to the hospital in his final days. Does he want life-sustaining support measures? Does he want to donate any of his organs? Use his answers to initiate a full discussion of what lies ahead.

Discuss plans for any memorial service or funeral with your loved one. Does he want burial or cremation? He may want to help prepare an obituary or eulogy.

Consult a laywer if your loved one has no will or wants to change an existing will to ensure the legal validity of the document. Drawing up a will is the only way the patient can be assured that last wishes will be carried out as he plans and that property will be distributed according to his desires. This is especially important if the patient wants to provide for a loved one who is not legally related.

The patient should authorize another person to act in his behalf if he becomes incapacitated.

This power of attorney can include routine authorization to write checks, pay bills, and make investments, but it also can include making medical decisions when the patient is unable. The person with power of attorney should be told the location of banking and checking accounts, safe deposit boxes, deeds, life insurance policies, and other important documents.

Check with your lawyer about the legality of a "living will" in your state. This document is used to stipulate that the patient does not want life-sustaining measures if he becomes so ill that he cannot survive without them. If your patient has some say in exercising his right to die, it may save the family from making painful decisions about disconnecting life-support equipment.

Death at Home

Talk with your doctor and the health care team about what the final days or hours may be like, so that you and your family are prepared. Your social worker or another member of the health care team may be able to help you anticipate problems and provide support. Families often do well right until the end and then panic because of fear they will do the wrong thing when their loved one dies. If you are concerned, call your doctor or nurse for reassurance before calling the paramedics or an ambulance. If your patient is taken to the hospital, it will be more difficult for you to control the patient's natural course of death.

Even in the home, health care professionals must carry out their duty to sustain life unless the family has made its wishes clear. If life-saving measures are not desired, get a written order from the doctor stating "Do Not Resuscitate" and include it with the patient's chart. If there is no specific order, the nurse will be legally obligated to begin life-saving measures when the patient is near death. If possible, have the patient and a witness sign the document, as well.

When the patient dies, call the following in this order: the physician, funeral home director, and relatives. The physician will notify the coroner or medical examiner if an autopsy is planned. If notifying officials will be too difficult, make sure someone is designated to make these calls.

If a nurse is present, have her do post-mortem care before she is dismissed. Remove the patient's valuables; take them to the funeral home later. If he wears dentures, put them in. Send clothes for the burial to the funeral home along with the body. The funeral home director usually will have the doctor sign the death certificate. Get a copy of this document; it will be useful for closing bank accounts, settling insurance claims, and other details.

The Death Process

Many people want to know what dying will be like, but they are afraid to ask. Your doctor may even find this type of discussion difficult; he or she may appear cold and distant, but actually the physician is experiencing feelings of defeat and loss.

As the end draws near, your patient is likely to spend much of his time sleeping. If he is taking pain medication, he may be unaware of his surroundings. One of the last senses to leave the patient is hearing; do not say anything in front of the patient that you do not want him to hear. Even if your loved one is unconscious, talk to him, hold his hand, and let him know that someone is there. As death becomes imminent, you may want others to share in your vigil. Most families fear leaving the dying patient alone during the final days. Accept offers from others to take turns sitting with the patient. Give yourself some time away from the patient, hard as it may be. Some patients will be alert right up to the end; others fall into a restful sleep; and some become agitated as breathing becomes more difficult.

Most patients ultimately die not from the disease, but from the complications of the disease as vital organs are affected. Pneumonia is a common cause of death. As these complications develop, the family, perhaps the patient, and the physician will have to determine if and how they will be treated.

The dying person may lose his desire to eat, maybe taking only sips of liquid. He may wish to be alone, or he may ask to see friends. The patient is sometimes alert, other times disoriented. Make your patient as comfortable as possible. Some dying patients will not want heavy covers; provide only a light sheet. Keep the environment restful and try to meet your loved one's requests; he may want light and fresh air, or perhaps quiet and dark.

What physical changes will take place as death approaches? The patient's breathing may become more rapid and increased initially, then slow down and become more shallow and labored. There may be irregular breathing that starts and stops. The patient's skin color may change and the pulse can be quite weakened and slow. His skin may feel cool and damp; cover him with a light blanket. Your patient is apt to be breathing through his mouth and you may offer ice chips or a lemon glycerine swab for moisture; don't give a drink to an unconscious patient.

His eyes may be open and in a fixed stare. Wipe away secretions with a damp, warm cloth. You can close his eyelids and tape two gauze pads over them to decrease eye irritation. The patient may be incontinent as he loses consciousness.

If your patient has trouble breathing, raise the head of the bed. Administer a low level of oxygen if he is on oxygen therapy. Sometimes the patient becomes restless and has trouble breathing because he is frightened or anxious. Stay with him; speak with a gentle, calm voice. Let your loved one hold your hand and reassure him that someone will stay with him at this time. If breathing problems continue, report them to your doctor; he or she may order something to make breathing less difficult.

In most cases, your patient will appear rested and peaceful as he slowly lapses into a deeper and deeper sleep. Most patients are not in pain at the end. The actual transition from life to death usually is subtle. How do you determine that the patient has died? The patient's eyes will most likely be open and in a fixed stare; the chest shows no signs of movement; there is no pulse; and if you place your face or hand over the patient's mouth, you will feel no breath.

When death comes, your family may want some time alone with the patient to say their final goodbyes. This time alone, while the patient is still at home, may be important in the final separation from a loved one.

After the Death

When your loved one is taken from the home, you will feel a tremendous loss. Make arrangements to dispose of or return all medical equipment as soon as possible; it serves only as a reminder of what the family has been through. The removal of the patient's personal belongings can wait until the family is able to deal with this.

You may find consolation in the fact that the family was able to offer the patient a dignified and loving death. If this was impossible, and in the end the patient had to die in the hospital, family members may be disappointed because they could not provide the kind of death the patient wanted. You can do only your best; don't blame yourself or perceive this as a failure.

Accept help and love from those around you. Do not shut them out; they can be your life preservers. Get out and enjoy life again. If you feel you cannot do it alone, seek help. Some counselors specialize in grief and bereavement; there are support groups of widows and widowers; and other networks to support someone who has experienced a loss.

Life goes on, and you must return to the business of living. Grief knows no boundaries. Only time will heal these wounds. Just as your patient had rights, so do his loved ones. They have a right to mourn. Know that each passing day will be a little easier. Slowly, your memories of the final days will fade and you will cherish thoughts of the vital, healthy person you loved.

Care Giver's Checklist

1. Many families want to protect their loved one from the knowledge that his condition is incurable. However, your patient may need this information to put his affairs in order and make his final days more comfortable.
2. If you want your loved one to die at home, talk with the health care team. Many communities have hospice organizations that will help you deal with this burden.
3. Psychologists have identified emotional stages that most patients go through when they learn they are terminally ill. Help your patient through these hard times by understanding his emotional state and allowing him to discuss his thoughts and fears.
4. You must plan for the inevitable. See that your patient's legal affairs are in order; discuss plans for a funeral or burial; discuss your loved one's last wishes so they may be carried out.
5. Give youself time to grieve when the end has come. But just as you dedicated your time to a dying loved one, you must now dedicate yourself to living. Seek support groups or professional help as you struggle with this deep loss.

Appendix

Table of Weights and Measures
Liquid Measurement and Approximate Metric Equivalents

1000 milliliters/l liter = 1 quart
500 milliliters/0.5 liters = 1 pint
250 milliliters/0.25 liters = ½ pint or 8 fluid ounces
30 milliliters = 1 fluid ounce
15 milliliters = 4 fluid drams or ½ fluid ounce

Common Household Equivalents:

60 drops = l teaspoon = 1 fluid dram = 4 milliliters
2 tablespoons = 1 fluid ounce = 30 milliliters
1 cup = 8 fluid ounces = 250 milliliters or 0.25 liter
1 pint = 500 milliliters or 0.5 liter
1 quart = 1,000 milliliters or 1 liter
1 gallon = 4,000 milliliters or 4 liters

Weights:

1 kilogram = 2.2 pounds
30 grams = 1 ounce
4 grams = 1 dram
1 gram = 15-16 grains
0.75 gram = 12 grains
1 grain = 60 milligrams
1/60 grain = 1.0 milligram
1000 grams = 1 kilogram
1000 micrograms = 1 milligram
1000 milligrams = 1 gram
500 milligrams = 0.5 grams

To change from Grains to Grams: Divide by 60.
To change from Grams to Grains: Multiply by 15.
To change from Grams to Ounces: Divide by 30.
To change from Ounces to Grams: Multiply by 30.
To change from Milligrams to Grains: Divide by 60.
To change from Grains to Milligrams: Multiply by 60.

Converting From Celsius to Fahrenheit

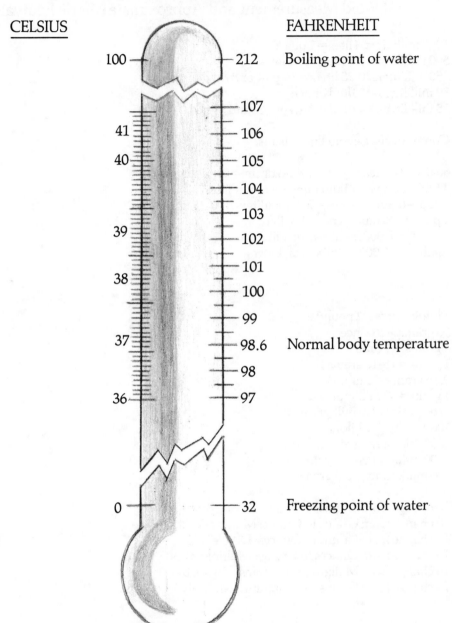

CELSIUS   FAHRENHEIT

100 — 212   Boiling point of water

— 107

41 — 106

40 — 105

— 104

— 103

39 — 102

— 101

38 — 100

— 99

37 — 98.6   Normal body temperature

— 98

36 — 97

0 — 32   Freezing point of water

Note: To convert Fahrenheit to Celsius, subtract 32 degrees and multiply by 5, then divide by 9; to convert Celsius to Fahrenheit, multiply by 9, divide by 5, then add 32 degrees.

Social service organizations and community groups can be valuable resources when caring for a loved one at home. Members of the health care team may be able to provide additional resources. Don't forget about support groups at your local hospital; fellow home care givers will have useful tips about services in your community.

Home Care and General Health

American Red Cross
17th and D Streets NW
Washington, DC 20006
202-734-8300

Medic Alert Foundation International
(bracelets & medallions)
P.O. Box 1009
Turlock, CA 95381
1-800-344-3226
209-668-3333

Sears Home Health Care Catalog
(for mail order supplies)
4640 Roosevelt Boulevard
Philadelphia, PA 19132

Aging

American Geriatric Society
10 Columbus Circle
New York, NY 10019

National Institute on Aging
National Institutes of Health
Building 31, Room 5C35
Bethesda, MD 20205
301-496-1752

Insurance

Group Health Association of America
(HMO information)
624 Ninth Street NW
Washington, DC

Healthcare Financing Administration
Bureau of Eligibility, Reimbursement, and Coverage
High Rise East, Room 100
6325 Security Boulevard
Baltimore, MD 21207

Health Insurance Association of America
1850 K Street NW
Washington, DC 20006

Hospice

National Hospice Organization
1901 North Fort Myer Drive, Suite 307
Arlington, VA 22209
703-243-5900

Cancer

National Cancer Information Service Hotline
1-800-638-6694

American Cancer Society
777 Third Avenue
New York, NY 10017

Cancer Counseling and Research Center
6060 North Central Expressway, Suite 140
Dallas, TX 75206

Leukemia Society of America
Public Education and Information
800 Second Avenue
New York, NY 10017

Ostomy

International Association for Enterostomal
Therapy
5000 Birch Street
Newport Beach, CA 92660

National Foundation for Ileitis and Colitis
444 Park Avenue South
New York, NY 10016
212-685-3440

United Ostomy Association
2001 West Beverly Boulevard
Los Angeles, CA 90057
213-413-5510

Heart Disease and Stroke

American Heart Association
7320 Greenville Avenue
Dallas, TX 75231
214-750-7300

Stroke Club of America
805 12th Street
Galveston, TX 77550

Respiratory Disease

American Lung Association
1740 Broadway
New York, NY 10019

Emphysema Association
P.O. Box 66
Fort Myers, FL 33902

Kidney Disease

American Kidney Fund
P.O. Box 975
Washington, DC 20044

National Association of Patients on
Hemodialysis and
Transplantation
505 Northern Boulevard
Great Neck, NY 11021

National Kidney Foundation
Two Park Avenue
New York, NY 10016

Office of End Stage Renal Disease
6401 Security Boulevard
1-C-C Dogwood West
Baltimore, MD 21235
301-934-6533

Diabetes

American Diabetes Association
505 Eighth Avenue
New York, NY 10018

Joslin Clinic Diabetic Foundation
1 Joslin Place
Boston, MA 02215

Miscellaneous Associations

American Parkinson's Disease Foundation
116 John Street
New York, NY 10038
212-732-9550

Arthritis Foundation
3400 Peachtree Road NE
Atlanta, GA 30326

Committee on Pain Therapy and
Acupuncture
American Society of Anesthesiologists
1515 Busse Highway
Park Ridge, IL 60068

Multiple Sclerosis Society National
Headquarters
205 East 42nd Street
New York, NY 10017
212-986-3240

National Committee on the Treatment of
Intractable Pain
P.O. Box 9553
Friendship Station
Washington, DC 20016-1353

Parkinson's Disease Foundation
William Black Medical Research Building
Columbia Presbyterian Medical Center
640 West 168th Street
New York, NY 10032
212-673-3850

Rehabilitation

American Association for Rehabilitation
Therapy
P.O. Box 83
North Little Rock, AR 72116

American Occupational Therapy
Association
1383 Piccard Drive
Rockville, MD 20850

American Physical Therapy Association
1156 15th Street NW
Washington, DC 20005

Barrier-Free Environments
(home design for handicapped)
P.O. Box 30334
Raleigh, N.C. 27622
919-782-7823

Eastern Paralyzed Veterans Association c/o
Barrier-Free Design Department (home
design for disabled)
432 Park Avenue South
New York, NY 10016
212-686-6770

Information Center for Individuals with
Disabilities
20 Park Plaza, Room 330
Boston, MA 02116
617-727-5540

National Foundation of Dentistry for the
Handicapped
Suite 422
1726 Champa
Denver, CO 80202
303-573-0264

National Paraplegia Foundation
333 North Michigan Avenue
Chicago, IL 60601

National Spinal Cord Injury Association
149 California Street
Newton, MA 02158

Sex Information and Education Council for
the United States
715 Broadway, Suite 213
New York, NY 10003

Society for the Advancement of Travel for
the Handicapped
International Head Office, Suite 1110
26 Court Street
Brooklyn, NY 11242

Veterans Association
810 Vermont Avenue NW
Washington, DC 20420

Whirlpool Appliance Information Service
Administration Center (appliances for the
disabled)
Benton Harbor, MI 49022

Organ Donor Programs

American Society for Artificial Internal
Organs
P.O. Box 777
Boca Raton, FL 33432

Committee on Donor Enlistment
2022 Lee Road
Cleveland Heights, OH 44118

The Living Bank (donor bank for organs)
P.O. Box 6725
Houston, TX 77265

AIDS

AIDS Medical Foundation
230 Park Avenue, Room 1266
New York, NY 10169
212-949-9411

AIDS Action Council
729 Eighth Street SE Suite 200
Washington, DC 20003
202-574-3101

Red Cross AIDS Education Office
1730 D Street NW
Washington, DC 20006
202-737-8300

Centers for Disease Control
AIDS Activity Bldg. 3, Room 5B-1
1600 Clifton Road
Atlanta, GA 30333
Hotline 1-800-342-AIDS in Atlanta:
404-329-3534

Gay Men's Health Crisis Center
P.O. Box 274
132 West 24th Street
New York, NY 10011
212-807-6655

Mothers of AIDS Patients
c/o Barbara Peabody
3403 East Street
San Diego, CA 92102
619-234-3432

U.S. Public Health Service
Public Affairs Office
Hubert H. Humphrey Building
Room 724-H
200 Independence Ave. SW
Washington, DC 20201
202-245-6867

National Association of People with AIDS
P.O. Box 65472
Washington, DC 20035

National AIDS Network
729 Eighth Street SE
Suite 300
Washington, DC 20003
202-546-2424

If you want to know more about home health care, consult some of these books and pamphlets. Ask someone on your home health care team for additional suggested reading materials.

Home Health Care

National Home Caring Council. *All About Home Care: A Consumers Guide.* New York, 1982.
American Red Cross. *Family Health and Home Nursing.* New York: Doubleday & Co., 1977.
Baulch, E. *Home Care: A Practical Alternative to Extended Hospitalization.* Millbrae, CA: Celestial Arts, 1980.
Beer, M., and Covell, H.E. *The Home Alternative to Hospitals and Nursing Homes.* New York: Holt, Rinehart & Winston, 1982.
MacLean, H. *Caring for Your Parents.* New York: Doubleday & Co., 1987.
Murphy, P. *The Home Hospital.* New York: Basic Books, 1982.

Caring for the Elderly

Citizens for Better Care. *How to Choose a Nursing Home: A Shopping and Rating Guide.* Detroit: The Institute of Gerontology, University of Michigan, Ann Arbor, and Wayne State University, Detroit, 1974.
Office of Consumer Services. *Nursing Home Care.* Washington, DC: Medical Services Administration, 1977. Stock No. 017061- 00040-2.
Willington, F.L. *Incontinence in the Elderly.* New York: Academic Press, 1976.

Insurance

Bloom, J. *Health Maintenance Organizations.* Tucson, AZ: The Body Press, 1987.
Fein, R. *Medical Care, Medical Costs: The Search for a Health Insurance Policy.* Cambridge: Harvard University Press, 1986.

Emergencies

Advanced First Aid and Emergency Care. American Red Cross. New York: Doubleday & Co., 1986.
Standard First Aid and Personal Safety. American Red Cross. New York, Doubleday & Co., 1986.

Nutrition

American Diabetes Association. *The American Diabetes Association Family Cookbook, Vol. III.* New York: Prentice Hall Press, 1987.
American Heart Association. *The American Heart Association Cookbook.* New York: David McKay Co., Inc., 1984.
Coleman Family, and Davidson, B. *The Gourmet Renal Nutrition Book.* New York: Coward, McCann & Geoghegan, 1983.
DeBakey, M., Gotton, A., Scott, L., and Foreyt, J. *The Living Heart Diet.* New York: Raven Press, 1984.
Hunt, J., and Margie, J. *Living with High Blood Pressure: The Hyptertension Diet Cookbook.* Bloomfield, N.J.: HLS Press, Inc., 1978.
Calories and Carbohydrates. Krause, B. New York: New American Library, 1987.
Complete Guide to Sodium. Krause, B. New York: New American Library, 1987.
Winick, M., ed. *Nutrition and Cancer.* New York: J. Wiley and Sons, 1977.

Medical References

Carper, J. *Health Care U.S.A.: Where to Find the Best Answers to Your Family Medical and Health Problems.* New York: Prentice Hall Press, 1987.

The Columbia University College of Physicians and Surgeons Complete Home Medical Guide. New York: Crown Publishing, 1985.

Eron, C., and Horn, C. *The Family Handbook of Medical Tests.* New York: Perigee Books, 1985.

Nilsson, L. *The Body Victorious.* New York: Delacorte Press, 1985.

Stedman's Medical Dictionary. New York: Prentice Hall Press, 1987.

Medications

Consumers Union. *Drug Information for the Consumer.* New York: Consumer Reports Books, 1987.

Graedon, J. *The Peoples Pharmacy.* New York: St. Martin's Press, 1985.

Long, J. *The Essential Guide to Prescription Drugs.* New York: Harper & Row, 1987.

Morgan, B. *The Food and Drug Interaction Book.* New York: Simon & Schuster, 1986.

Physicians Desk Reference. Oradell, N.J.: Medical Economics Books, 1987.

Pain Management

Caprino, F. *Better Health with Self-Hypnosis.* New York: Parker Publishing Co., 1985.

Manaka, Y., and Urguahart, I. *The Layman's Guide to Acupuncture.* New York: Weatherhill, 1986.

Melzack, R. *The Puzzle of Pain.* New York: Basic Books, 1973.

Sternbach, R. *Mastering Pain.* New York: G.P. Putnam's Sons, 1987.

Zborowski, R. *People in Pain.* San Francisco: Jossey-Bass, 1969.

Cancer

Cancer Facts and Figures. American Cancer Society. New York, 1985.

Brody, J.E., and Holleb, A.I. *You Can Fight Cancer and Win.* New York: McGraw-Hill, 1977.

Cancer Book. The American Cancer Society. New York: Doubleday & Co., 1986.

National Institutes of Health. *Coping with Cancer: An Annotated Bibliography.* Bethesda, MD: Cancer Information Clearing House, 1980. Number 80-2129.

National Cancer Institute. *Chemotherapy and You.* Bethesda, MD: U.S. Department of Health and Human Services, 1987.

The Breast Cancer Digest: A Guide to Medical Care, Emotional Support, Education Programs, and Resources. Bethesda, MD: U.S. Department of Health and Human Services, 1980.

Ostomy

Mahoney, J.M. *Guide to Ostomy Care.* Boston: Little, Brown & Co., 1976.

Heart Disease

Cohn, K., and Duke, D. *Coming Back: A Guide to Recovering from Heart Attack.* Reading, MA: Addison-Wesley Publishing Co., 1987.

Khan, G. *Heart Attacks, Hypertension, and Heart Drugs.* Emmaus, PA: Rodale Press, 1986.

Diabetes

Dolger, H., and Seeman, B. *How to Live with Diabetes.* New York: W.W. Norton & Co., 1985.

American Diabetes Association. *Exchange Lists for Meal Planning.* rev. ed. New York, 1976.

Foot Care for the Diabetic Patient. Washington, DC: U.S. Department of Health and Human Services, 1977 (Number 017- 001-000264).

Krall, L., ed. *Joslin Diabetic Manual.* Philadelphia: Lea & Febiger, 1978.

Rehabilitation

Basmajian, J.V., ed. *Therapeutic Exercise.* 3d ed. Baltimore: Williams & Wilkins, 1978.

Crickmay, M.C. *Helping the Stroke Patient to Talk.* Springfield, IL: Charles C. Thomas, 1977.

Gilbert, A. *You Can Do It From a Wheelchair.* New Rochelle, NY: Arlington House Publications, 1973.

Chartered Society of Physiotherapy. *Handling the Handicapped: A* Eckhart, E., Waggoner, N., and Hotte, E. *Independent Living for the Handicapped and the Elderly.* Boston: Houghton Mifflin Co., 1974.

O'Brien, M.T., and Pallet, P.J. *Total Care of the Stroke Patient.* Boston: Little, Brown & Co., 1978.

Perske, R., et. al. *Mealtimes for Severely and Profoundly Handicapped Persons.* Baltimore: University Park Press, 1977.

Pierce, D.S., and Nickel, V.H. *Total Care of Spinal Cord Injuries.* Boston: Little, Brown & Co., 1977.

Rosner, L., and Ross, S. *Multiple Sclerosis: New Hope and Practical Advice for People with Multiple Sclerosis and their Families.* New York: Prentice Hall, 1987.

Sargent, J.V. *An Easier Way: Handbook for the Elderly and Handicapped.* Ames, IA: Iowa State University Press, 1981.

Sexuality

Greengross, W. *Entitled to Love: The Sexual and Emotional Needs of the Handicapped.* London: Malaby Press, 1976.

Heslinga, K., Schellen, A., and Verkuyla, A. *Not Made of Stone: The Sexual Problems of Handicapped People.* Springfield, IL: Charles C. Thomas, 1974.

Psychology

Benjamin, H. *From Victim to Victor.* Los Angeles: Jeremy Tarcher, 1987.

Register, C. *Living with Chronic Illness.* New York: Free Press, 1987.

Papolus, D., and Papolus, J. *Overcoming Depression.* New York: Harper & Row, 1987.

AIDS

Black, D. *The Plague Years: A Chronicle of AIDS, the Epidemic of Our Times.* New York: Simon & Schuster, 1985.

Gong, V., and Rudnick, N. *AIDS: Facts and Issues.* New Brunswick, NJ: Rutgers University Press, 1986.

Gong, V. *Understanding AIDS: A Comprehensive Guide.* New Brunswick, NJ: Rutgers University Press, 1985.

Leonard, B., and Gregory, S. *Conquering AIDS Now with Natural Treatment: A Non-Drug Approach.* New York: Warner Books, 1986.

Martelli, L., Peltz, F. *When Someone You Know Has AIDS, A Practical Guide.* New York: Crown Publishers, 1987.

Hospice

Hamilton, M., and Reid, H. *A Hospice Handbook: A New Way to Care for the Dying.* Grand Rapids, MI: William B. Eerdmans Publishing Co., 1980.

Rossman, P. *Hospice.* New York: Fawcett Book Group, 1979.

Death and Dying

Downing, A.B., *Euthanasia and the Right to Die.* New York: Humanities Press, 1970.

Jackson, E. *Telling a Child About Death.* New York: Channel Press, 1965.

On Death and Dying. Kubler-Ross, E. New York: Macmillan Publishing Co., 1969.

Questions and Answers on Death and Dying. Kubler-Ross, E. New York: Macmillan Publishing Co., 1974.

Lamerton, R. *Care for the Dying.* New York: Penquin Books, 1981.

Little, M. *Home Care of the Dying.* New York: Dial Press, 1985.

Grief and Bereavement

Grollman, E. *Living When a Loved One Has Died.* Boston: Beacon Press, 1977.

Morris, S. *Grief and How to Live With It.* New York: Grossett & Dunlap, 1972.

Raphael, B. *The Anatomy of Bereavement.* New York: Basic Books, 1983.

Westbert, G. *Good Grief.* Philadelphia: Fortress Press, 1977.

Glossary

Nursing a Loved One at Home was written in clear, common language for the home care giver with no medical training. Health care professionals sometimes use confusing technical terms, so this glossary was prepared to help you understand discussions of your loved one's medical condition.

Abdominal Thrust. Upward thrust to the abdomen given in an emergency to clear an obstructed airway. Also called the Heimlich Maneuver.

Abscess. A localized collection of pus.

Acetaminophen. A non-aspirin pain reliever.

Acupuncture. Puncture with needles for diagnostic and therapeutic purposes.

Acquired Immune Deficiency Syndrome (AIDS). A deadly virus that attacks the body's ability to fight infection or disease.

Acute. Sharp, severe. Acute conditions usually have rapid onset and last a short time.

Addiction. Physical or psychological dependence on a substance.

AIDS-Related Complex (ARC). A condition in which the patient has been exposed to the AIDS virus and suffers some of the same symptoms, but has not developed any of the diseases associated with AIDS.

Airway. The passageway through which air enters the body to the lungs. Also an artificial device passed through the mouth and into the trachea to maintain a clear passageway.

Airway Obstruction. Blockage of the airway. When obstruction is complete, the choking victim is unable to breathe, cough, or speak due to blockage of the windpipe.

Ambulate. To walk.

Ampule. A sealed glass container that holds medicine.

Analgesia. Absence of the sense of pain.

Analgesic. A medicine that relieves pain.

Anemia. An insufficiency of red blood cells, hemoglobin, or both. It exists when hemoglobin content is less than 13-14 gm per 100 ml for men; 11-12 gm per 100 ml for women.

Angina. A disease marked by brief attacks of chest pain caused by deficient oxygenation of the heart muscle.

Ankylosis. Abnormal immobility of a joint.

Anorexia. Loss of appetite.

Anoxia. Oxygen deficiency.

Antacid. An agent that neutralizes acidity.

Antibody. A protein substance developed by the body, usually in response to foreign matter and working to resist disease.

Anticoagulant. An agent that hinders blood clotting.

Antidote. A substance that neutralizes or counteracts poisons or adverse effects of medications.

Antigen. A foreign substance that induces the formation of antibodies.

Anuria. Complete urinary suppression.

Aphasia. Loss of verbal expression or comprehension.

Apical Pulse. The pulse felt at the apex of the heart.

Arrythmia. Irregular heart rhythm.

Artificial Respiration. Emergency first aid breathing into the lungs of a person who has stopped breathing. Also called rescue breathing.

Ascites. Abnormal accumulation of fluid in the abdominal cavity.

Aseptic. Free of germs or bacteria.

Aspirate. To remove by suction.

Ataxia. An inability to coordinate muscle movement.

Atelectasis. A collapsed or airless lung.

Atrophy. Shrinking or wasting away of a body part.

Axillary. Pertaining to the armpit.

Barbiturate. Any of a group of chemical compounds used primarily as sedatives or to produce sleep.

Bedsore. An ulcer of the skin and underlying tissues produced by prolonged pressure. Also called pressure sore or decubitus ulcer.

Binder. An encircling support of the abdomen or chest.

Biofeedback. Technique of making unconscious or involuntary body processes perceptible to the senses in an effort to mentally manipulate them.

Biopsy. Removal of tissue, cells, or fluids for microscopic examination.

Blood Clot. A thickened lump of blood.

Blood Count. A laboratory test to count and classify the number of red and white blood cells in a measured sample in order to gain information about a patient's health.

Blood Pressure. The force of the circulating blood pulsing against the walls of the blood vessels.

Body Mechanics. The coordinated use of muscles, joints, and ligaments to produce motion and maintain balance.

Bradycardia. Slow heart rate.

Cannula. A tube inserted into the body for infusion or drainage of fluids, or to keep the opening accessible.

Cardiac Arrest. Cessation of heartbeat.

Cardiopulmonary Resuscitation (CPR). A lifesaving rescue technique using artificial stimulation of the heart and lungs.

Carotid Pulse. The beat felt at the side of the neck when the carotid artery is pressed.

Cathartic. An active agent that initiates bowel evacuation.

Catheter. A tube inserted into the body for evacuating or injecting fluids.

Cerebral Hemorrhage. See Stroke.

Chest Compression. Pressing the breastbone to manually circulate blood in a person whose heart has stopped beating.

Chest Thrust. A thrust to the middle of the breastbone used to clear airway obstruction in a person who is obese or in the late stages of pregnancy.

Chronic. Long and drawn out or frequently occurring. Chronic conditions often have a slow, progressive course.

Clysis. A slow injection of fluid into the superficial tissues of the body for purposes of hydration.

Colostomy. Surgical formation of an artificial anus by making an opening from the colon through the abdomen.

Comatose. A state of unconsciousness caused by illness or injury. A comatose person cannot be aroused by external stimuli.

Congestive Heart Failure. A condition in which the heart is unable to pump effectively, resulting in inefficient circulation.

Constipation. Delayed or infrequent passage of dry, hard stools for an abnormal period of time.

Continuous Ambulatory Peritoneal Dialysis. A form of kidney dialysis in which impurities are removed from the blood by instilling a solution into the peritoneal cavity through a catheter.

Contracture. Permanent shortening or tightening of a muscle.

Convulsion. An involuntary, usually violent, contraction or spasm of the muscles.

CPR. See Cardiopulmonary Resuscitation.

Crutch Palsy. Weakness of the hand, wrist, and forearm induced by prolonged pressure of a crutch on the nerves in the armpit.

Decubitus Ulcer. An ulcer of the skin and underlying tissues produced by prolonged pressure. Also called pressure sore or bedsore.

Deep Breathing Exercises. Inhaling and exhaling maximum amounts of air to expand the lungs and prevent accumulation of secretions. This is prescribed when a patient is confined to bed or has limited movement.

Dehiscence. A splitting open or rupture, usually along sutures.

Dehydrated. Insufficient fluid in the body.

Depressant. A drug that acts on the central nervous system to lower the level of body activity and produce relaxation.

Diagnosis. The process of identifying a disease.

Diagnostic Related Groups. A Medicare cost-cutting measure classifying hundreds of diagnoses and setting a fee to be paid to the hospital for each. This acts as an incentive for hospitals to discharge Medicare patients more quickly.

Dialysate. A solution used in dialysis that contains electrolytes and salts.

Dialysis. The separation of subtances in solution by passing them through a porous membrane. This process functions as an artificial kidney.

Diarrhea. Frequent evacuation of liquid feces.

Diastolic Pressure. The pressure of the blood against the arterial walls when the ventricles of the heart are at rest.

Distension. Swelling of the abdomen.

Diuretic. An agent that increases the production of urine.

Drawsheet. A sheet folded in half that is placed under the body's trunk. It provides extra protection for other bed linens and can be used to move the patient.

Edema. Excessive accumulation of fluid in the tissues.

Electrolyte. A chemical substance that plays a critical role in the body's fluid balance. Common electrolytes are sodium, potassium, calcium, and chloride.

Embolus. A clot, air bubble, or other foreign substance obstructing blood circulation.

Enterostomy. An opening through the abdominal wall into the intestines.

Evisceration. Protrusion from a surgical incision.

Exudate. Fluid and cells that have escaped from blood vessels into the tissues.

Febrile. Pertaining to fever.

Fecal Impaction. A mass of hardened feces in the folds of the rectum.

Finger Sweep. A technique used to remove a piece of food or an object from the airway of a choking victim.

Flatus. Gas in the stomach or intestines.

Foley Catheter. A urinary catheter inserted through the urethra and into the bladder. Also called an indwelling or retention catheter.

Foot Drop. Extension of the foot with permanent contracture of the muscle and tendon. This is a hazard of bed rest.

Foreskin. A skin fold that covers the glans of the penis.

Fracture. A break in the bone.

Fracture Reduction. Setting broken bones back into proper alignment.

Gastrostomy. A surgical opening through the abdominal wall into the stomach for the introduction of food.

Generic. In drugs, pertaining to the chemical identity of the substance and not protected by trademark. For example, acetaminophen is the generic; Tylenol is the brand name.

Genitalia. The external reproductive organs.

Glycosuria. Abnormal amount of sugar in the urine.

Guided Imagery. The use of a mental image to create a form of distraction to relieve pain or produce relaxation.

Health Care Team. Physicians, therapists, nurses, social workers, technicians, and others who will be advising you while you care for your loved one at home.

Heimlich Maneuver. Upward thrust to the abdomen given in an emergency to clear an obstructed airway. Also called abdominal thrust.

Hematoma. A collection of blood in a tissue or organ due to a broken blood vessel.

Hemiplegia. Paralysis on one side of the body.

Hemodialysis. An artificial means of cleansing the blood of waste products and excess fluids.

Hemoglobin. The red pigment in red blood cells that carries oxygen.

Hemorrhage. Copious bleeding, either internally or externally.

Hemorrhoids. Varicose veins in the rectum or anus.

Heparin. An anticoagulant. Heparin is injected after any intravenous infusion to prevent blood clots in the IV line or catheter. This procedure is known as a heparin lock.

Home Health Agency. An agency or service that provides health care in the home.

Hydration. The act of providing the body with adequate fluids.

Hyperalimentation. A method of supplying the body with nourishing solutions through a catheter inserted into the superior vena cava. Also called total parenteral nutrition

Hyper-extension. Extreme or abnormal extension.

Hyperglycemia. Increased blood sugar.

Hypertension. High blood pressure.

Hypoglycemia. Decreased blood sugar.

Hypotension. Abnormally low blood pressure.

Hypoxia. Lack of oxygen.

Ileostomy. An artificial opening of the small intestine through the abdomen.

IM. Intramuscular; often used as a designation for intramuscular injection.

Incontinence. Inability to control the passage of urine or feces.

Indwelling Catheter. A urinary catheter inserted through the urethra and into the bladder. Also called a Foley catheter or retention catheter.

Infusion. Administration of a solution into a vein.

Inhalant. A medication administered by inhalation.

Ingestion. Taking a substance by mouth.

Insulin. An essential hormone secreted in the pancreas. Commercially produced insulin is administered in the treatment of diabetes.

Inspiration. Inhaling.

Internal Fixation. Surgical immobilization of a fracture.

Intramuscular Injection. Injecting into muscle tissue.

Intravenous (IV). Passage of fluids directly into the blood vessels.

Intravenous Infiltration. The leakage of a drug or substance from a blood vessel and into surrounding tissues.

IV. See Intravenous.

Jaundice. A disease or condition giving the skin, tissues, or body fluids a yellow tinge.

Labia. The fleshy folds of the female genitalia.

Lavage. Irrigation or washing out of a body organ.

Laxative. An agent that promotes bowel evacuation.

Lethargy. A condition of weakness and slowness.

Ligament. A broad, fibrous band that holds bones together or supports organs.

Malaise. A sense of physical ill-being.

Malignancy. An abnormal tissue or growth, usually cancerous and having a tendency to progress and invade other tissues.

Medicaid. Federal plan paying for health care for the indigent.

Medicare. Federal plan paying some health care costs for persons over 65, or those under 65 who meet certain requirements. Medicare Plan A pays for hospitalization; Medicare Plan B, which requires subscription, covers physicians' bills, medical equipment, and some other costs.

Mitered Corner. A method of folding bed sheet corners to secure them in place.

Mucous Membrane. Membranes full of mucous glands that line passages and cavities of the body.

Mucus. A sticky substance secreted by mucous membranes and glands that moistens and protects them.

Myocardial Infarction. Heart attack.

Narcotic. A powerful drug that induces insensibility while relieving pain.

Nasogastric Tube. A tube passed down through the nose and into the stomach for the introduction of fluids or nutrients.

Necrosis. Tissue or bone death usually caused by lack of blood.

Needlestick. Accidental puncture with a hypodermic needle.

Neuropathy. Disturbance of the nerves.

Nocturia. Excessive need to urinate during the night.

Non-productive Cough. Cough without producing secretions.

Occult Blood. Bleeding in minute quantities that is recognized by microscope or chemical means.

Ostomy. An operation to create an artificial outlet for body wastes.

Overbed Trapeze. A triangular bar suspended over the bed to help in patient lifting and positioning.

Palpation. Medical examination of the body exterior by applying pressure with fingers or hands.

Paralysis. Temporary or permanent loss of sensation or voluntary motion.

Paroxysmal. A sudden attack or recurrence of disease symptoms.

Patent. Open, accessible.

Pathogen. A microorganism or substance capable of causing disease.

Perineum. The area between the anus and the posterior of the genitals.

Peripheral Vascular Disorders. Diseases of the blood vessels, usually in the lower extremities.

Peristalsis. A wavelike movement in the intestines to help move contents along the digestive tract.

Peristomal. Referring to the skin around a stoma.

Peritoneal Cavity. The area between the layers of the peritoneum in the abdomen.

Peritonitis. Inflammation of the peritoneum.

Peritoneum. The membrane lining the abdominal wall.

Petechiae. Pinpoint purplish-red dots on the skin.

pH. A symbol used to express the relative alkalinity or acidity of a substance.

Phlebitis. Inflammation of a vein.

Placebo. An inactive substance used to satisfy a patient's demand for medication.

Plasma. The liquid part of the blood.

Platelets. A blood component that promotes clotting.

Pleura. The membrane that enfolds the lungs.

Pleurisy. Inflammation of the pleura.

Pressure Sore. An ulcer of the skin and underlying tissues produced by prolonged pressure. Also called bedsore or decubitus ulcer.

Productive Cough. A cough in which mucus is raised.

Prognosis. Prediction of the course or end of a disease.

Pulmonary. Concerning the lungs.

Pulmonary Embolus. A blood clot that has moved to the lungs.

Pulse. The wave of blood within an artery.

Pulse Rate. The number of pulse beats per minute.

Pulse Rhythm. The pattern of pulse beats.

Quadriplegia. Paralysis affecting all four limbs.

Radial Pulse. The pulse felt over the radial artery in the wrist.

Range of Motion. The degree of motion possible for each joint.

Red Blood Cell. A blood component containing hemoglobin that delivers oxygen to the tissues.

Renal. Pertaining to the kidneys.

Rescue Breathing. The process of breathing air into the lungs of a person who has stopped breathing. Also called artificial respiration.

Respiration. Breathing.

Respiratory Arrest. The cessation of breathing.

Respiratory Distress. Labored breathing.

Restraints. Ties or devices applied to a patient to keep him from injuring himself or others.

Resuscitate. To restore life.

Retention Catheter. A urinary catheter inserted through the urethra and into the bladder. Also called a Foley or indwelling catheter.

Sanguineous. Relating to blood.

Secretion. The product of a gland, such as saliva.

Sedative. An agent that calms or tranquilizes.

Shock. Acute circulatory failure, usually seen in excessive bleeding.

Skin Breakdown. A condition in which the skin's integrity is compromised. Poor diet and inattention to the hazards of bed rest are common causes of skin breakdown.

Sphygmomanometer. An instrument used to measure blood pressure.

Sputum. Saliva, mucus, or sometimes pus ejected from the mouth.

Stasis. Stagnation of normal flow of fluids.

Sterile. Free of microorganisms.

Sterile Abscess. An abscess caused by improper technique at an injection site.

Sterile Field. A sterile pad or other sterile area upon which sterile instruments and supplies are deposited during a sterile medical procedure.

Sterile Technique. A method for medical procedures that keeps objects free from microorganisms or bacteria.

Stimulants. Drugs that affect the central nervous system and increase body activity.

Stoma. An artificial opening in the abdomen.

Stool. Fecal matter.

Stroke. A condition in which one or more of the blood vessels to the brain becomes clogged or bursts, causing part of the brain to die from lack of oxygen.

Subcutaneous Injection. An injection into the subcutaneous tissues just beneath the skin, and not into the muscle.

Sublingual. Under the tongue.

Superior Vena Cava. The central vein into the heart.

Suppository. A solid, cone-shaped medication that melts when inserted into the rectum, vagina, or urethra.

Suture. A surgical stitch used to close wounds.

Syringe. An instrument used to inject or withdraw fluids.

Systolic Pressure. The pressure of the blood against the arterial walls when the heart contracts.

Tachycardia. An excessively rapid pulse or heart rate; over 100 beats per minute in an adult.

Tendon. A fibrous cord that attaches muscle to bone.

Thrombophlebitis. Inflammation of a vein followed by formation of a blood clot.

Thrombus. A blood clot.

Topical. Applied to the skin.

Total Parenteral Nutrition (TPN). A method of supplying the body with nourishing solutions through a catheter inserted into the superior vena cava. Also called hyperalimentation.

Trachea. A membraneous tube in the neck and descending into the right and left bronchi of the lungs.

Tracheostomy. A procedure in which an opening is made in the trachea and a cannula is introduced into the opening.

Traction. Application of force in a horizontal position to align broken bones, usually in the lower extremities.

Tranquilizer. A drug that quiets patients.

Turgor. Normal fullness and elasticity of the skin.

Ulcer. An open lesion on the skin or mucous membrane of the body.

Unresponsive. A condition in which a patient does not react to verbal or physical stimuli.

Uremia. Toxic condition associated with serious kidney problems.

Ureterostomy. An opening into the urinary tract that permits the drainage of urine.

Urinalysis. Laboratory analysis of urine.

Urinary Retention. Inability to urinate.

Vacuum Vial. Medication vial with its contents in a vacuum.

Vasoconstriction. A narrowing of the blood vessels.

Vasodilatation. A widening of the blood vessels.

Vital Signs. Measurement of respiration, pulse, blood pressure, and temperature.

White Blood Cells. The infection-fighting component of blood.

Index